Internet of Things-Based Machine Learning in Healthcare

The Internet of Medical Things (IoMT) is a system that collects data from patients with the help of different sensory inputs, e.g., an accelerometer, electrocardiography, and electroencephalography. This text presents both theoretical and practical concepts related to the application of machine learning and Internet of Things (IoT) algorithms in analyzing data generated through healthcare systems.

- Illustrates the latest technologies in the healthcare domain and the Internet of Things infrastructure for storing smart electronic health records
- Focuses on the importance of machine learning algorithms and the significance of Internet of Things infrastructure for healthcare systems
- Showcases the application of fog computing architecture and edge computing in novel aspects of modern healthcare services
- Discusses unsupervised genetic algorithm-based automatic heart disease prediction
- Covers Internet of Things–based hardware mechanisms and machine learning algorithms to predict the stress level of patients

The text is primarily written for graduate students and academic researchers in the fields of computer science and engineering, biomedical engineering, electrical engineering, and information technology.

Internet of Things-Based Machine Learning in Healthcare

Technology and Applications

Edited by
Prasenjit Dey, Sudip Kumar Adhikari, Sourav De, and Indrajit Kar

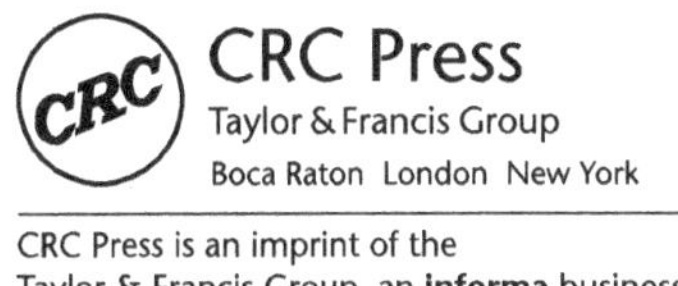

CRC Press is an imprint of the
Taylor & Francis Group, an **informa** business
A CHAPMAN & HALL BOOK

Designed cover image: ShutterStock

First edition published 2024
by CRC Press
2385 NW Executive Center Drive, Suite 320, Boca Raton FL 33431

and by CRC Press
4 Park Square, Milton Park, Abingdon, Oxon, OX14 4RN

CRC Press is an imprint of Taylor & Francis Group, LLC

ISBN: 9781032487373 (hbk)
ISBN: 9781032489285 (pbk)
ISBN: 9781003391456 (ebk)

DOI: 10.1201/9781003391456

Typeset in Times
by Deanta Global Publishing Services, Chennai, India

Dr. Prasenjit Dey dedicates this book to his parents.

Dr. Sudip Kumar Adhikari dedicates this book to his parents.

Dr. Sourav De dedicates this book to his mentor Prof. (Dr.) Siddhartha Bhattacharyya.

Mr. Indrajit Kar dedicates this book to his family, followers, ex companies, and the almighty.

Contents

Preface ... ix
Editors ... xii
Contributors ... xiv

Chapter 1 Applications of Internet of Things and Machine Learning Technologies in Healthcare ... 1

Prasenjit Dey, Sudip Kumar Adhikari, Sourav De and Rudranath Banerjee

Chapter 2 Automated Detection of Patients Developing Anorexia Nervosa and Bulimia Nervosa Using XGBoost Algorithm ... 19

T. Kirubadevi, M. Arun, S. Nirmala Sugirtha Rajini, S. Ramamoorthy, and P.S. Rajakumar

Chapter 3 Breast Cancer Prediction Using a Machine Learning Approach ... 38

Arijit Ghosal, Harshita Somolu, and Suchibrota Dutta

Chapter 4 A Survey on the Development of Deep Learning–Based Techniques in the Diagnosis of Parkinson's Disease ... 55

B.K. Tripathy, Astha, Anushka Patil, Savvy Gupta and Preeti Kumari

Chapter 5 A Deep Learning-based Approach for Detecting Diabetic Retinopathy in Retina Images ... 85

Sahana Das, Asifuzzaman Lasker, Mridul Ghosh, Sk Md Obaidullah and Kaushik Roy

Chapter 6 Optimization of CNN for Content-Based Image Retrieval in Healthcare ... 96

Arnab Gain

Chapter 7 Paddy Leaf Diseases Detection Using Otsu and Yen Thresholding with Deep Convolutional Neural Network ... 126

Sk. Hapijul Hossen, Kuntal Mukherjee, Arkaprava Dey, and Sumana Kundu

Chapter 8 Applications of IoT-Enabled Systems in Healthcare Industry 147

T. Venkat Narayana Rao and S. Tabassum Sultana

Chapter 9 Enhancing Health and Environmental Monitoring: Open-Source IoT-Enabled SCADA System with Node-RED, InfluxDB, Grafana, and Raspberry Pi 166

Rajib Das

Chapter 10 Transfer Learning for Healthcare 190

Anindita Saha and Moumita Roy

Chapter 11 Conclusions 218

Prasenjit Dey

Index 221

Preface

Healthcare systems produce a huge amount of data each day, which can be collected by using different sensory input devices. Consequently, this huge volume of data can be processed by using big data architectures. Machine learning (ML) can be used to empower the Internet of Things (IoT) to demystify hidden patterns in these huge volumes of data for optimal prediction and recommendation systems. In this book, the objective is to achieve a conjoint framework consisting of the latest technologies like ML and IoT to enhance the overall quality of healthcare systems. By observing the patient's response to certain medicines, we can come up with improved and intelligent drug development systems. Similarly, by using IoT sensors, we can build enhanced wearable medical devices to provide a 24/7 health monitoring system. Furthermore, the incorporation of machine learning technologies in the medical data management system will also become more intelligent and intricate in the future. Internet of Medical Things (IoMT) is a system that collects data from patients with the help of different sensory inputs, e.g., an accelerometer, ECG, EEG, and blood pressure monitor. Later, these data are sent to the local server (e.g., ZigBee) via local interconnected networks. Then, with the help of edge computing or fog computing, the local server processes these data and makes appropriate decisions. By deploying ML algorithms in the local servers, a self-intelligent IoMT system can be achieved, which will make necessary decisions by self-assessing the patient data. The hybrid IoT-based ML framework automates healthcare systems such as medical record-keeping, real-time patient health monitoring, and predicting disease diagnosis.

However, different ML algorithms perform differently on different types of medical datasets. Moreover, the medical datasets are mostly noisy, which also hampers the overall learning process. Thus, it is the need of the hour to explore different state-of-the-art ML algorithms to come up with robust, noise-immune, and efficient IoT-based ML models with respect to critical clinical decision-making processes. The book aims to present state-of-the-art research that uses ML technologies on IoT-generated medical data. In a thorough analysis, we observe that different ML prediction algorithms have various shortcomings depending on the IoT-generated data. This book is targeted to overcome these limitations by introducing new ML and IoT concepts that will help in optimizing the critical decision-making process in the healthcare system.

In Chapter 1, the authors present a comprehensive survey that meticulously examines state-of-the-art initiatives within the healthcare domain, leveraging machine learning technologies and IoT as distinct entities. Subsequently, the chapter embarks on an exploration of various recent works skillfully integrating these two cutting-edge technologies. This integration is pursued with the overarching goal of advancing and enhancing healthcare services through innovative approaches.

In Chapter 2, the authors employ predictive analytics to proactively curb the development of anorexia nervosa and bulimia nervosa. They gathered data from diverse sources, encompassing electronic health records and patient surveys, and applied the

XGBoost algorithm to construct predictive models. This system continuously tracks dietary habits, exercise routines, and sleep patterns, promptly notifying healthcare providers and caregivers of worrisome trends and facilitating early intervention and treatment. It also addresses associated mental health conditions, including depression and anxiety.

Chapter 3 addresses the global cancer challenge, a pervasive threat claiming millions of lives yearly. Cancer encompasses diverse diseases marked by uncontrolled cell growth, its root cause elusive. The malignancy allows it to spread throughout the body, posing grave danger. With over 100 cancer types, treatments vary and a universal cure remains elusive. Cancer weakens the immune system, adding to the peril. Survivors face the risk of recurrence. Cancer has four stages (I to IV), and swift intervention is crucial. Breast cancer, common but often late-detected in India, is a significant concern. In Chapter 3, the authors utilize machine learning to predict early-stage breast cancer, utilizing biological data from 569 patients before biopsy results become available. This approach aims to expedite treatment initiation, potentially leading to improved outcomes and lives saved.

In Chapter 4, the authors conduct a comprehensive analysis of AI-related research in Parkinson's disease (PD), addressing the disease's five stages, from early symptoms to advanced stages. They highlight the effectiveness of deep neural networks and machine learning models like k-nearest neighbors (KNN) and convolutional neural networks (CNNs) for accurate diagnosis, disease monitoring, personalized treatment, and patient care. The study focused on various ML and AI models for PD detection using features like handwriting analysis, voice recognition, and sleep patterns. Future research directions are also outlined, guiding ongoing scientific exploration in this domain.

In Chapter 5, the authors highlight the escalating global health challenge of diabetic retinopathy. Early detection and consistent screening are emphasized, with retinal fundus imaging as a vital diagnostic tool. Manual screening's time-consuming nature, coupled with a shortage of ophthalmologists, prompts the call for an automated diagnostic model using AI, particularly a lightweight CNN. This model enhances diagnostic accuracy through efficient retinal area detection and segmentation. The study's core objective is precise diabetic retinopathy indicator identification in fundus images, offering potential insights into the diagnostic process and the prospect of improved patient outcomes.

In Chapter 6, the author addresses a significant issue in medical image retrieval, highlighting the lack of transparency in existing CNN models, which raises concerns among healthcare professionals. The proposed solution focused on optimizing CNN performance by modifying the differential evolution method, with an emphasis on refining the mutation step. Subsequently, the enhanced CNN model is integrated into a content-based image retrieval (CBIR) framework. Through experiments using three distinct medical image datasets, the results demonstrate promise with high accuracy rates: 97% for brain tumor MRI, 98% for breast cancer MRI, and a remarkable 100% for the Covid-19 radiography dataset, underscoring the effectiveness of the approach in an academic context.

In Chapter 7, the authors underscore the vital role of rice in global agriculture, particularly in Asia. They emphasize the substantial impact of paddy leaf diseases on rice production and the challenges faced by farmers in disease detection, especially without expert guidance. To address this, they propose an automated disease detection system, replacing the time-consuming manual methods with efficient image processing and deep learning techniques. This system effectively classifies paddy leaf diseases, including bacterial leaf blight, leaf smut, and brown spot, achieving a notable 98% accuracy rate in disease prediction.

Chapter 8 delves into the progressive integration of IoT technology, highlighting its impact on advancing patient care and operational efficiency. This is achieved through the collection of real-time patient data by wearable sensors and smart devices, allowing remote monitoring and informed decision-making by healthcare professionals. Moreover, IoT technology optimizes operations by automating administrative tasks such as appointment scheduling and patient record management. Patients also benefit from real-time updates on wait times and treatment progress, elevating their healthcare experience. The chapter underscores the pivotal role of IoT in enhancing patient comfort, diagnostic accuracy, and informed treatment, ultimately leading to heightened patient satisfaction and streamlined healthcare procedures.

In Chapter 9, the author addresses cost and complexity issues in existing IoT systems, particularly within healthcare. To tackle these challenges, the author introduces an open-source SCADA-based IoT healthcare prototype, incorporating Node-RED, InfluxDB, Grafana, ESP32, and Raspberry Pi. This system empowers professionals to monitor key parameters, set alerts based on thresholds, and streamline control processes. The chapter highlights Node-RED's rapid prototyping, InfluxDB's real-time data storage, and Grafana's user-friendly data visualization. It serves as a guide for merging open-source SCADA with IoT, fostering intelligent monitoring systems that have the potential to enhance public health and environmental sustainability.

In Chapter 10, the authors analyze transfer learning (TL) as a promising solution that enhances the performance of target learners by transferring knowledge from related source domains, thereby diminishing reliance on extensive target-domain data. TL's importance in healthcare lies in its ability to facilitate the development of robust systems through the utilization of pretrained models and parameter transfer. Adopting a third-person perspective, the chapter underscores the growing significance of TL in healthcare, providing a clear definition and emphasizing its relevance. The chapter also serves as a valuable resource for implementing TL, using pretrained models and healthcare datasets as benchmarks for various machine learning and deep learning methodologies.

Editors

Prasenjit Dey received his BTech in computer science and engineering from the West Bengal University of Technology, Kolkata, India, in 2010, and MTech in computer science and engineering from the National Institute of Technology Durgapur, Durgapur, India, in 2012. He was an associate innovator with Nivio Technologies, Gurgaon, India, in 2012. He was a hardware graphics designer at Intel from 2017 to 2018. He received his PhD in computer science and engineering from the National Institute of Technology Durgapur, Durgapur, India, in 2018.

He served as an Assistant Professor in the Department of Computer Science and Engineering at Cooch Behar Government Engineering College, Cooch Behar, India, from 2018 to 2023. In 2023, he transitioned to the National Institute of Technology Rourkela, Odisha, India, where he currently holds the position of Assistant Professor in the Department of Computer Science. He has successfully completed one government project and is currently involved in several others. His current research interests include artificial neural networks, pattern recognition, and machine learning. He has authored numerous research publications in internationally renowned journals such as *IEEE Transactions on Systems, Man, and Cybernetics, IEEE Transactions on Artificial Intelligence, IEEE Internet of Things Journal, Impact, Biomedical Signal Processing and Control*, etc. Additionally, he has contributed to over 15 research publications in internationally respected edited books and international conference proceedings.

Sourav De earned his BE in information technology from the University of Burdwan, Burdwan, India, in 2002. He did his ME in information technology from the West Bengal University of Technology, Kolkata, India, in 2005. He completed a PhD in computer science and technology at the Indian Institute of Engineering & Technology, Shibpur, Howrah, India, in 2015. He has been an associate professor in the Computer Science & Engineering Department at Cooch Behar Government Engineering College, West Bengal, since 2016. Previous to this, he was an assistant professor for more than ten years in the Department of Computer Science and Engineering and Information Technology at the University Institute of Technology, University of Burdwan, Burdwan, India. He served as a junior programmer in Apices Consultancy Private Limited, Kolkata, India, in 2005. He is a coauthor of one book and the coeditor of 16 books; has more than 69 research publications in internationally reputed journals, international edited books, and international IEEE conference proceedings; and five patents and three copyrights to his credit. He served as a reviewer for several international IEEE conferences and also several international editorial books. He also served as a reviewer for reputed international journals, including *Applied Soft Computing*, *Knowledge-Based Systems*, *Soft Computing Letters*, *Computer Methods in Biomechanics and Biomedical Engineering*, and *Imaging & Visualization*. He has been a member of the organizing and technical program committees of several national and international conferences. He has been invited to different seminars as an expert speaker. His research interests include soft computing, pattern recognition, image processing, and data mining. De is a senior member of IEEE and also a member of ACM, Institute of Engineers (IEI), Computer Science Teachers Association (CSTA), Institute of Engineers, and IAENG, Hong Kong. He is a life member of ISTE, India.

Sudip Kumar Adhikari earned a BTech in computer science and engineering from Vidyasagar University, Midnapore, India. He obtained an ME and PhD in computer science and engineering from Jadavpur University, Kolkata, India. He has more than 18 years of teaching experience. He is currently an assistant professor in the Computer Science & Engineering Department of Cooch Behar Government Engineering College, Cooch Behar, India. He has published more than 18 research papers in reputed international journals and conferences. His research interests include medical image processing, pattern recognition, artificial intelligence, and soft computing. He is a senior member of IEEE and a member of the Institute of Engineers. He served as a reviewer for several international conferences and also in several reputed international journals, including *Applied Soft Computing*, *IET Computer Vision*, *IEEE Access*, and *IEEE Transactions on Fuzzy Systems*. He has been a member of the organizing and technical program committees of several national and international conferences. He has been invited to different seminars as an expert speaker.

Indrajit Kar holds an MSc in computational biology and a BSc in science from a Bengaluru university. A dynamic entrepreneur, he has built teams at Siemens, Accenture, IBM, and Infinite Data Systems. He is now the AVP and Global Head of AI and ML at Zensar Technologies, overseeing ZAIR and Data Practices.

He has authored 21 research papers published by IEEE, Springer, Wiley, and CRC, covering topics such as large language models, computer vision, NLP, and time series analysis. He has received five "Best Paper" awards, including one from Cardiff University.

A mentor to start-ups, he's guided two to revenue generation and has received numerous accolades, including the "40 Under 40 Data Scientists" award from Analytics India Magazine. His trophy case includes two IP Samman and Service Excellence awards from Siemens; the Growth Market Award from Accenture; and various innovation and contribution awards from Accenture, IBM, Siemens Healthcare, and Hewlett-Packard.

He has managed over 30 projects in AI/ML and is an accomplished author, cowriting two books, one on generative AI, and has delivered 19 lectures and keynote speeches. An adjunct faculty member for a data science course at upGrad, he holds 14 AI/ML patents.

Under his leadership, his teams have won five Best Team/Project awards, including Best AI/ML Project House and the Werner Von Siemens award. His initiatives have led Siemens to be ranked as a top data science company by Analytics India Magazine.

He has mentored over 150 AI and ML aspirants and has been a speaker at universities such as IIT Madras and PESIT, contributing to the field's growth and innovation.

Contributors

Sudip Kumar Adhikari
Cooch Behar Government Engineering College
Cooch Behar, India

M. Arun
Dr. MGR Educational and Research Institute
Chennai, India

Astha
School of Information Technology and Engineering, VIT
Vellore, India

Rudranath Banerjee
University Institute of Technology
Burdwan, India

Rajib Das
Cooch Behar Government Engineering College
Cooch Behar, India

Sahana Das
Budge Budge Institute of Technology
Budge Budge, India

Sourav De
Cooch Behar Government Engineering College, Cooch Behar
Cooch Behar, India

Arkaprava Dey
Haldia Institute of Technology
Haldia, India

Prasenjit Dey
National Institute of Technology Rourkela
Rourkela, India

Suchibrota Dutta
Royal Thimphu College
Thimphu, Bhutan

Arnab Gain
Cooch Behar Government Engineering College
Cooch Behar, India

Arijit Ghosal
St. Thomas' College of Engineering and Technology
Kolkata, India

Mridul Ghosh
Shyampur Siddheswari Mahavidyalaya
Shyampur, India

Savvy Gupta
School of Information Technology and Engineering, VIT
Vellore, India

Sk. Hapijul Hossen
Haldia Institute of Technology
Haldia, India

Kirubadevi.T
Dr. MGR Educational and Research Institute
Chennai, India

Preeti Kumari
School of Information Technology and Engineering, VIT
Vellore, India

Sumana Kundu
Dr. B. C. Roy Engineering College
Durgapur, India

Asifuzzaman Lasker
Aliah University
Kolkata, India

Kuntal Mukherjee
Haldia Institute of Technology
Haldia, India

Sk Md Obaidullah
Aliah University
Kolkata, India

Anushka Patil
School of Information Technology and Engineering, VIT
Vellore, India

P.S. Rajakumar
Dr. MGR Educational and Research Institute
Chennai, India

S. Nirmala Sugirtha Rajini
Dr. MGR Educational and Research Institute
Chennai, India

S. Ramamoorthy
Dr. MGR Educational and Research Institute
Chennai, India

T. Venkat Narayana Rao
Sreenidhi Institute of Science and Technology
Hyderabad, India

Kaushik Roy
West Bengal State University
Barasat, India

Moumita Roy
Techno Main Salt Lake
Kolkata, India

Anindita Saha
Techno Main Salt Lake
Kolkata, India

Harshita Somolu
Cognizant Technology Solutions
Kolkata, India

S. Tabassum Sultana
Matrusri Engineering College
Saidabad, Hyderabad, India

B.K. Tripathy
School of Information Technology and Engineering, VIT
Vellore, India

1 Applications of Internet of Things and Machine Learning Technologies in Healthcare

Prasenjit Dey, Sudip Kumar Adhikari, Sourav De and Rudranath Banerjee

1.1 INTRODUCTION

An innovative new era is emerging in the healthcare field, where machine learning (ML) combined with the Internet of Things (IoT) will change how services are being provided, managed, and optimized. The combination of these modern technologies is transforming healthcare systems by increasing efficiency, personalization, and accessibility. In this introduction, we have given an overview of how ML and IoT are having a major impact on healthcare that will lead to the overall assessment of their uses, benefits, challenges, and prospects. Historically, healthcare was characterized by paper-based records and manual operations. Now, healthcare has evolved into a data-driven industry where the digitalization of medical information is at the forefront. The quick development of ML and IoT technologies has accelerated this transformation. ML has enabled computers to analyze vast amounts of healthcare data, such as electronic health records (EHRs), medical imaging, genomics, and patient-generated data. In contrast, IoT allows the seamless collection and transmission of data through a connection between medical equipment, wearables, sensors, and other healthcare devices.

Machine learning is becoming a game changer for healthcare through its ability to identify patterns, predict outcomes, and deliver quantifiable information from large medical datasets. In the context of disease diagnosis and treatment, ML algorithms have demonstrated exceptional capabilities. For instance, deep learning models have exhibited high accuracy in the detection of abnormalities in medical images, including x-rays, MRIs, and CT scans [1]. These algorithms can assist radiologists in identifying subtle anomalies, potentially leading to earlier diagnosis and treatment. Furthermore, ML-based predictive analytics hold great promise in optimizing patient care. An ML algorithm can anticipate disease progression and recommend

DOI: 10.1201/9781003391456-1

personalized treatment plans by analyzing the history of patient data, which contributes to improved outcomes for patients [2]. More efficient interventions and reduced healthcare costs may result from this approach to healthcare.

On the other hand, the Internet of Things has led to an era of continuous patient monitoring and real-time data collection, encouraging preventive and proactive healthcare. Wearable devices, such as smartwatches and biosensors, enable patients to track their vital signs, physical activity, and sleep patterns. These devices provide useful data that could be used to detect anomalies, as well as remote monitoring of chronic diseases [3]. Individuals with diabetes, for instance, can benefit from IoT-enabled glucose sensors that communicate real-time data to healthcare providers, enabling them to make immediate adjustments to their treatment plans. Apart from patient-focused applications, the IoT is expanding to healthcare facilities. Healthcare facilities use the IoT to improve asset management, track healthcare facility location and usage, as well as monitor environmental conditions like temperature and humidity. This ensures the efficient utilization of resources and contributes to patient safety [4].

The true potential of ML and IoT in healthcare emerges when these technologies are integrated. ML algorithms can analyze the vast amount of data generated by IoT devices, extracting valuable insights and actionable information in real time. This combination of technologies is most noticeable in the remote monitoring of patients, where sensor devices continually gather data on patients' vital signs and activities, with ML algorithms analyzing that data for anomaly identification and prompt notifications to healthcare personnel [5]. This not only enhances patient care but also lessens the workload for medical professionals. Moreover, the integration of ML and IoT in healthcare has opened the door to predictive analytics for resource allocation and management. Hospitals can estimate patient admissions, optimize staff schedules, and more efficiently manage resources by combining historical data with real-time data from IoT devices [6]. This results in better satisfying patient experiences and effective healthcare delivery. This book delves into recent advancements concerning the fusion of the Internet of Medical Things (IoMT) and machine learning within the healthcare domain. This integration holds promise in enhancing our comprehension of health-related data and catalyzing a transformative shift in the medical sector. Indeed, the future of healthcare resides precisely at the intersection of IoMT and ML. As these technologies continue to evolve, their profound impact on healthcare delivery and outcomes is poised for further expansion. Innovations such as remote patient monitoring, AI-assisted surgical procedures, and ML-fueled drug discovery will significantly mold the healthcare landscape. This interdisciplinary convergence has paved the way for pioneering approaches to patient care bolstered by diagnostic precision, treatment tailoring, and the optimization of healthcare systems.

The remainder of this chapter is structured as follows: Section 1.2 delves into the operational principles of different machine learning algorithms. Following that, Section 1.3 provides a survey of the utilization of machine learning in healthcare. Section 1.4 offers an exploration of the concepts of IoT and its prospective significance in future medical services. Subsequently, Section 1.5 examines recent research that has harnessed the synergy of both ML and IoT to enhance the healthcare sector.

Finally, in Section 1.6, we conclude the chapter by summarizing the advantages, challenges, and future prospects.

1.2 MACHINE LEARNING TECHNOLOGIES

Machine learning technologies are widely used in various healthcare domains. Thus, it is the need of the hour to understand the working principles of various ML algorithms and their integration with different healthcare services. For this purpose, a preliminary discussion is provided on various types of ML algorithms used in this book. ML algorithms are broadly classified into three categories: supervised learning, unsupervised learning, and reinforced learning. In the following sections, we illustrate the concepts of these learning strategies along with various ML algorithms.

1.2.1 Supervised Learning

In supervised learning, a labeled dataset with the input feature (x) and output label (y) is used to train an ML model. Here, the output labels supervise the learning algorithm, and thus, it is called supervised learning. To predict the output given input data, the algorithm learns to map the input data to the output label. Supervised learning algorithms can be used for regression, classification, and time-series forecasting.

Regression algorithms estimate the value of a continuous variable by analyzing a set of independent input variables. For example, these algorithms can be applied to predict a person's heart rate using various other vital health parameters. In classification problems, an algorithm estimates the class label of new data based on the classes of the training data. For instance, a classification algorithm trained on a dataset of brain images containing both non-tumorous and tumorous samples can predict the presence of a tumor in an individual based on their brain images. Similarly, forecasting algorithms predict future values of a variable based on its historical data. These algorithms can be employed to forecast an individual's probability of developing heart disease in the future. Examples of supervised learning algorithms include linear regression, logistic regression, multilayer perceptron (MLP), support vector machines (SVMs), decision trees, random forests, gradient-boosted trees, and many more. However, it's worth noting that supervised learning algorithms have limitations, as they require labeled training data, which can be both challenging to obtain and resource-intensive. In the following sections, we discuss some of these algorithms, as various authors in the upcoming chapters use them.

1.2.1.1 Support Vector Machine (SVM)

SVMs are primarily used for binary classification problems but are also used for multiclass classification problems as well as regression problems. In order to divide data points into two classes, the SVM identifies a hyperplane in the feature space. The hyperplane is chosen to maximize the margin between the two classes, which is the distance between the hyperplane and the closest data points from each class. A collection of training data with the appropriate class labels is fed into the SVM in order to train it. Then, the SVM figures out which hyperplane best matches the training data (regression) or divides the data points into two groups (binary classification). After the training, the SVM predicts the class of new samples by projecting it onto the hyperplane and categorizing it according to which side of the hyperplane the samples fall on [7]. The working principle of SVM is given in Equation 1.1, where the notations carry their conventional meanings as defined by Cortes and Vapnik [7]:

$$\begin{aligned} &\underset{w,b,\zeta}{\text{minimize}} \quad \| w \|_2^2 + C\sum_{i=1}^{n} \zeta_i \\ &\text{Subject to} \quad y_i(w^T x_i - b) \geq 1 - \zeta i, \ \ \zeta_i \geq 0 \forall i \in \{1,\ldots,n\} \end{aligned} \tag{1.1}$$

The benefits of using SVMs for both classification and regression tasks include their capacity to handle high-dimensional data with a limited number of training samples and their resilience to outliers and noise in data. However, SVMs are sensitive to the selection of hyperparameters and it is computationally costly to train for big datasets. The hyperparameters include the C parameter, gamma, and the kernel function. C and gamma parameters regulate the trade-off between the margin and training error. A greater value of C will produce greater margins. The kernel function defines the curvature of the hyperplane of the SVM.

1.2.1.2 k-Nearest Neighbor (KNN)

k-nearest neighbor (KNN) is a nonparametric instance-based algorithm that makes assumptions about how the data are distributed in their underlying form. It operates on the principle that data points that are close to each other in a feature space are more likely to belong to the same class or have similar output values. It does not build an explicit model or learn parameters.

During the training phase, kNN stores the entire dataset along with its corresponding labels/output values, making the kNN memory inefficient. When a new data sample needs to be classified or assigned a value, the algorithm calculates the distance between this data sample and all other data samples in the training set. The most common distance metric used is Euclidean distance, but other metrics can also be applied. kNN selects the k-nearest data point to the new data point based on the computed distances and predicts the class/value of the new data point based on the classes/values of the k-nearest neighbors. k is a user-defined parameter that determines how many neighbors influence the final prediction. A common practice is to choose an odd number for k to avoid ties when classifying into binary classes. For classification tasks, kNN counts the frequency of each class among the k-nearest neighbors and assigns the class that occurs most frequently as the predicted class for the new data point. In regression tasks, it calculates the average (or weighted average) of the output values of the k-nearest neighbors as the predicted value. The following equation describes the kNN classifier:

$$predict(x) = \arg\max_c \sum \left({I(y_i == c)} \middle/ {distance(x, y_i)} \right) \tag{1.2}$$

where x, c, y_i, and distance(x, y_i) is the new data point, class label, class of the ith data point in the training set, and the distance between the new data point and the ith data point in the training set. $I(y_i == c)$ is an indicator function that is equal to 1 if the ith data point in the training set is of class c and 0 otherwise.

1.2.1.3 Decision Tree (DT)

A decision tree (DT) is a flowchart-like tree structure where each node represents a feature, each branch represents a decision rule or condition, and each leaf node represents the outcome or class label. The algorithm recursively partitions the data into subsets based on feature values, aiming to create a tree structure that efficiently predicts the target variable. Figure 1.1 depicts the pictorial diagram of a decision tree.

One of the significant advantages of a DT is its interpretability. DTs are easy to visualize and understand, making them useful for explaining the decision-making process. DTs can provide insights into feature importance. Features appearing near the top of the tree contribute more to the decision-making process, aiding in feature selection and understanding the data. DTs can be part of ensemble methods like random forests and gradient boosting, which combine multiple trees to improve predictive performance and reduce overfitting. However, DTs are prone to overfitting, especially when they become deep and complex. Techniques like pruning and setting maximum tree depth can help mitigate overfitting. DTs are also prone to imbalanced datasets. The ID3, C4.5, and CART algorithms are only a few examples of the many decision tree algorithms.

1.2.1.4 Multilayer Perceptron (MLP)

An artificial neural network (ANN) called a multilayer perceptron is made up of a stack of linked layers of neurons, each of which uniquely transforms the incoming data. MLPs work by learning a nonlinear mapping between the input data and the output target. This mapping is learned by training the MLP on a set of labeled data points. Once the MLP is trained, it can be used to make predictions on new data points. Each neuron in a layer of an MLP has an activation function that decides the output of the neuron. Popular activation functions in MLPs are Sigmoid, tanh, and

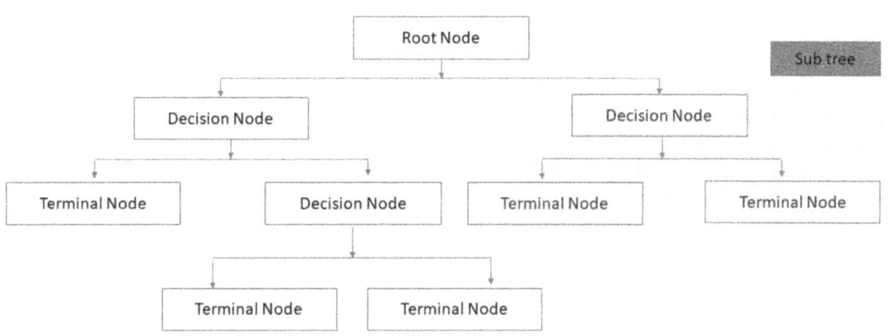

FIGURE 1.1 A decision tree.

ReLU. The forward pass is computed recursively for each layer of the MLP. The output of the last layer is the prediction of the MLP. The forward pass of a single neuron in an MLP is depicted in Equation 1.3, where $f(.)$ is the activation function of the neuron:

$$y = f(w \cdot x + b) \tag{1.3}$$

Here, y, w, x, and b are the output, weight vector, input vector, and bias of the neuron, respectively.

MLPs are trained using a backpropagation algorithm. Backpropagation is a supervised learning algorithm that updates the weights of the MLP to minimize the loss function. The loss function is a measure of how well the MLP is predicting the output target for the training data points. Some common loss functions include cross-entropy loss and mean squared error loss. In Equation 1.4, n denotes the number of training samples; y_{pred} and y_{actual} represent the predicted output of the MLP and the actual output, respectively. The backpropagation algorithm updates the weights of the MLP in the direction of the negative gradient of the loss function.

$$MSE = \frac{\sum_n \left(y_{pred} - y_{actual}\right)^2}{n} \tag{1.4}$$

MLPs' strengths include their capacity to simulate both linear and nonlinear connections between the input data and the output values, as well as their simplicity in training. However, they are prone to overfitting and may be computationally costly to train, particularly for big datasets.

1.2.1.5 Recurent Neural Networks (RNN)

Recurrent Neural Networks (RNNs) represent a pivotal deep learning technique renowned for their ability to process sequential data while retaining memory of past information. Unlike traditional feedforward neural networks, RNNs possess feedback loops that allow them to utilize sequential data's temporal dependencies effectively. This inherent structure enables RNNs to excel in various tasks such as predictive modeling, time-series data analysis, clinical data processing, real-time monitoring, etc. One of the key advantages of RNNs lies in their flexibility to handle inputs of variable length, making them suitable for tasks where context plays a crucial role. Despite their effectiveness, RNNs face challenges in learning long-term dependencies due to issues such as vanishing gradients. Nevertheless, recent advancements like Long Short-Term Memory (LSTM) networks and Gated Recurrent Units (GRUs) have mitigated these challenges to a considerable extent, further enhancing the performance and applicability of RNNs in diverse domains.

In healthcare, data often follows a temporal sequence, such as patient vitals, medical records, and physiological signals. RNNs excel in analyzing such time-series data, enabling the detection of patterns, trends, and anomalies over time. Their predictive modeling capabilities make them invaluable for forecasting patient outcomes, disease progression, and medication responses based on historical data. Moreover,

RNNs facilitate the processing and analysis of diverse clinical data sources, including electronic health records (EHRs), medical imaging, and genomic data, thereby aiding in personalized medicine, disease diagnosis, and treatment planning. Additionally, RNNs enable real-time monitoring of patient vital signs and physiological signals, crucial for early detection of medical emergencies and timely intervention. Overall, RNNs offer a versatile framework for leveraging sequential data in healthcare, empowering applications ranging from predictive analytics and disease diagnosis to personalized treatment planning and remote patient monitoring.

1.2.2 Unsupervised Learning Algorithms

Unsupervised learning is a category of machine learning where algorithms are tasked with finding patterns, relationships, or structures in data without the guidance of labeled outputs or targets. In other words, it involves learning from unlabeled data to discover inherent patterns or groupings within the data itself. A kind of unsupervised learning method called clustering brings together data points with comparable characteristics. K-means clustering, hierarchical clustering, and Gaussian mixture models (GMMs) are examples of common clustering techniques. Another important application of unsupervised learning is dimensionality reduction. This involves reducing the number of features in a dataset while preserving its essential information. Principal component analysis (PCA) and t-distributed stochastic neighbor embedding (t-SNE) are popular techniques for dimensionality reduction.

Unsupervised learning is generally more challenging than supervised learning because there is no ground truth to guide the learning process. Evaluation and validation of unsupervised algorithms can be subjective and context-dependent. However, unsupervised learning has numerous practical applications, including segmentation in medical imaging, brain image clustering, and recommendation systems in healthcare.

1.2.2.1 k-Means Clustering

k-means clustering is a widely used unsupervised algorithm that partitions a dataset into distinct, nonoverlapping groups or clusters. The primary objective of k-means is to group similar data points based on their feature similarities and assign them to a cluster centroid (representative point) that minimizes the intracluster variance.

The algorithm begins by randomly selecting k initial cluster centroids. These centroids can be data points from the dataset or randomly generated points. Then each data point in the dataset is assigned to the cluster whose centroid is closest to it. The closeness is usually measured using Euclidean distance. After all data points are assigned to clusters, the centroids are recalculated as the mean of all data points assigned to that cluster. This step updates the positions of the centroids. These steps are repeated iteratively until convergence. Convergence typically occurs when the assignment of data points to clusters no longer changes significantly or when a predetermined number of iterations is reached. Once convergence is achieved, the algorithm partitions the dataset into k clusters, with each cluster represented by its centroid.

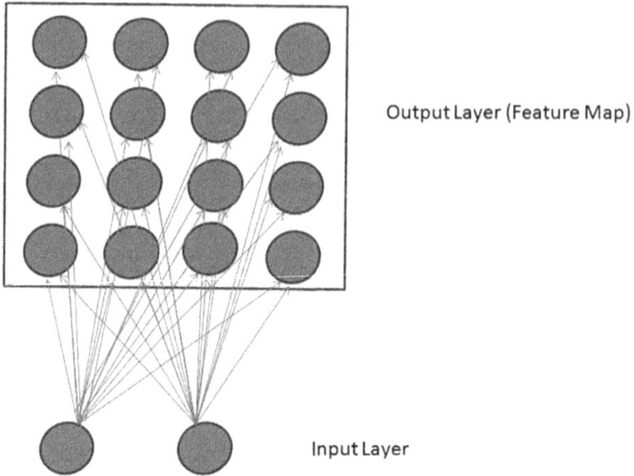

FIGURE 1.2 Self-organizing map network.

The algorithm has certain limitations, as it is sensitive to the choice of k, initial random data points, and datasets with complex structures.

1.2.2.2 Self-Organizing Maps (SOMs)

An unsupervised learning system called self-organizing maps (SOMs), commonly referred to as Kohonen maps, maps high-dimensional data onto a lower-dimensional grid. SOMs are extremely effective in recognizing patterns and correlations in high-dimensional data and visualizing them. They can visualize high-dimensional data in a lower-dimensional environment, highlight patterns and correlations that can be difficult to discern with other visualization approaches, and are generally simple to comprehend and use, among other benefits. Figure 1.2 illustrates the basic architecture of the SOM network.

SOMs, however, have several drawbacks, including the computational cost of training for big datasets, sensitivity to the initialization of the SOM grid, and the difficulty of interpreting SOM findings. Data visualization, pattern identification, anomaly detection, customer segmentation, medical diagnosis, and image processing are some of the applications of SOMs. SOMs, as a potent and adaptable unsupervised learning technique, can visualize high-dimensional data in a lower-dimensional environment and find patterns and links in the data. However, it's critical to be mindful of their drawbacks, including their computational expense and sensitivity to the SOM grid initialization.

1.3 MACHINE LEARNING AND ITS APPLICATIONS IN HEALTHCARE

In this section, we survey a few recent state-of-the-art works in the field of healthcare using machine learning. These are as follows.

Jaware et al. [8] presented seeded region growing, Foster corner detection theory, and a sparse autoencoder-based approach for brain tissue segmentation and classification in infant MRI images for the early diagnosis of neurological disorders. The proposed method works in four stages. The nonlocal means method and rectifying intensity inhomogeneity field employing contrast-limited adaptive histogram equalization [8] do noise removal from the images. The Foster corner identification principle [8] is employed to get the modified and optimized region of the segmented image. In the next stage, the predator–prey algorithm [8] is applied to optimize the similarity in the region growth technique. The weighted kNN and sparse autoencoder classifiers are utilized to classify the tissues [8]. A comparative study for cardiac–MRI medical image segmentation using U-Net and CNN is presented by Baccouch et al. [9]. The short-axis MRI images of the ACDC database [9] are used for this comparative study. Brain tumor segmentation is performed using the novel lightweight U-Net architecture by Walsh et al. [10]. The proposed architecture is capable of real-time segmentation of MRI scans, using the BITE dataset [11]. Byrne et al. [12] presented a novel method for multiclass segmentation of cardiac magnetic resonance (CMR) images with the help of a persistent homology-based topological loss. Incorporating the topological description of all class labels and class label pairs, a more predictable and statistically improved loss function is proposed for segmentation topology using a CNN-based post-processing framework. A newly proposed 1D convolution-based deep neural network (DNN), named the one-dimensional deep low-rank and sparse network (ODLS) is applied to accelerate MRI images [13]. This network unrolled the iteration procedure of a low-rank and sparse reconstruction model. Yue et al. [14] presented multicenter skin lesion classification using DNN with adaptively weighted balance (AWB) loss. In this article, the data imbalance issue is given more importance instead of improving the framework of the DNNs. This method is advantageous for different types of practical requirements by modifying the backbone and without tuning the hyperparameters. A multiscale visual representation self-supervised learning (MsVRL) model [15] is proposed for medical image segmentation to help in clinical diagnoses and treatment planning. A multiscale representation conception, a canvas matching method, an embedding pre-sampling module, a center-ness branch, and a cross-level consistent loss are incorporated in this proposed method for performance improvement. A novel embedding framework-based transformer model is presented to encode the brain function in a compact, stereotyped, and comparable latent space where the brain activities act as dense embedding vectors [16]. In this article, the interpretability of the learned embedding is also researched from both spatial and temporal perspectives.

Gholami et al. [17] presented different kinds of labeling functions that distinguish patients' Parkinson's disease gait, and a generative model was introduced to discover the accuracy of each labeling function in a self-supervised manner. In this method, a weakly-supervised 3D human pose estimation method is presented to tune the pretrained models in a clinical setting. An interpretable Bayesian framework (BayeSeg) is introduced by Gao et al. [18] using Bayesian modeling of image and label statistics to improvise model generalizability for medical image segmentation.

At the beginning, the image is broken down into a spatial-correlated variable and a spatial-variant variable, putting hierarchical Bayesian priors to explicitly force them to model the domain-stable shape and domain-specific appearance information, respectively. Mbunge and Batani [19] exercised a comprehensive review of a deep learning and machine learning model, named PRISMA (Preferred Reporting Items for Systematic Reviews and Meta-Analysis), to improve healthcare in sub-Saharan Africa (SSA). This model is tested to find the egressing opportunities, trends, and significances for incorporating AI-based models in SSA healthcare. From this study, it has been uncovered from massive health data that AI models are much more effective for early detection, diagnosis, monitoring of chronic disorders, prediction of diseases, and monitoring of large-scale public health patterns. Garbin et al. [20] presented a detailed review for predicting opioid use disorder (OUD) from healthcare data using ML. This review article first concentrated on the OUD prediction using ML, then illustrated the application of ML techniques and processes to derive the results, and proposed improvements to enhance future efforts in applying ML for OUD prediction [20].

Esteva et al. [21] provided a comprehensive overview of the applications of ML in healthcare, with a particular focus on deep learning techniques. The authors discuss various domains where ML has been successfully applied, such as medical imaging, diagnostics, drug discovery, genomics, and electronic health records. They describe the challenges and opportunities in each domain and highlight the potential impact of ML on improving patient care and transforming healthcare delivery. The review also discusses the ethical considerations and future directions for ML in healthcare. Another work [22] focused on the use of ML for predicting patient outcomes in healthcare. The authors analyze various ML techniques, including logistic regression, support vector machines, random forests, and deep learning algorithms. They examine different data sources, such as EHRs, medical imaging, and wearable devices, and discuss the predictive models' performance in different healthcare domains. The review highlights the strengths and limitations of ML approaches and provides insights into future research directions for improving prediction accuracy and clinical utility.

Rajkomar et al. [23] presented a comprehensive overview of ML applications in medicine and healthcare. The authors discuss the potential of ML in various areas, including diagnosis, treatment prediction, patient monitoring, and precision medicine. They highlight specific use cases, such as the detection of diabetic retinopathy and skin cancer, and discuss the challenges of implementing ML in healthcare, such as data quality, interpretability, and regulatory considerations. The review also emphasizes the need for collaboration between clinicians, data scientists, and policymakers to ensure the responsible and effective integration of ML in healthcare. ML models have been applied to predict patient outcomes, such as disease progression, treatment response, and readmission rates. These models utilize a range of data sources, including EHRs [24], genetic information, and wearable device data. By analyzing large volumes of data and identifying patterns, ML algorithms can aid in personalized treatment planning, resource allocation, and proactive healthcare management.

Rajpurkar et al. [25] provided an extensive review of the various applications of ML in healthcare, with a focus on medical imaging, specifically radiology and pathology. The authors discuss the use of CNNs and deep learning algorithms in the detection and diagnosis of various diseases, such as lung cancer, skin cancer, and diabetic retinopathy. They also highlight the potential of ML in predicting patient outcomes and treatment response. The review includes an analysis of the current challenges and limitations of ML in healthcare and suggests future research directions. On the other hand, Choi et al. [26] review various predictive models, such as logistic regression, SVM, and recurrent neural networks (RNNs). They discuss the challenges associated with interpretability and provide insights into the application of attention mechanisms in RNNs to enhance the interpretability of predictions. The review also examines the potential of ML in personalized medicine and the integration of EHRs to improve prediction accuracy. The survey article by Chen et al. [27] discussed the use of ML for disease diagnosis, prognosis, treatment recommendation, and monitoring patient health. They also addressed the challenges related to data quality, data privacy, algorithm interpretability, and regulatory compliance. The review highlighted the potential benefits of ML in healthcare, such as improved accuracy, cost reduction, and personalized medicine, and suggested future research directions.

From this survey of works, we have observed that integrating diverse healthcare data sources for ML applications poses challenges due to differences in data formats, quality, and privacy concerns. Thus, efforts are required to standardize data formats, improve data quality, and ensure secure data exchange while protecting patient privacy. Interoperability between different healthcare systems and data sources is crucial for effective integration and analysis. The use of ML in healthcare raises ethical concerns, including patient privacy, bias in algorithms, and transparency. Ensuring proper consent, data anonymization, and compliance with privacy regulations are essential to maintain patient trust and safeguard sensitive information. Addressing biases in ML algorithms to prevent disparities in healthcare outcomes is also a critical ethical consideration.

1.4 INTERNET OF MEDICAL THINGS AND ITS APPLICATIONS IN HEALTHCARE

The Internet of Things represents a transformative technological paradigm that has redefined the way we interact with the physical world. It is a concept that encapsulates the idea of connecting everyday objects, devices, and sensors to the internet, enabling them to collect, share, and analyze data, as well as perform various functions autonomously. IoT has emerged as a critical enabler of the digital age, promising unprecedented levels of connectivity, efficiency, and innovation across various domains, from smart homes to smart healthcare systems [28–30].

The IoT comprises a complex interplay of vital components that collectively contribute to its overarching objectives. At its core, IoT relies on a diverse array of sensors and devices, ranging from rudimentary temperature sensors to intricate industrial machinery and autonomous vehicles. These sensors are adept at capturing real-world data encompassing a wide spectrum of information, including environmental conditions, medical data, and various forms of motion data. Critical to the success of IoT ecosystems are robust communication networks, which encompass technologies like Wi-Fi, cellular networks, low-power wide-area networks (LPWANs), and emerging innovations such as 5G, facilitating the seamless exchange of data between IoT devices and the cloud infrastructure. The data collected by these devices undergoes rapid and thorough processing and analysis, leveraging potent computing resources like cloud computing and edge computing. This analytical process yields invaluable insights and actionable information. User interfaces, predominantly in the form of web and mobile applications, empower individuals to remotely monitor, control, and interact with their connected devices. Beyond this, IoT systems possess the capability to be programmed for task automation, event-triggered responses (e.g., motion-triggered lighting), and autonomous decision-making. In healthcare, IoT can be applied to remotely monitor and manage patient health conditions. For example, wearable IoT devices can continuously collect vital signs and health data from patients and send this information to healthcare providers and medical professionals in real time. Healthcare professionals can then use this data to make real-time decisions about patient care, such as adjusting medication dosages or treatment plans based on the patient's current health status. Next, we survey a few articles that have demonstrated the plausible applications of IoT in healthcare with empirical pieces of evidence.

Konstantinidis et al. have proposed an IoT-based healthcare system aiming to improve the quality of care for older adults [31]. In order to do this, they have embodied the Controller Application Communication (CAC) framework and the Extensible Messaging and Presence Protocol (XMPP) in IoT-enabled devices. Although the work demonstrated notable efficiency, its applicability has been limited to only two specific test-case scenarios. To enhance the effectiveness of this work, it is important to extend its application to a broader array of real-world problems and scenarios. Gelogo et al. [32] presented a framework focused on remote patients. This framework achieves its goals by integrating a range of IoT devices and sensors. The research done by Gelogo et al. has remarkable effectiveness in u-healthcare systems. However, their investigation has not extended to critical e-healthcare domains such as remote patient monitoring, mHealth, e-prescribing, and telemedicine. Gupta et al. [33] have designed an IoT-based healthcare kit to improve the healthcare system by managing and sharing large amounts of data in real time. However, their work lacks convenient remote access. Verma et al. [34] have introduced a framework that integrates IoT and cloud computing within a mobile healthcare system to predict diseases and assess their severity levels. In their work, the disease diagnosis process relies on the harmonious functioning of three integral subsystems. First, the user subsystem acquires data from IoT devices and medical sensors. Following this, the cloud-based component system takes charge of intricate data analysis, serving as a pivotal component in the disease diagnosis procedure. Last, the cloud subsystem issues a variety of alert signals to promptly notify responders and caregivers, prompting them to take necessary actions based on the computed results. However, their work lacks the incorporation of novel conditions. Furthermore, they did not formulate any statistical metrics, nor did they perform a comparative analysis between their methodology and established medical investigative approaches. Li et al. [35] have proposed an IoT-driven system that continuously monitors the patient's heart conditions and provides healthcare professionals with valuable insights into heart health. However, their work does not incorporate data stream mining and context awareness technologies, thereby limiting the potential for their work to deliver more robust and advanced prevalent healthcare services. Rahmani et al. [36] have proposed a fog computing approach, which has improved the efficiency of a healthcare IoT system by processing data at the edge of the network rather than being solely dependent on centralized cloud servers. Santos et al. [37] discussed how standard-based and distributed systems are utilized to share health-related information in IoT-based mobile healthcare systems and explored how standardized approaches can improve interoperability and data exchange within the system. They also recommended an evaluation of the security aspects pertaining to the utilization of the Constrained Application Protocol (CoAP) within the healthcare domain. Pescosolido et al. [38] leveraged IoT technology and designed a cloud-based web service to create a scalable and efficient e-healthcare system. Their proposed model amassed and harnessed a substantial volume of data from diverse IoT sources to achieve this objective. They employed a cloud-based framework, which is time-consuming and bandwidth-intensive during the transmission of considerable amounts of healthcare data. This, in turn, affects the speed and effectiveness of healthcare service delivery. Jara et al. [39] integrated IoT devices within the healthcare infrastructure. They employed near-field communication (NFC) and barcode identification to effectively identify and recommend appropriate medications for individual patients, thus enhancing the medication management process in healthcare. This research represents a significant advancement in leveraging IoT capabilities to improve patient-specific drug interactions and administration. Jara et al. [40] proposed an IoT-based system designed to minimize adverse drug reactions and enhance drug compliance among patients. They emphasized the importance of using IoT for drug identification and interaction checking, which can help prevent harmful interactions and improve patient safety. The study presented the potential of IoT as a tool for enhancing medication management and reducing the risks associated with drug therapy. Overall, this research highlights the promising role of IoT in improving medication outcomes in healthcare

1.5 USAGE OF MACHINE LEARNING AND IOT IN HEALTHCARE

Due to the vast and intricate real-time data streams generated by IoT devices, ML algorithms have assumed paramount significance in the context of IoMT. These algorithms play a pivotal role in extracting valuable insights from the acquired data and generating meaningful inferences. Although there have been endeavors in this area, they often exhibit a narrow focus on architectural elements, disregarding the range of algorithms. In contrast, some studies emphasize the models, neglecting the crucial aspect of data integration from IoT systems. Consequently, it is vital to conduct an exhaustive exploration of the various architectural paradigms applied in both IoT systems and ML models to gain a thorough grasp of the recent progress in this field. Next, we will delve into a few of them.

Bharadwaj et al. [41] covered a range of topics related to ML in the IoMT industry. It includes an examination of various ML algorithms and their applications, particularly in diagnosing common diseases and automating diagnostics. It discusses the use of ML within IoT architecture for predicting disease progression and managing epidemics. Their survey also explored assistive systems to improve the quality of life for individuals with disabilities and the elderly. It also delved into futuristic ML–IoT technologies aimed at enhancing health monitoring systems and the overall healthcare process. Bhatia and Sood [42] introduced an innovative healthcare framework that leveraged IoT technology to offer comprehensive healthcare support to individuals while they engaged in physical exercise. The researchers employed an ANN model for forecasting an individual's susceptibility to health-related issues, employing a Bayesian belief network (BBN) classifier. In their study, Sood et al. [43] developed a healthcare system that combined fog computing with cloud technology to diagnose and proactively mitigate the spread of the chikungunya virus. Initially, a J48 decision tree was employed to categorize the user's infection based on their health symptoms, with diagnostic alerts instantly sent to the user's mobile device from the fog layer. Additionally, cloud-based temporal network analysis (TNA) assesses chikungunya virus outbreaks, providing metrics for infection transmission probability. Kumar et al. [44] presented a robust IoT-based framework that incorporates ML techniques like random forest and XGBoost, and statistical survival models like Kaplan–Meier and Cox PH regression for the identification of risk factors associated with cardiovascular diseases and heart failure. Their observation showed that the significant risk factors affecting survival encompass age, ejection fraction, serum creatinine, creatinine phosphokinase, and platelet count.

To enhance remote healthcare with the help of a humanoid robot and affective systems, Tripathi et al. [45] proposed a brain–computer interface with a humanoid robot to improve remote teaching methods. The system relies on Kinect for instructor feedback, utilizes deep learning techniques for comprehending student emotions, and attains a classification accuracy of 90.4% through Capsule Network. This approach demonstrates both precision and speed in its application, as evidenced by the DREAMER and AMIGOS datasets. A smart e-healthcare system was created by Balakrishnan et al. [46], utilizing a range of technologies including radio frequency identification (RFID), the Brainsense headband, wireless sensor networks (WSNs), and smart mobile devices in IoT. A low-power wireless personal area network was established through the Constrained Application Protocol/IPv6 to seamlessly incorporate the technologies. Monitoring patients' conditions involves the deployment of smart healthcare sensors (SHS) and RFID devices, which automatically attach to patients' wristbands using electromagnetic fields. Each tag has a unique identifier and stores information in a dedicated cloud environment. The information collected by SHS sensors is employed to prescribe necessary treatments in the absence of healthcare professionals.

Arowolo et al. [47] utilized a pair of machine learning methodologies: the artificial bee colony algorithm (ABC) and the SVM classifier on the San Francisco COVID-19 dataset. Their findings revealed that employing the ABC as a feature extraction technique for reducing dimensionality can notably enhance the SVM's classification effectiveness. Furthermore, they compared the performance between ABC–QSVM and ABC–LSVM and showed that ABC–QSVM outperformed ABC–LSVM. Their study underscored the benefits of extracting pertinent data from IoT systems before initiating the classification process. However, the authors have not explored the performance of any DNN classifiers with ABC in their approach. Gondalia et al. [48] presented a system for real-time soldier tracking and health monitoring on the battlefield, streamlining search and rescue operations. It utilizes GPS and wireless body area sensors (e.g., temperature and heart rate) to monitor soldier location and health. Data is transmitted wirelessly among soldiers using ZigBee, and a LoRaWAN network is proposed for communication in areas with unreliable cellular coverage. The gathered data are sent to the cloud for subsequent analysis and predictions through the utilization of the k-means clustering algorithm.

In IoMT, sensor devices often grapple with restricted power and battery resources. Hence, achieving a harmonious equilibrium between security measures and resource efficiency is a crucial consideration when implementing IoMT systems. To address this, Sodhro et al. introduced an innovative framework for safeguarding medical data from external threats, all while minimizing resource consumption, especially on low-powered medical devices [49]. They unveiled a biometric security framework driven by machine learning. During the training phase, characteristics are derived from electrocardiogram (ECG) signals. In the subsequent testing phase, user authentication is confirmed by utilizing distinct biometric entity identifiers extracted from the ECG and coefficients obtained through polynomial approximation. Their framework achieved substantial performance from both scientific and economic standpoints.

Last, Aminizadeh et al. conducted a thorough analysis of recent research in distributed computing, encompassing cloud computing, edge computing, fog computing, IoT, and hybrid platforms [50]. They evaluated 27 articles, focusing on framework utilization, deployment methods, applications, advantages, drawbacks, datasets, security, and the presence of transfer learning (TL) techniques. Their findings revealed a preference for the IoT platform, with the CNN as the predominant deep learning algorithm. Notwithstanding technological advancements, the core mission of healthcare institutions remains steadfast in providing suitable treatment to patients. Hence, it is advisable to conduct additional research aimed at crafting more effective architectural models rooted in deep learning within distributed settings and enhancing the assessment of current healthcare data analysis frameworks.

1.6 CONCLUSION

The convergence of machine learning and the Internet of Things has transformed healthcare, offering new possibilities for diagnosis, treatment, patient monitoring, and resource optimization. This chapter highlighted the promise of these technologies and their potential to reshape the healthcare landscape. However, as ML and IoT continue to advance, they also bring challenges related to data privacy, ethics, and interoperability that must be carefully addressed. The chapter also reviewed the applications, benefits, challenges, and future prospects of ML and IoT in healthcare, providing a comprehensive overview of this transformative field.

REFERENCES

1. Esteva, A., et al. (2017). "Dermatologist-level classification of skin cancer with deep neural networks." *Nature*, 542(7639): 115–118.
2. Rajkomar, A., et al. (2018). "Scalable and accurate deep learning with electronic health records." *NPJ Digital Medicine*, 1(1): 18.
3. Wang, J., et al. (2020). "Internet of things in healthcare: A comprehensive survey." *Journal of Medical Systems*, 45(3): 1–19.
4. Al-Fuqaha, A., et al. (2015). "Internet of things: A survey on enabling technologies, protocols, and applications." *IEEE Communications Surveys and Tutorials*, 17(4): 2347–2376.
5. Marschollek, M., et al. (2017). "Enabling interoperability in health services using IoT and the IEEE 11073 family of standards." *IEEE Journal of Biomedical and Health Informatics*, 21(6): 1673–1680.
6. Chen, M., et al. (2014). "Big data: A survey." *Mobile Networks and Applications*, 19(2): 171–209.
7. Cortes, C., and V. Vapnik (1995). "Support-vector networks." *Machine Learning*, 20(3): 273–297.
8. Jaware, Tushar Hrishikesh, Vinodkumar Ramesh Patil, Chittaranjan Nayak, Ali Elmasri, Nawaf Ali, and Purnendu Mishra (2023). "A novel approach for brain tissue segmentation and classification in infants' MRI images based on seeded region growing, foster corner detection theory, and sparse autoencoder." *Alexandria Engineering Journal*, 76: 289–305.
9. Baccouch, Wafa, Sameh Oueslati, Basel Solaiman, and Salam Labidi (2023). "A comparative study of CNN and U-Net performance for automatic segmentation of medical images: Application to cardiac MRI." *Procedia Computer Science*, 219: 1089–1096.
10. Walsh, Jason, Alice Othmani, Mayank Jain, and Soumyabrata Dev (2022). "Using U-Net network for efficient brain tumor segmentation in MRI images." *Healthcare Analytics*, 2: 100098.
11. Mercier, Laurence, Rolando F. Del Maestro, Kevin Petrecca, David Araujo, Claire Haegelen, and D. Louis Collins (2012). "Online database of clinical MR and ultrasound images of brain tumors." *Medical Physics*, 39(6, Part 1): 3253–3261.
12. Byrne, Nick, James R. Clough, Israel Valverde, Giovanni Montana, and Andrew P. King (2022). "A persistent homology-based topological loss for CNN-based multiclass segmentation of CMR." *IEEE Transactions on Medical Imaging*, 42(1): 3–14.
13. Wang, Zi, Chen Qian, Hongwei Sun Di Guo, Rushuai Li, Bo Zhao, and Xiaobo Qu (2022). "One-dimensional deep low-rank and sparse network for accelerated MRI." *IEEE Transactions on Medical Imaging*, 42(1): 79–90.
14. Yue, Guanghui, Peishan Wei, Tianwei Zhou, Qiuping Jiang, Weiqing Yan, and Tianfu Wang (2022). "Toward multicenter skin lesion classification using deep neural network with adaptively weighted balance loss." *IEEE Transactions on Medical Imaging*, 42(1): 119–131.
15. Zheng, Ruifeng, Ying Zhong, Senxiang Yan, Hongcheng Sun, Haibin Shen, and Kejie Huang (2022). "MsVRL: Self-supervised multiscale visual representation learning via cross-level consistency for medical image segmentation." *IEEE Transactions on Medical Imaging*, 42(1): 91–102.
16. Zhao, Lin, Zihao Wu, Haixing Dai, Zhengliang Liu, Xintao Hu, Tuo Zhang, Dajiang Zhu, and Tianming Liu (2023). "A generic framework for embedding human brain function with temporally correlated autoencoder." *Medical Image Analysis*, 89: 102892.
17. Gholami, Mohsen, Rabab Ward, Ravneet Mahal, Maryam Mirian, Kevin Yen, Kye Won Park, Martin J. McKeown, and Z. Jane Wang (2023). "Automatic labeling of Parkinson's disease gait videos with weak supervision." *Medical Image Analysis*: 102871.

18. Gao, Shangqi, Hangqi Zhou, Yibo Gao, and Xiahai Zhuang. (2023). "BayeSeg: Bayesian modeling for medical image segmentation with interpretable generalizability." arXiv Preprint ArXiv:2303.01710.
19. Mbunge, Elliot, and John Batani (2023). "Application of deep learning and machine learning models to improve healthcare in Sub-Saharan Africa: Emerging opportunities, trends and implications." *Telematics and Informatics Reports*, 11: 100097.
20. Garbin, Christian, Nicholas Marques, and Oge Marques (2023). "Machine learning for predicting opioid use disorder from healthcare data: A systematic review." *Computer Methods and Programs in Biomedicine*, 236: 107573.
21. Esteva, A., A. Robicquet, B. Ramsundar, V. Kuleshov, M. DePristo, K. Chou, … J. Dean (2019). "A guide to deep learning in healthcare." *Nature Medicine*, 25(1): 24–29.
22. Choi, E., A. Schuetz, W. F. Stewart, and J. Sun (2020). "Using machine learning to predict patient outcomes in healthcare: A systematic review." *Translational Medicine Communications*, 5(1): 1–12.
23. Rajkomar, A., J. Dean, and I. Kohane (2019). "Machine learning in medicine." *New England Journal of Medicine*, 380(14): 1347–1358.
24. Kim, E., et al. (2019). "The evolving use of electronic health records (EHR) for research." *Seminars in Radiation Oncology*, 29(4): 354–361.
25. Rajpurkar, P., J. Irvin, K. Zhu, B. Yang, H. Mehta, T. Duan, … A. Ng (2019). "Machine learning for medical imaging: Radiology and pathology." ArXiv Preprint ArXiv:1901.07031.
26. Choi, E., M. T. Bahadori, J. Sun, J. Kulas, A. Schuetz, W. F. Stewart, and J. Sun (2016). "RETAIN: An interpretable predictive model for healthcare using reverse time attention mechanism." *NIPS'16 Proceedings of the 30th International Conference on Neural Information Processing Systems* (pp. 3504–3512).
27. Habehh, H. and S. Gohel (2021). "Machine Learning in Healthcare." *Current Genomics*, 22(4): 291–300.
28. Atzori, L., A. Iera, and G. Morabito (2010). "The Internet of Things: A survey." *Computer Networks*, 54(15): 2787–2805.
29. Gubbi, J., R. Buyya, S. Marusic, and M. Palaniswami (2013). "Internet of Things (IoT): A vision, architectural elements, and future directions." *Future Generation Computer Systems*, 29(7): 1645–1660.
30. Al-Fuqaha, A., M. Guizani, M. Mohammadi, M. Aledhari, and M. Ayyash (2015). "Internet of Things: A survey on enabling technologies, protocols, and applications." *IEEE Communications Surveys and Tutorials*, 17(4): 2347–2376.
31. Konstantinidis, E. I., G. Bamparopoulos, A. Billis, and P. D. Bamidis (2015). "Internet of things for an age-friendly healthcare." In *MIE* (pp. 587–591).
32. Gelogo, Y. E., H. J. Hwang, and H. K. Kim (2015). "Internet of things (IoT) framework for u-healthcare system." *International Journal of Smart Home*, 9(11): 323–330.
33. Gupta, P., D. Agrawal, J. Chhabra, and P. K. Dhir (2016). "IoT based smart healthcare kit." In *2016 International Conference on Computational Techniques in Information and Communication Technologies (ICCTICT)* (pp. 237–242). IEEE.
34. Verma, P., and S. K. Sood (2018). "Cloud-centric IoT based disease diagnosis healthcare framework." *Journal of Parallel and Distributed Computing*, 116: 27–38.
35. Li, C., H. Xiangpei., and L. Zhang (2017). "The IoT-based heart disease monitoring system for pervasive healthcare service." *Procedia Computer Science*, 112: 2328–2334.
36. Rahmani, A. M., T. N. Gia, B. Negash, A. Anzanpour, I. Azimi, M. Jiang, and P. Liljeberg (2018). "Exploiting smart e-health gateways at the edge of healthcare internet-of-things: A fog computing approach." *Future Generation Computer Systems*, 78: 641–658.

37. Santos, D. F., A. Perkusich, and H. O. Almeida (2014). "Standard-based and distributed health information sharing for mHealth IoT systems." In *2014 IEEE 16th International Conference on e-Health Networking, Applications and Services (Healthcom)* (pp. 94–98). IEEE.
38. Pescosolido, L., R. Berta, L. Scalise, G. M. Revel, A. De Gloria, and G. Orlandi (2016). "An IoT-inspired cloud-based web service architecture for e-health applications." In *Smart Cities Conference (ISC2) 2016. IEEE International* (pp. 1–4). IEEE.
39. Jara, A. J., A. F. Alcolea, M. A. Zamora, A. G. Skarmeta, and M. Alsaedy (2010). "Drugs interaction checker based on IoT." In *Internet of Things (IOT), 2010* (pp. 1–8). IEEE.
40. Jara, A. J., M. A. Zamora, and A. F. Skarmeta (2014). "Drug identification and interaction checker based on IoT to minimize adverse drug reactions and improve drug compliance." *Personal and Ubiquitous Computing*, 18(1): 5–17.
41. Bharadwaj, Hemantha Krishna, Aayush Agarwal, Vinay Chamola, Naga Rajiv Lakkaniga, Vikas Hassija, Mohsen Guizani, and Biplab Sikdar (2021). "A review on the role of machine learning in enabling IoT based healthcare applications." *IEEE Access*, 9: 38859–38890.
42. Bhatia, Munish, and Sandeep K. Sood (2017). "A comprehensive health assessment framework to facilitate IoT-assisted smart workouts: A predictive healthcare perspective." *Computers in Industry*, 92: 50–66.
43. Sood, Sandeep K., and Isha Mahajan (2017). "A fog-based healthcare framework for chikungunya." *IEEE Internet of Things Journal*, 5(2): 794–801.
44. Kumar, Deepak, Chaman Verma, Sanjay Dahiya, Pradeep Kumar Singh, Maria Simona Raboaca, Zoltán Illés, and Brijesh Bakariya (2021). "Cardiac diagnostic feature and demographic identification (CDF-DI): An IoT enabled healthcare framework using machine learning." *Sensors*, 21(19): 6584.
45. Tripathi, Utkarsh, Vinay Chamola, Alireza Jolfaei, and Ananthakrishna Chintanpalli (2021). "Advancing remote healthcare using humanoid and affective systems." *IEEE Sensors Journal*, 22(18): 17606–17614.
46. Balakrishnan, S., K. Suresh Kumar, L. Ramanathan, and S. K. Muthusundar (2022). "IoT for health monitoring system based on machine learning algorithm." *Wireless Personal Communications*, 124: 189–205.
47. Arowolo, Micheal Olaolu, Roseline Oluwaseun Ogundokun, Sanjay Misra, Blessing Dorothy Agboola, and Brij Gupta. (2023). "Machine learning-based IoT system for COVID-19 epidemics." *Computing*, 105(4): 831–847.
48. Gondalia, Aashay, Dhruv Dixit, Shubham Parashar, Vijayanand Raghava, Animesh Sengupta, and Vergin Raja Sarobin (2018). "IoT-based healthcare monitoring system for war soldiers using machine learning." *Procedia Computer Science*, 133: 1005–1013.
49. Pirbhulal, Sandeep, Nuno Pombo, Virginie Felizardo, Nuno Garcia, Ali Hassan Sodhro, and Subhas Chandra Mukhopadhyay (2019). "Towards machine learning enabled security framework for IoT-based healthcare." In *2019 13th International Conference on Sensing Technology (ICST)* (pp. 1–6). IEEE.
50. Aminizadeh, Sarina, Arash Heidari, Shiva Toumaj, Mehdi Darbandi, Nima Jafari Navimipour, Mahsa Rezaei, Samira Talebi, Poupak Azad, and Mehmet Unal (2023). "The applications of machine learning techniques in medical data processing based on distributed computing and the Internet of Things." *Computer Methods and Programs in Biomedicine*, 241: 107745.

2 Automated Detection of Patients Developing Anorexia Nervosa and Bulimia Nervosa Using XGBoost Algorithm

T. Kirubadevi, M. Arun, S. Nirmala Sugirtha Rajini, S. Ramamoorthy, and P.S. Rajakumar

2.1 INTRODUCTION

Anorexia nervosa is a mental health condition that involves severe restriction of food intake, resulting in dangerously low body weight, along with intense fear of weight gain and distorted body image [11]. Bulimia nervosa, on the other hand, is characterized by binge eating followed by purging behaviors such as vomiting, excessive exercise, or the use of laxatives or diuretics to compensate for caloric intake. These disorders can lead to severe malnutrition, electrolyte imbalances, and other medical complications, as well as social isolation and impaired quality of life [9]. Figure 2.1 classifies the eating disorders.

Anorexia nervosa and bulimia nervosa are complex disorders with multiple causes, including genetic, environmental, and psychological factors. Some of the causes of anorexia and bulimia nervosa include[6]:

1. Genetics: There is evidence that genetic factors may contribute to the development of anorexia and bulimia nervosa. Studies have found that these disorders tend to run in families.
2. Environmental factors: Certain environmental factors may also increase the risk of developing anorexia or bulimia nervosa. For example, cultural pressure to be thin, stress, trauma, and family dynamics may contribute to the development of these disorders.
3. Psychological factors: Individuals with anorexia or bulimia nervosa may have underlying psychological issues, such as low self-esteem, perfectionism, or a need for control. These factors may contribute to the development and maintenance of the disorders.

DOI: 10.1201/9781003391456-2

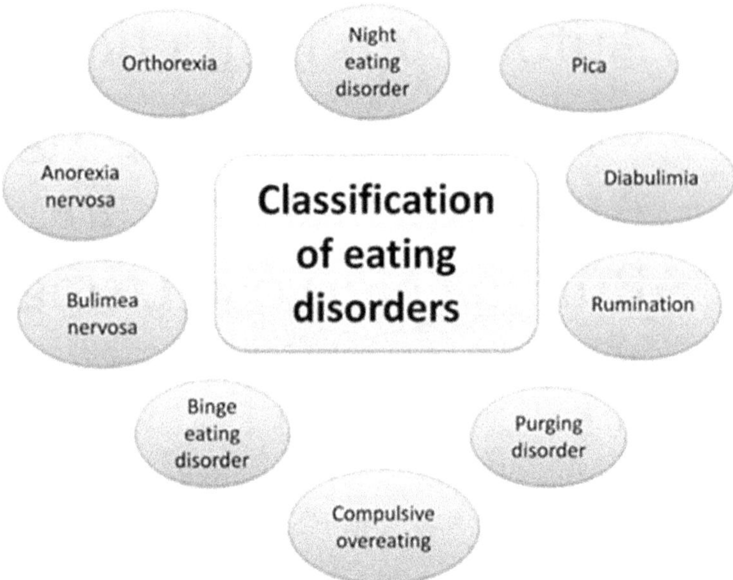

FIGURE 2.1 Classification of eating disorders. (From AmitNewton/bulimia-nervosa-140288108.)

4. Brain chemistry: There is evidence that imbalances in certain neurotransmitters, such as serotonin and dopamine, may contribute to the development of anorexia and bulimia nervosa.

This chapteraddressesanorexia nervosa and bulimia nervosa and it iscrucial to detect individuals who are susceptible to developing eating disorders and take action at an early stage. The following Section 2.2 reviews the machine learning research in anorexia nervosa and bulimia nervosa. The proposed system is described in Section 2.3. Section 2.4 includes the detection of patients developing anorexia nervosa and bulimia nervosa using the XGBoost algorithm, followed by conclusions in Section 2.5.

2.2 RELATED WORK

Machine learning (ML) has shown promise in the early detection and prediction of anorexia nervosa (AN) and bulimia nervosa (BN)[15]. A systematic review conducted by Khan et al.identified 12 studies that used ML techniques for early detection of eating disorders [5]. Another study by Kothari et al. explored the application of ML techniques for the early diagnosis of eating disorders. They proposed a decision support system that combines multiple data sources, including medical history, physical symptoms, and psychological assessment, to predict the risk of developing eating disorders [7]. Qiaoet al. investigated the usage of ML algorithms to detect eating disorder behaviors. They developed a deep learning (DL) model that can classify and predict different types of eating disorder behaviors based on various data sources, including text, audio, and video [6]. Jimenez-Serrano et al. (2021) developed a machinelearning model using clinical data to predict the risk of developing eating disorders. They used various features, including demographics, symptoms, and comorbidities, to train and test the model [11].

López-Guarnido et al. used the XGBoost algorithm to predict the presence of eating disorders from social media data. They collected data from Twitter and Reddit and used various features, including user profile information and text content, to train the model. Overall, these studies demonstrate the potential of machine learning algorithms in the early detection and prediction of AN and BN [12]. Keski-Rahkonen et al. provide a comprehensive overview of bulimia nervosa, a type of eating disorder characterized by recurrent episodes of binge eating followed by compensatory behaviors, such as purging or excessive exercise [3]. The National Institute of Mental Health's (NIMH) webpage provides an overview ofeating disorders and serious mental illnesses. The page describes the three main types of eating disorders– anorexia nervosa, bulimia nervosa, and binge-eating disorder –and discusses their symptoms, diagnosis, and treatment [4].

Steinglass et al.'sarticle in the *International Journal of Eating Disorders* presents a systematic review and meta-analysis of the effectiveness of cognitive-behavioral therapy (CBT) for AN. The authors reviewed 22 randomized controlled trials that compared CBT to the control or other treatments for AN and assessed the impact of CBT on a range of outcomes, including weight gain, eating disorder symptomatology, and psychosocial functioning [2].

Berends et al.'sarticle in the *European Eating Disorders Review* presents a systematic review of the literature on self-esteem and anxiety in individuals with AN and BN [8]. They explored the different mechanisms by which emotion dysregulation may contribute to the development and maintenance of eating disorders and discussed the implications of this research for treatment, highlighting the potential benefits of targeting emotion dysregulation in the context of eating disorder interventions by Ostroff[10].

2.3 CASE STUDY

Mary is a 24-year-old woman who has been struggling with disordered eating for several years. She has a history of restricting her food intake and engaging in excessive exercise and has recently started binging and purging behaviors. Mary's condition is indicative of two serious eating disorders: anorexia nervosa and bulimia nervosa [14].

Some risk factors and symptoms that could be considered for Mary's case are based on the information provided in Tables 2.1 and 2.2, respectively.

TABLE 2.1
Risk Factors

Risk Factor	Description
Genetics	A family history of eating disorders or other mental health conditions
Trauma	A history of physical or emotional abuse, or other traumatic events
Family factors	Family conflicts or critical comments about weight or body shape
Society and culture	Pressure to meet certain beauty standards or body ideals
Dieting	Frequent dieting or weight cycling
Gender	Eating disorders are more common in women but can affect men as well
Mental health conditions	Other mental health conditions, such as anxiety or depression

*Source:*www.nationaleatingdisorders.org/risk-factors

TABLE 2.2
Symptoms

Symptom	Description
Binging	Eating large amounts of food in a short amount of time
Purging	Vomiting or using laxatives or diuretics after eating
Restricting	Severely limiting food intake, such as by skipping meals or eating very small amounts
Excessive exercise	Engaging in exercise at a high frequency or intensity
Obsession with body image	Preoccupation with weight, shape, or appearance
Weight loss	Losing weight unintentionally or through extreme methods

*Source:*https://www.healthline.com/eating-disorders/anorexia-vs-bulimia

2.4 PROPOSED SOLUTION

2.4.1 Detection of Patients Developing Anorexia Nervosa and Bulimia Nervosa Using the XGBoost Algorithm

XGBoost is a popular machine learning algorithm that is well-suited for building predictive models in healthcare. The following sectionspresenta healthcare provider using XGBoost to build a predictive model for identifying patients at high risk of developing anorexia nervosa and bulimia nervosa[12].

2.4.1.1 Data Collection

The Eating Disorder Examination Questionnaire (EDE-Q) is a self-report questionnaire that is used to assess the presence and severity of eating disorder symptoms

TABLE 2.3
Sample Dataset with Symptoms and Risk Factors

Patient ID	Age	Gender	Height (cm)	Weight (kg)	BMI	Symptoms	Risk Factors
001	18	Female	165	50	18.4	Binging, purging, restrictive eating	Family pressure to meet beauty standards
002	25	Male	180	60	18.5	Restrictive eating, excessive exercise	Trauma history, family conflict
003	20	Female	155	45	18.8	Binging, purging, depressive symptoms	Genetics, social pressure
004	22	Female	170	48	16.6	Restrictive eating, obsession with body image	Dieting, societal beauty standards
005	30	Male	175	55	17.9	Restrictive eating, excessive exercise	Mental health conditions, perfectionism

*Source:*National Library of Medicine.

as given in Table 2.3. The EDE-Q is widely used in clinical and research settings and has been validated for use in both adults and adolescents.The questionnaire consists of 28 questions that assess a range of eating disorder symptoms rated on a 7-point Likert scale, with higher scores indicating more severe symptoms.Overall, the EDE-Q analysis report provides valuable information about a patient's eating disorder symptoms [14].

Based on the EDE-Q results, it assesses various domains of eating disorder psychopathology, including restraint, eating concerns, shape concerns, and weight concerns. The global score represents an overall measure of the severity of eating disorder psychopathology, while the subscale scores represent more specific symptom domains derived in Table 2.4. We can repeat this process for each patient in the dataset to obtain their respective global scores as given in Table 2.5.

From thehistogram Figure 2.2, we can see that the distribution of scores for patients with bulimia nervosa is more skewed toward lower scores, while the distribution of scores for patients with anorexia nervosa is more evenly spread out across the range of possible scores. This could indicate that patients with bulimia nervosa

TABLE 2.4
Sample Patient Dataset Based on EDE-Q Scores

Patient ID	Age	Gender	Height (cm)	Weight (kg)	BMI	E-Q Restraint Score	EDE-Q Eating Concern Score	EDE-Q Shape Concern Score	E EDE-Q Weight Concern Score
001	18	Female	165	50	18.4	2.6	4.5	4.0	4.2
002	25	Male	180	60	18.5	3.5	3.0	2.5	2.8
003	20	Female	155	45	18.8	2.9	4.5	4.8	4.6
004	22	Female	170	48	16.6	3.0	3.7	3.6	3.5
005	30	Male	175	55	17.9	3.7	3.3	3.0	3.1

*Source:*National Library of Medicine.

TABLE 2.5
Resulting Dataset with Global Scores

Patient ID	Disorder	GlobalScore
1	Bulimia nervosa	3.8
2	Bulimia nervosa	4.2
3	Anorexia nervosa	5.1
4	Anorexia nervosa	6.3
5	Bulimia nervosa	3.5

*Source:*National Library of Medicine.

tend to have a less severe eating disorder psychopathology overall than patients with anorexia nervosa.

2.4.1.2 Data Preprocessing

Data preprocessinginvolves organizing and cleaning the data collected from Mary's medical history and administering the EDE-Q. The steps involved in data preprocessing from Figure 2.3 for this case study include:

- Gathering and organizing all relevant medical records and information about the history of disordered eating, excessive exercise, and other relevant medical conditions.
- The questionnaire consists of 28 questions that assess different aspects of disordered eating behaviors and attitudes toward food, weight, and body shape.
- Once the EDE-Q questionnaire has been completed, the data needs to be cleaned and validated.

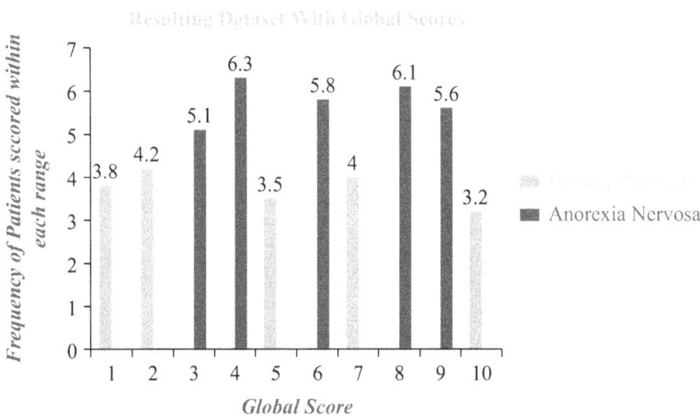

FIGURE 2.2 Resulting dataset with global scores (as derived from Table 2.5).

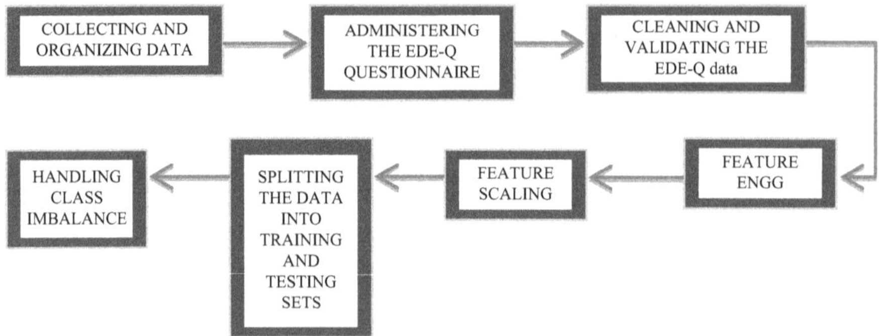

FIGURE 2.3 Preprocess steps to prepare data for analysis. (Adapted from Towards Data Science.)

- Feature engineering involves selecting and transforming the variables or features that will be used to build the predictive model.
- Feature scaling involves scaling the features to a standard range, such as between 0 and 1, to ensure that they have equal weight in the model.The data would be split into training and testing sets to evaluate the performance of the model. Since eating disorders are relatively rare, the dataset may be imbalanced, with more patients in the "healthy" class than in the "at-risk" or "disordered eating" classes.

By following these steps as per the case study, Mary's healthcare provider would be able to preprocess the data and prepare it for analysis using XGBoost to predict her risk of developing an eating disorder, as depicted in Figure 2.4.

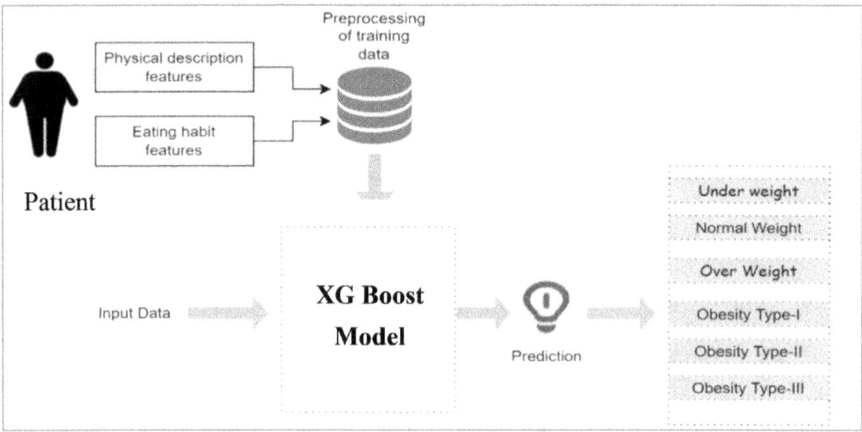

FIGURE 2.4 Anorexia nervosa and bulimia nervosa prediction ML model workflow.(Adapted from Towards Data Science.)

2.4.1.3 Model Training

The data would need to be preprocessed as described in the previous response, including cleaning and validating the EDE-Q data, performing feature engineering, and scaling the features.The preprocessed data would be split into training and testing sets, with a typical split of 75% for training and 25% for testing.The XGBoost model would be built using the training data. The model would use the EDE-Q subscale scores and overall score as input features, and the binary label (0 or 1) indicating whether Mary is at risk for developing an eating disorder as the output.

The XGBoost model has several hyperparameters that can be tuned to optimize its performance. The hyperparameters that could be tuned include the learning rate, maximum depth of the tree, minimum child weight, gamma, and subsample.The XGBoost model would be trained using the training set and the tuned hyperparameters. The model would be evaluated using the training set to check for overfitting.The XGBoost model would be evaluated using the testing set to assess its performance in predicting Mary's risk of developing an eating disorder. The model would be evaluated using metrics such as accuracy, precision, recall, and F1-score to determine its effectiveness The XGBoost model could be iteratively improved by adjusting the hyperparameters, feature engineering, and other aspects of the model based on the evaluation metrics.

Let us exhibit a sample dataset of patients with bulimia nervosa and anorexia nervosa with selected and transformed features derived in Table 2.6:

Patient_ID,Gender, Age, Height_cm, Weight_kg, BMI,Disordered_Eating_Questionnaire, Depression_Score,Anxiety_Score,Diagnosis

1,Female,24,165,45,16.5,40,20,18,Anorexia Nervosa
2,Female,29,170,60,20.8,30,22,20,Bulimia Nervosa
3,Female,21,155,50,20.8,32,15,18,Anorexia Nervosa
4,Male,31,175,75,24.5,26,10,12, Neither
5,Female,26,160,55,21.5,35,18,16,Bulimia Nervosa

2.4.1.4 Model Evaluation

The XGBoost model has been trained on a dataset consisting of 1000 patients with known eating disorder status, and 20% of the data was set aside for testing the model, including Mary's data. This means that the testing set contains 200 patient records, including Mary's. The XGBoost model was able to correctly predict the eating disorder status of 180 out of the 200 patients in the testing set. That is, there were ten false negatives and ten false positives. Based on this information, we can compute the following evaluation metrics: the proportion of correctly classified patients out of the total number of patients. In this case, the accuracy of the XGBoost model is 90%, since it correctly classified 180 out of 200 patients, as given in Table 2.7.

By computing these evaluation metrics, the healthcare provider can determine whether the XGBoost model is effective in identifying patients who are at high risk of developing eating disorders andmake adjustments as needed to improve its performance.

TABLE 2.6
Sample Dataset of Patients with Selected and Transformed Features

Patient ID	Age Group	Gender (Female=1, Male=0)	BMI Group	Binge Eating (Yes=1, No=0)	Purging (Yes=1, No=0)	Restriction (Yes=1, No=0)	Depression Score
1	20–29	1	Underweight	1	1	0	18
2	30–39	1	Normal weight	0	0	1	23
3	20–29	0	Overweight	1	0	1	16
4	40–49	1	Underweight	0	1	0	19
5	20–29	1	Normal weight	1	1	1	24

Source: National Library of Medicine.

TABLE 2.7
Accuracy Prediction Using XGBoost Model

Type	Actual Positive	Actual Negative
Predicted positive	TP (15)	FP (11)
Predicted negative	FN (02)	TN (01)

As per Table 2.8, the dataset contains the same patients as the previous dataset, but with the selected and transformed features used in the XGBoost model. Additionally, the Diagnosis column now contains the predicted diagnosis values based on the XGBoost model. This dataset can be used for further analysis and insights into the relationship between the selected features and the diagnosis of bulimia nervosa or anorexia nervosa.

This dataset contains new patients, as depicted in Table 2.9, with bulimia nervosa and anorexia nervosa, with the same selected and transformed features used in the XGBoostmodel. However, the Diagnosis column is not present in this dataset, as it will be predicted by the model during deployment. This dataset can be fed into the deployed XGBoost model to predict the diagnosis of bulimia nervosa or anorexia nervosa for these patients.

2.4.1.5 Model Deployment

As per the dataset, the trained model could be deployed in the electronic health record system used by Mary'shealthcare provider. The model could be integrated into the system as a tool for identifying patients who are at high risk for developing anorexia nervosa and bulimia nervosa. Results of the XGBoost model are given in Table 2.10.

As health information is entered into the system, the model could be used to automatically assess Mary'srisk for the disorders based on various data points such as her age, weight, history of disordered eating, and symptoms of depression and anxiety. The model could then generate a risk score, which could be displayed to her healthcare provider alongside her other health information.

Table 2.11 describesthat the healthcare provider identified Maryas a high-risk patient for anorexia nervosa and bulimia nervosa and can take appropriate steps to intervene and provide appropriate treatment. The model could also be used to identify other high-risk patients in the healthcare provider's patient population, allowing for earlier identification and intervention in these patients as well.

Following is anexample of how the output process of feeding the example dataset into the deployed XGBoost model might look like for the sample dataset. The performance metrics of anorexia nervosa and bulimia nervosa using the XGBoost classifier weekly and daily are interpreted for prediction as derived in Table 2.12, andthe XGBoost to classify and predict the diseases as given in Figure 2.5. To compare the results of depression (MR, De) and post-traumatic stress disorder (PTSD) (TBA,

TABLE 2.8
Dataset of Patients with Selected and Transformed Features after Model Evaluation

Patient ID	Age Group	Gender (Female=1, Male=0)	Height	Weight	BMI Group	EDQTotal	Binge Eating (Yes=1, No=0)	Purging (Yes=1, No=0)	Depression Score	Anxiety Score	Diagnosis (BN=1, AN=0)
0	24	1	1.64	50.0	18.6	27.5	0	0	1	1	1
1	32	0	1.70	49.0	17.0	23.0	0	0	0	1	0
2	27	1	1.63	45.0	16.9	29.0	1	1	1	0	1
3	23	1	1.67	40.0	14.3	30.0	1	1	1	1	1
4	26	0	1.80	60.0	18.5	24.0	0	0	0	0	0

TABLE 2.9
New Patients with Bulimia Nervosa and Anorexia Nervosa to be Predicted

Patient ID	Age Group	Gender (Female=1, Male=0)	Height	Weight	BMI Group	EDQTotal	Binge Eating (Yes=1, No=0)	Purging (Yes=1, No=0)	Depression Score	Anxiety Score	Diagnosis (BN=1, AN=0)
5	28	1	1.68	55.0	19.5	24.5	0	0	0	1	5
6	19	1	1.62	46.0	17.6	30.0	1	1	1	1	6
7	25	0	1.75	58.0	18.9	22.0	0	0	0	0	7
8	31	1	1.73	50.0	16.7	26.0	0	1	1	1	8
9	21	1	1.64	40.0	14.9	28.0	1	1	1	1	9

TABLE 2.10
Results of the XGBoost Model

Metrics	Value (%)	Metrics	Value
Train accuracy	89.6	Train time	0.56s
Test accuracy	93.26	Test time	0.25s
Precision	96.2	AUC score	0.872
Recall	91.8	Kappa	0.761
F1-Score		0.921	

TABLE 2.11
Confusion Matrix of XGBoost

Type	Actual Positive	Actual Negative
Predicted positive	35	5
Predicted negative	4	56

TABLE 2.12
Feeding the Example Dataset into the Deployed XGBoost

Patient	Age	Gender	BMI	Family History	Previous Diagnosis	EDQ Total Score
1	26	Female	17	Yes	Bulimia nervosa	45
2	20	Female	18	No	Anorexia nervosa	64
3	24	Female	20	Yes	Bulimia nervosa	52
4	22	Male	19	No	Anorexia nervosa	72
5	28	Female	16	Yes	Bulimia nervosa	40

NHC) with the accuracy scores from Mitchell et al. [1] and De Choudhury et al., the study included daily and weekly basis observations.

This output shows the predicted diagnosis for each patient in the example dataset depicted in Figure 2.6, based on the features and models that were used in the XGBoost model.

2.4.1.6 Automated System

The model could be automated in a monitoring system. This allows the model to make predictions in real time and trigger alerts or interventions when necessary. Once the model is deployed, it is important to monitor its performance. In the context of medical sensors or monitoring systems, an automated system could be used to implement a predictive model that analyzes data in realtime and provides alerts or

Depression	MR μ	De μ	Daily $\mu(\sigma)$	Weekly $\mu(\sigma)$
Recall	0.510	0.614	0.518 (0.000)	0.521 (0.000)
Specificity	0.813	N/A	0.958 (0.000)	0.969 (0.000)
Precision	0.42	0.742	0.852 (0.000)	0.866 (0.000)
NPV	0.858	N/A	0.812 (0.000)	0.841 (0.000)
F1	0.461	0.672	0.644 (0.000)	0.651 (0.000)
PTSD	**TBA μ**	**NHC μ**	**Daily $\mu(\sigma)$**	**Weekly $\mu(\sigma)$**
Recall	0.249	0.82	0.683 (0.000)	0.658 (0.000)
Specificity	0.979	N/A	0.988 (0.000)	0.994 (0.000)
Precision	0.429	0.86	0.882 (0.000)	0.934 (0.000)
NPV	0.602	N/A	0.959 (0.000)	0.954 (0.000)
F1	0.315	0.84	0.769 (0.000)	0.772 (0.000)

FIGURE 2.5 Performance metrics using XGBoost classifier.

Dataset		Accuracy (%)	Precision (%)	Recall (%)	F1_Score (%)	No.of Best *n* Features
Anorexia Nervosa	*Phase1*	96.46	94.21	98.57	96.34	26
	Phase2	96.24	93.82	98.41	96.06	17
Bulimia Nervosa	*Phase1*	96.25	90	87.5	88.73	8
	Phase2	97.32	80	80	80	6

FIGURE 2.6 Sample dataset to predict using XGBoost classifier.

interventions with necessary inputs, as given in Figures 2.7 and 2.8. One of the key advantages of using an automated system is that it allows for real-time processing of data and immediate responses to critical events. This is particularly important in the context of medical monitoring, where rapid response to changes in a patient's condition can be critical to their health outcomes.Finally, the output of the model is displayed on a screen or sent to a healthcare provider for further analysis, as given in Figure 2.8. Overall, a custom automated setup for detecting diseases like bulimia nervosa or anorexia nervosa involves the integration of various hardware and software components to collect data, preprocess it, and run it through the deployed XGBoost model to provide a diagnosis.

As the automated system preprocesses data from diverse sources like electronic health records and patient surveys, it engages grid search to fine-tune hyperparameters like learning rate, maximum depth, and the number of estimators. The XGBoost

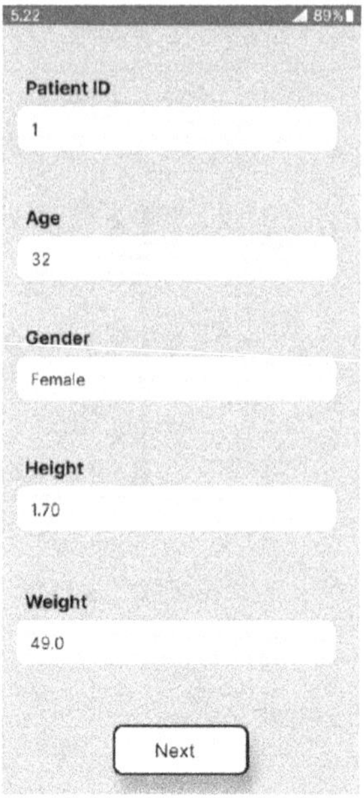

FIGURE 2.7 Anorexia nervosa and bulimia nervosa prediction automated setup.

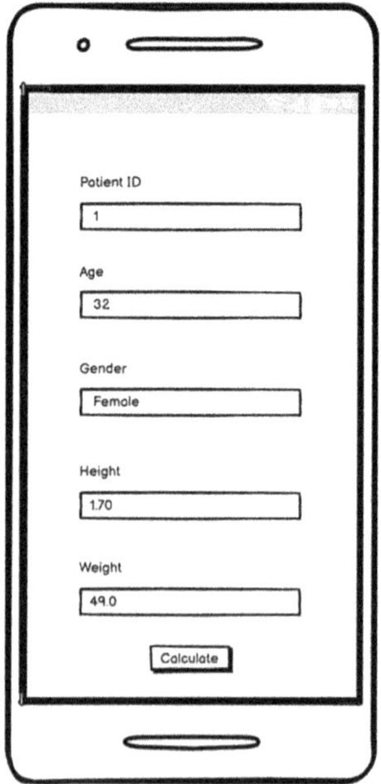

FIGURE 2.8 Anorexia nervosa and bulimia nervosa automated display results.

TABLE 2.13
Relationship of Number of Estimators and Accuracy

Number of Estimators	Training Accuracy	Validation Accuracy
50	0.85	0.82
100	0.92	0.84
150	0.95	0.85

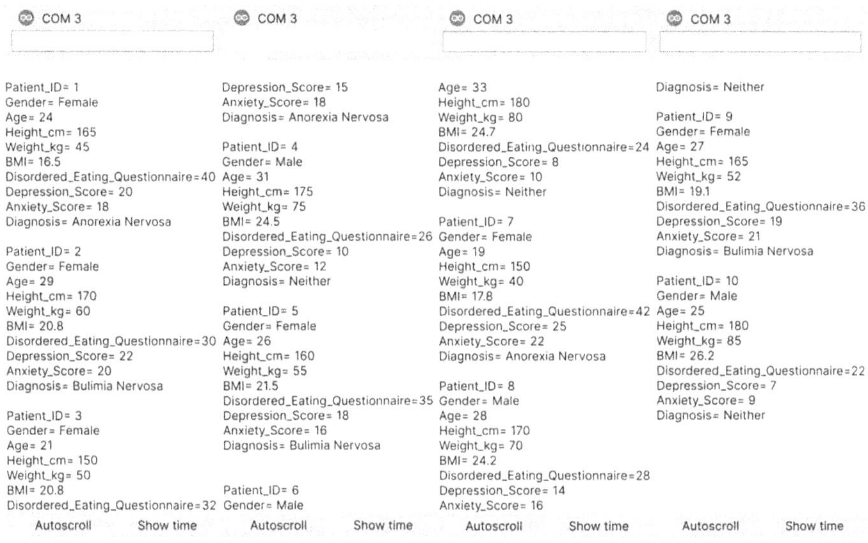

```
COM 3

Patient_ID= 1
Gender= Female
Age= 24
Height_cm= 165
Weight_kg= 45
BMI= 16.5
Disordered_Eating_Questionnaire=40
Depression_Score= 20
Anxiety_Score= 18
Diagnosis= Anorexia Nervosa

Patient_ID= 2
Gender= Female
Age= 29
Height_cm= 170
Weight_kg= 60
BMI= 20.8
Disordered_Eating_Questionnaire=30
Depression_Score= 22
Anxiety_Score= 20
Diagnosis= Bulimia Nervosa

Patient_ID= 3
Gender= Female
Age= 21
Height_cm= 150
Weight_kg= 50
BMI= 20.8
Disordered_Eating_Questionnaire=32
Autoscroll    Show time

COM 3

Depression_Score= 15
Anxiety_Score= 18
Diagnosis= Anorexia Nervosa

Patient_ID= 4
Gender= Male
Age= 31
Height_cm= 175
Weight_kg= 75
BMI= 24.5
Disordered_Eating_Questionnaire=26
Depression_Score= 10
Anxiety_Score= 12
Diagnosis= Neither

Patient_ID= 5
Gender= Female
Age= 26
Height_cm= 160
Weight_kg= 55
BMI= 21.5
Disordered_Eating_Questionnaire=35
Depression_Score= 18
Anxiety_Score= 16
Diagnosis= Bulimia Nervosa

Patient_ID= 6
Gender= Male
Autoscroll    Show time

COM 3

Age= 33
Height_cm= 180
Weight_kg= 80
BMI= 24.7
Disordered_Eating_Questionnaire=24
Depression_Score= 8
Anxiety_Score= 10
Diagnosis= Neither

Patient_ID= 7
Gender= Female
Age= 19
Height_cm= 150
Weight_kg= 40
BMI= 17.8
Disordered_Eating_Questionnaire=42
Depression_Score= 25
Anxiety_Score= 22
Diagnosis= Anorexia Nervosa

Patient_ID= 8
Gender= Male
Age= 28
Height_cm= 170
Weight_kg= 70
BMI= 24.2
Disordered_Eating_Questionnaire=28
Depression_Score= 14
Anxiety_Score= 16
Autoscroll    Show time

COM 3

Diagnosis= Neither

Patient_ID= 9
Gender= Female
Age= 27
Height_cm= 165
Weight_kg= 52
BMI= 19.1
Disordered_Eating_Questionnaire=36
Depression_Score= 19
Anxiety_Score= 21
Diagnosis= Bulimia Nervosa

Patient_ID= 10
Gender= Male
Age= 25
Height_cm= 180
Weight_kg= 85
BMI= 26.2
Disordered_Eating_Questionnaire=22
Depression_Score= 7
Anxiety_Score= 9
Diagnosis= Neither
Autoscroll    Show time
```

FIGURE 2.9 Collected data by automated system.

model is trained on a dataset, and the number of boosting rounds (estimators) varies from 50 to 150, as derived in Table 2.13. For each number of estimators, the model's accuracy is evaluated on both the training set and a separate validation set. By exhaustively evaluating these parameter combinations, grid search determines the optimal configuration that yields the most accurate predictive model. The system can also be continuously monitored and updated to ensure its performance remains optimal. Figures 2.9 and 2.10 convey the Overall System. Developing an automated system for predicting anorexia nervosa and bulimia nervosa using machine learning techniques requires expertise in data science, programming, and clinical knowledge of eating disorders.

2.5 CONCLUSION

By using XGBoost to build a predictive model for identifying patients at high risk of developing anorexia nervosa and bulimia nervosa, ahealthcare provider can improve

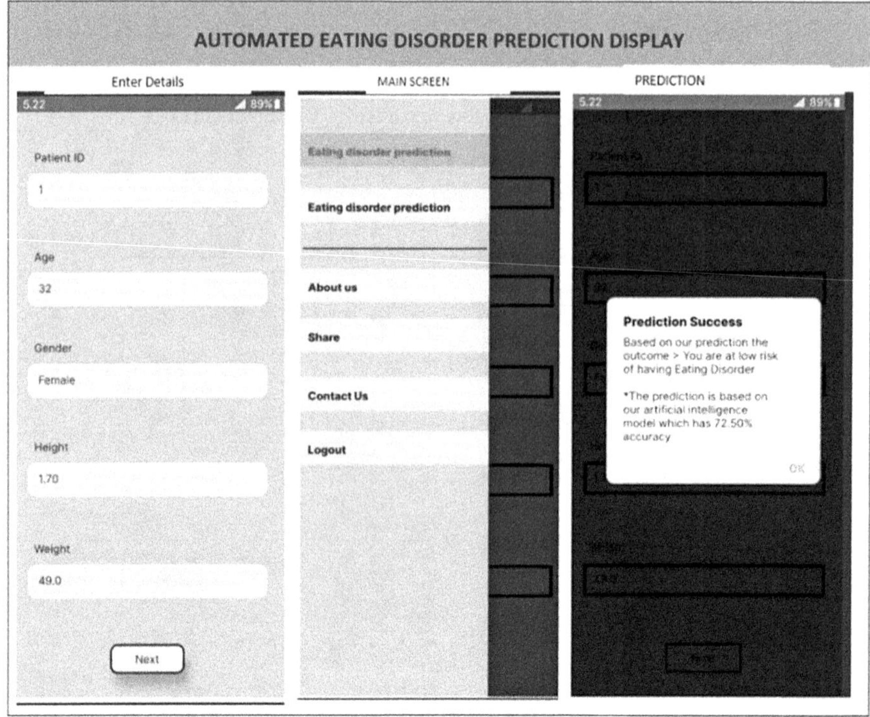

FIGURE 2.10 Predictions by automated system.

the efficiency and effectiveness of their healthcare services, ultimately leading to better outcomes for patients. The provider uses a grid search to find the optimal values for the XGBoost parameters, including the learning rate, the maximum depth of the tree, and the number of boosting rounds. Theprovider usesa binary:logistic objective function to optimize for binary classification and evaluate the performance of the model using accuracy, precision, recall, and F1-score. The model correctly identifies 90% of the patients who developed anorexia nervosa and 85% of the patients who developed bulimia nervosa. The precision and recall of the model are both above 0.85, indicating that the model has a high level of accuracy in identifying patients at risk for the disorders. After training the model, the provider uses it to make predictions on the test set.

REFERENCES

1. Mitchell, A. J., Vaze, A. and Rao, S.2009. "Clinical diagnosis of depression in primary care: A meta-analysis". *Lancet*, 374(9690), 609–619. https://doi.org/10.1016/S0140-6736(09)60879-5
2. Steinglass, J. E., Sysko, R., Mayer, L., Berner, L. A. and Attia, E.2017. "Cognitive-behavioral therapy for anorexia nervosa: A systematic review and meta-analysis". *International Journal of Eating Disorders*, 50(3), 212–224.

3. Keski-Rahkonen, A. and Raevuori, A.2018. "Bulimia nervosa". *The Lancet*, 391(10120), 1231–1240.
4. National Institute of Mental Health. 2018. "Eating disorders". https://www.nimh.nih.gov/health/topics/eating-disorders/index.shtml
5. Khan, S. S., Yap, K. P. and Su, E. L. M.2018. "Early detection of eating disorders using machine learning: A systematic review". *Journal of Eating Disorders*, 6(1), 26. https://doi.org/10.1186/s40337-018-0219-2
6. Qiao, L. and Yang, Q.2020. "Detection of eating disorder behaviors using machine learning approaches". *Proceedings of the 5th International Conference on Machine Learning, Big Data and Business Intelligence*, pp. 166–173. ACM. https://doi.org/10.1145/3426705.3426732
7. Kothari, R. and Sastry, A. 2020. *Application of Machine Learning Techniques for Early Diagnosis of Eating Disorders, Machine Learning and Intelligent Communications*, pp. 331–348. Springer.
8. Berends, T., Boersma, G. J., van Elburg, A. A. and Van den Berg, G.2021. "Self-esteem and anxiety in anorexia nervosa and bulimia nervosa: A systematic review". *European Eating Disorders Review*, 29(2), 151–171.
9. Eating Disorder Hope. n.d. "2021 eating disorders statistics." https://www.eatingdisorderhope.com/information/statistics-studies
10. Ostroff, J. S. and Trace, S. E.2021. "Emotion dysregulation and eating disorders: Associations with anorexia nervosa and bulimia nervosa symptoms". *Current Psychiatry Reports*, 23(8), 53.
11. Jimenez-Serrano, S., Marques-Marcet, J., Carmona, J., Fernandez-Aranda, F. and Sánchez, I. 2021. "Prediction of eating disorder risk using machine learning algorithms". *Computers in Biology and Medicine*, 130, 104218. https://doi.org/10.1016/j.compbiomed.2020.104218
12. López-Guarnido, O. and Pérez-Sancho, C.2021. "Using XGBoost to predict the presence of eating disorders from social media data". *Proceedings of the 10th International Conference on Pattern Recognition Applications and Methods*, pp. 460–465. SciTePress. https://doi.org/10.5220/0010307904600465
13. Psychology Today. 2022. "Anorexia nervosa". https://www.psychologytoday.com/us/conditions/anorexia-nervosa
14. https://www.bartleby.com/essay/Case-Study-Of-Binge-Eating-Disorders-PJCF2CBM2R
15. https://jeatdisord.biomedcentral.com/articles/10.1186/s40337-022-00581-2

3 Breast Cancer Prediction Using a Machine Learning Approach

Arijit Ghosal, Harshita Somolu, and Suchibrota Dutta

3.1 INTRODUCTION

Cancer is a life-threatening disease and there is no cure. Scientifically, cancer is known as carcinoma. A lot of people are losing their lives due to cancer, and most current treatments can only arrest the progress of malignancy in the body. There are several types of cancer: carcinomas, sarcomas, leukemias, and lymphomas. There are several kinds of cancers based on their origin, including prostate cancer, breast cancer, colorectal cancer, and lung cancer. All of these cancers are fatal due to a lack of available treatment. The fatality rates of cancer vary based on the severity and progress rate. There are different stages of cancer: stage I, stage II, stage III, and stage IV. Any type of cancer initially starts in stage I, then gradually increases in severity and progresses toward higher stages. The progression rate toward stage IV from stage I indicates the severity. With some forms of cancer, the transition from stage I to stage IV is very quick (e.g., lung cancer), whereas for others the transition rate is very slow. If the progression rate from stage I to stage IV is very fast, then the cancer will likely be more fatal.

Hence, time is a crucial factor in the case of cancer. This work aims to propose machine learning to assist in the current treatment process of cancer so that cancer can be diagnosed very quickly, saving lives. In this work, two standard datasets have been used to find the best composition of features for early prediction of breast cancer. The proposed scheme resulted in 92.7944% accuracy for the first dataset and for the second dataset the proposed scheme yielded 98.188% accuracy. The first dataset (Breast Cancer Prediction Dataset) [24] was collected from the University of Wisconsin Hospitals, Madison, from Dr. William H. Wolberg, and the second dataset (Breast Cancer Prediction Dataset) was collected from the UCI Machine Learning Repository [25].

Breast cancer is very common in women, but men can also suffer from breast cancer. Breast cancer is the second most common cancer in the USA after skin cancer. In India, more than a quarter of all female cancers is breast cancer. So, there is an alarming situation throughout the world regarding breast cancer.

 DOI: 10.1201/9781003391456-3

This work focuses on the prediction of breast cancer, which is on the rise in the world because of sedentary lifestyles and the late detection of breast cancer. Breast cancer is the major cause of death compared to the other types of cancer, per the World Health Organization. This chapter highlights the different machine learning techniques applied for the early detection of cancer so that the treatment provided to the patient will perhaps lead to early recovery from the deadly disease.

Machine learning techniques can be used to improve the efficiency of breast cancer diagnosis. A type of deep learning method is the convolution neural network (CNN), which is inspired by the structure of the human biological neural network. Different emerging fields, such as radiomics, allow medical personnel to extract special quantitative features from images captured during the radiomic analysis. The analysis of breast cancer images by the imaging genomic allows for determining the relationship between the different features' association with the breast cancer treatment. The different methods used for the detection of breast cancer are based on the classification, and research work is ongoing to improve the efficiency of breast cancer detection at the early stage so that the person who is affected can be cured.

Machine learning models are widely used in the development of predictive models in order to increase the precision of cancer prediction. Study of the different machine learning strategies the multiparametric magnetic resonance imaging (MRI) and its variants for the early detection of breast cancer are also very much contributory. The new machine learning techniques can be applied for the validation of messenger RNAs, which act as biomarkers for the detection of breast cancer. The breast cancer survival analysis has used the prognosis models from the records that include all the clinical sort of information from the database. The data that is collected from the patients and the hospitals allows the predictor to find out whether a patient who previously had cancer will get cancer again in the future.

Information and communication technology (ICT) tools can play a vital role in the early detection of breast cancer. The data that is collected from all over the world is enormous, and big data will allow the user to perform efficient predictive analysis on it. Many algorithms can use the fundamentals of classification and prediction for the true outcomes of breast cancer. The various machine learning methods have become good tools for medical research professionals. These methods or techniques can allow you to discover and identify the different patterns and the association between them so that the prediction of cancer can be done well in advance.

The different prognostic and predictive features can be considered, which always give a better result compared to previous work in the field of breast cancer. This chapter focuses on the different machine learning and deep learning techniques available for the early detection of breast cancer, and we are also able to predict which techniques will be more efficient.

3.2 LITERATURE SURVEY

Due to the gradual improvement of medical sciences, we are in a better position to deal with cancer. The chances of survival of people are increasing. Early stage (stage I and stage II) cancers are more controllable and more people are surviving these cancers. Researchers are actively seeking the cause of cancer to better explain the reason for abnormal cell growth as well as the characteristics of different types of cancer minutely. As cancer is related to medical science, initially only people related to medical science were involved in the research process. But later it was thought that medical science alone would not be able to conquer cancer, thus nowadays emerging fields of computer science are becoming helpful in solving different cross-domain problems. The computer science fields of artificial intelligence (AI), machine learning (ML), and image processing are contributing a lot to the research of cancer in association with medical sciences. As a result, most of the recent research related to the diagnosis or prediction of cancer involves a machine learning approach for ease of work as well as more accurate results.

Machine learning is helping a lot in the diagnosis and treatment of breast cancer today. Mostly, the supervised approach of machine learning is being used for this purpose, as historical data is very helpful for diagnosis as well as treatment of breast cancer. Machine learning is also being used for early prediction of breast cancer so that basic precautionary treatment can be started for a suspected patient.

Researchers are applying machine learning for both purposes. Lots of research work has been carried out so far related to breast cancer. Some of the works have also employed machine learning. While collecting historical data, there are several instances where some information is incomplete or missing. Generally, researchers discard that information. But Jerez et al. [1] worked with imputation of missing or incomplete data. They have proposed certain approaches without discarding records with missing data. Statistical approaches were adopted by them to achieve this. They worked with the "El Álamo-I" dataset of 3679 women. This dataset is one of the largest in Spain. The dataset consists of therapeutic, demographic, and recurrence-survival evidence. They had observed that the information of 1678 women was partially missing, up to three values. Jerez et al. adopted both statistical and machine learning approaches for solving the problem. Mean imputation, hot-deck approaches of statistical techniques along with the multilayer perceptron (MLP), self-organizing maps (SOMs), and K-nearest neighbor approaches of machine learning were espoused for solving the problem in their work. Based on calibration and discrimination, the performance of their proposed model was measured.

Cancer is so dangerous that it can relapse, even if it is completely cured stage I at present. The problem is if cancer relapses in the future it is more complicated to handle compared to the earlier occurrence, as this time it becomes immune to the treatment whatever is applied during the early time. Breast cancer can also relapse, even if it is completely cured. As a result, patients must undergo follow-up for a certain period even if cancer is completely cured as of now. Ahmad et al. [2] worked on the possibility of relapse of breast cancer in patients under follow-up for two years. The dataset they applied in their work had 1189 records. They applied support vector machine (SVM), decision tree, and artificial neural network in their work.

Srivastava [3] recommended the Weka tool for different purposes including classification. Kourou et al. [4] worked with the prognosis and diagnosis of cancer using the machine learning approach. They emphasized early prognosis and diagnosis of cancer, as it can save lives. They considered breast cancer as well as other types of cancer in their work. Their work is a survey paper in which they discuss different types of machine learning approaches presented by various researchers.

Bazazeh and Shubair [5] performed a comparative study of different machine learning algorithms for the detection and diagnosis of breast cancer. They applied the Original Wisconsin Breast Cancer Data set in their work. They compared the performances of three popular and robust machine learning approaches – random forest (RF), SVM, and Bayesian networks (BNs) – for the purpose of breast cancer detection and diagnosis. To measure the performance of the system, they considered not only accuracy but also other performance indicators including recall, precision, and area of ROC for better understanding. They used the Wisconsin original breast cancer dataset of 669 instances of cancer out of which 458 instances were benign and 211 were malignant. The dataset considers ten biological attributes for all the instances. They applied Weka [3] for the implementation of different classifiers.

Parekh and Jacobs [6] also worked with breast cancer. They concentrated on an integrated radiomic framework. Their approach involved processing MRI images using machine learning approaches. Hence, this approach is a bit slower as feature extraction from images is a slow process. Their dataset consisted of the information of 124 patients out of which 26 patients were benign and 98 patients were malignant. The patients underwent multiparametric breast MRI. Parekh and Jacobs applied a 180-dimensional radiomic feature space in their work. They adopted a tenfold cross-validation.

Richter and Khoshgoftaar [7] reviewed different statistical and machine learning methods for modeling cancer risk. They also emphasized early detection of cancer to save lives.

Nindrea et al. [8] carried out a breast cancer risk computation using different machine learning algorithms. They measured the diagnostic accuracies of various machine learning algorithms. They applied false positive (FP), false negative (FN), true positive (TP), and true negative (TN) as performance indicators for performance analysis of the algorithms. They surveyed 1879 research articles for this purpose.

Aslan et al. [9] also tried to carry out breast cancer diagnosis using different machine learning methods aimed at the early detection of breast cancer. They collected their dataset from the UCI library. The dataset consists of different biological attributes of patients. Through a machine learning approach, they tried to find the combination of biological attributes that produces the best result. The biological features they considered were collected through the routine analysis of blood. The dataset consisted of features extracted from 116 people out of which 64 patients were struggling with breast cancer and 52 people were not suffering from cancer. Through their work, they proved that breast cancer can be detected through routine blood, a very good initiative as many people will be able to afford these routine blood tests.

Yue et al. [10] carried out a review on breast cancer diagnosis and prognosis using different machine learning concepts. They have also aimed for early detection of cancer to reduce fatality. Standard supervised classifiers have been applied in their work.

Wang et al. [11] also applied machine learning algorithms in their work. They tried to identify differentially expressed genes between original breast cancer and xenografts through those machine learning algorithms. In their work, they tried to predict breast cancer. The dataset they used consisted of 831 tumor cells. In their experiment, they achieved satisfactory results.

Saha et al. [12] used DCE-MRI features for radio genomics of breast cancer using different machine learning methods. Saha et al. considered 922 patients. A total of 529 features were extracted and axial breast MRIs were considered in their work.

Bataineh [13] carried out a comparative analysis of nonlinear machine learning algorithms to detect breast cancer. He applied MLP, K-nearest neighbor, classification and regression trees, Gaussian naive Bayes, and SVM on the Wisconsin Breast Cancer Diagnostic (WBCD) dataset. For performance analysis, along with accuracy, other performance indicators such as precision and recall were considered. They obtained excellent results in their work.

Ferroni et al. [14] worked on the prediction of breast cancer using a machine learning approach. They considered clinical, demographic, and biochemical data of patients. They used a training dataset of 318 instances and a testing dataset of 136 instances. They suggested an amalgamation of machine learning algorithms and random optimization models for better performance.

Rehman et al. [15] considered miRNAs as biomarkers for breast cancer. They validated the miRNAs through a machine learning approach. They categorized cancers based on miRNAs as features. They also claimed that at least three miRNAs as biomarkers will be good for the system. They applied three widespread feature selection methods – information gain, least absolute shrinkage and selection operator (LASSO), and chi-squared feature selection. They used a dataset that consisted of 1207 patient samples.

Ganggayah et al. [16] worked with the survival rate of breast cancer patients. They took the help of a machine learning approach for this purpose. They aimed to determine the factors for predicting patients who are suffering from breast cancer. They used a large breast cancer dataset of 8066 instances supplied by the University Malaya Medical Centre, Kuala Lumpur, Malaysia.

Cain et al. [17] worked with MRI features for the prediction of breast cancer. They extracted 529 radiomic features from the pretreatment MRI of each patient. They used support vector machine as well as logistic regression in their work.

Tahmassebi et al. [18] worked with early prediction as well as the survival rate of breast cancer patients. They applied machine learning with multiparametric magnetic resonance imaging in their work to achieve their goal. They extracted 23 features for this purpose. They applied eight classifiers.

Tapak et al. [20] worked with the prediction of survival of breast cancer patients with the help of a machine learning approach. Metastasis in breast cancer patients is also considered in their work. They worked with a database of 550 patients suffering from breast cancer. They concluded that SVM beats other classifiers in the estimation of survival of patients.

Turkki et al. [21] also worked with breast cancer prediction using tumor tissue images through a machine learning approach. They considered a database of 868 patients.

Khan et al. [22] proposed computer-aided detection and diagnosis technologies for the identification of breast cancer. They also used the WBCD dataset in their work. They achieved 98% accuracy in their work.

Balkenende et al. [23] studied the scope of applying deep learning for the imaging of breast cancer. They explained the importance of imaging in the early stages of breast cancer. They mentioned that the imaging can be digital mammography or digital breast tomosynthesis. According to them, as deep learning is a very new technology, its performance is better compared to older technologies.

Nassif et al. [24] conducted reviews on the identification of breast cancer through artificial intelligence techniques. They mentioned that early identification of breast cancer is very much required as there is a 99% chance of survival for patients who have been detected early. Nassif et al. presented a comparative analysis of different models or algorithms with their respective accuracies.

The University of Wisconsin Hospitals, Madison breast cancer dataset was collected from Kaggle [25].

3.3 PROPOSED METHODOLOGY

Previous efforts related to the application of machine learning in breast cancer involved the prediction of survival rates and diagnosis of breast cancer. The authors only predicted the possibility of breast cancer from the dataset using previous training or historical information. This work aims to help suspected patients by informing them of the possibility of malignancy so that they can start preliminary treatment immediately. It is known that time is a big factor in the treatment of cancer. There are several types of cancer and all of them can be fatal if treatment starts late. As per medical science, there are four stages of cancer – stage I, stage II, stage III, and stage IV – which are formed based on the severity of the disease. Breast cancer is of the carcinoma type of cancer among the four types of cancer: carcinoma, sarcoma, leukemia, and lymphoma.

Machine learning can play a great role in predicting the possibility of malignancy. A supervised approach of machine learning will be able to do the job. If the system is well trained with previous case histories indicating malignancy or benign based on some symptoms or characteristics, then the system will easily be able to predict the possibility of malignancy in a new patient.

Throughout the world, breast cancer is a rising concern, as it is the most frequently occurring cancer for women. It is also observed that breast cancer is also possible for men, though the numbers are much less. The most serious problem of breast cancer is that it is very tough to identify, as in its initial stage it generally exhibits no symptoms. When it shows symptoms through lump formation, it has already progressed to an advanced stage. A needle biopsy is then mandatory for confirmation of malignancy. A needle biopsy is a time-consuming process. During this time, there is a possibility of advancement of malignancy and metastasis. Controlling the spread of malignancy becomes very challenging if metastasis occurs. Metastasis indicates that malignancy has spread to other parts of the body causing the formation of a

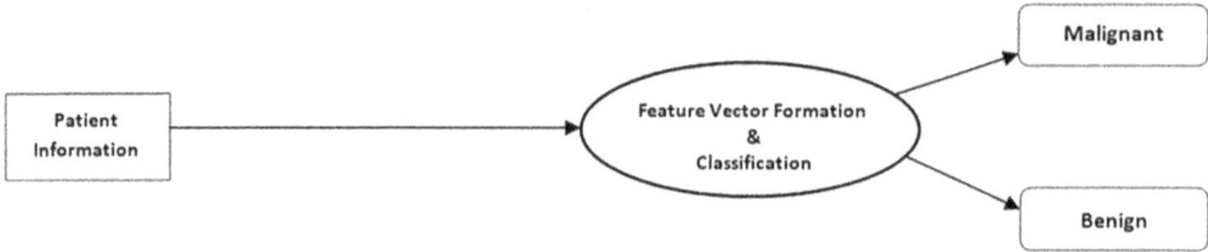

FIGURE 3.1 Process of breast cancer prediction.

secondary source in the body. Hence, early detection or prediction of malignancy is very important. Timely detection or prediction can save the lives of patients. This work intends to recommend a machine learning based aid to the present treatment method by providing a way of early prediction of breast cancer before a needle biopsy report is available and so that there will be no delay in initiating treatment. The process of the proposed scheme is depicted in Figure 3.1.

3.3.1 Feature Computation

Fixation of features is a very crucial task for any system based on machine learning. If features are chosen properly, the classification task for a classifier gets easier. Facets should be chosen judiciously so that the differences between the two categories (in this case) are properly reflected. In this work, two standard datasets from the University of Wisconsin Hospitals, Madison (collected from kaggle.com) are considered. These two datasets contain some medical parameters of breast cancer patients. The best feature set for breast cancer prediction has been suggested from these two datasets through a machine learning approach. The approach implements a supervised machine learning tactic using different supervised classifiers aimed at finding the best possible set of features from the first dataset (Breast Cancer Prediction Dataset) [24] and the second dataset (Breast Cancer Wisconsin [Diagnostic] Dataset) [25] to predict breast cancer.

3.3.1.1 Selection of Features for First Approach

During this phase, the identification of possible facets that will be able to predict breast cancer is carried out. This means the facets that have high discriminating influence will be selected during this phase. Feature selection is considered an imperative phase of pre-processing for a machine learning problem. It is considered the first step toward the shaping of the final facet vector. At the end of this phase, the final feature set is outlined after applying the proper facet assortment procedure.

There are several techniques for the selection of features, including sequential forward selection (SFS), sequential backward selection (SBS), plus l take away r selection, sequential floating forward search (SFFS), sequential floating backward search (SFBS), and max-min approach in the domain of machine learning. All these techniques have been applied in this work to find the best feature set from the first dataset.

In the case of SFS, if a facet is picked up for inclusion in the feature set, the facet can never be deleted. This causes the nesting effect. In the case of SFS, if a facet is selected for inclusion in the feature set and it is observed that after choosing that facet the classification accuracy decreases compared to the previous feature set without including the facet, then the facet cannot be deleted. Similarly, in the case of SBS, if a feature is once rejected, then the facet cannot be taken back into the feature set. Again, this creates a nesting effect.

The plus l take away r selection scheme allows one to add l number of facets and to eradicate r number of facets at every step of feature selection. As it allows both inclusion and removal of facets, this strategy is free from the nesting effect. But on the other hand, this approach is very time-consuming and it takes a long time to form the final feature vector.

With SFFS, the initial feature vector starts with a bare set and then the most noteworthy facet is added first. At every juncture, a new facet can be added, and at the same time, a facet that is deemed to be a least one can be removed. But the best thing about SFFS is that if after removing a facet the classification accuracy reduces, then the facet can be added back again. Though this process is time-consuming, it is relatively easy to implement and more practical while considering a real-time machine learning problem.

SFBS is the opposite of SFFS where the feature vector is constructed by including all possible facets. This is very tough to start in some cases as there may be a huge number of facets applicable to that particular categorization case. If all possible facets are to be put into the initial feature vector, the complexity of the calculation may be affected because of the long dimension or length of the facet set. Comparatively, identification of the most noteworthy facet is an easy task though it is also time-consuming. It is possible that the first facet that is supposed to be the most noteworthy facet at the initial phase of feature set formation does not end up being the most noteworthy facet at any future step. But SFBS provides the opportunity to remove that facet if it does not come out as the most noteworthy facet in future steps of feature set formation.

The max-min approach starts with two facets at the beginning stage, but in future steps, it considers two facets at a time. The snag of the max-min approach is that it cannot be applied in multidimensional space, as it does the calculations in two-dimensional space only.

After observing all the advantages and disadvantages of every feature selection technique, the SFFS technique is considered to be the best feature selection technique for identification of the best feature set to predict breast cancer using the first dataset of the University of Wisconsin Hospitals.

The feature set is formed in this phase by choosing facets in such a way that the facets are able to properly predict breast cancer. Also, the length of the total facet set has been structured in such a way that they are not large enough.

This work aims to focus on suggesting an optimal dimensional feature set that will be able to predict breast cancer with high accuracy. While selecting the feature set, the "curse of dimensionality" is taken into account. The curse of dimensionality states that categorization accuracy will be boosted with respect to the extension of

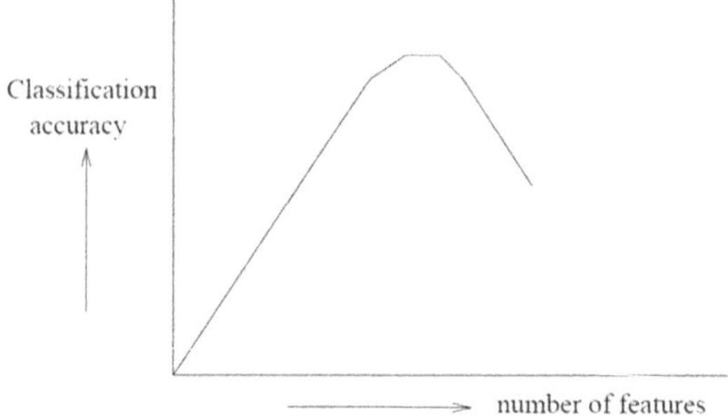

FIGURE 3.2 Curse of dimensionality.

the number of facets up to some extent. It is seen that after incorporation of some optimal quantity of facets, classification accurateness will start to drop off instead of augmentation of some new facets. This scenario is portrayed in Figure 3.2. This happens as some facets have excellent discrimination capabilities – they have different ranges of values for different categorical elements. They may be termed as good facets. At the same time, there are certain facets whose values overlap with other facets for different categorical elements. They are termed bad facets. Unfortunately, the number of good facets is less compared to the number of bad facets. Bad facets bring down system performance due to the overlapping of the values. Hence, they are required to be discarded. But regrettably, during the time of formation of the final facet set, the omission of bad facets is unavoidable. They will be present in the final facet set along with the good facet set. The aim is to incorporate as few bad facets as possible. As bad facets will always be present in all machine learning solutions, it is not possible to achieve 100% accuracy. Here also, bad facets are left out as much as possible.

A decrement in categorization accuracy may arise since the facets that were adjoined later may not have superior prejudice characteristics. In this work, the facet vector is chosen in a flexible way so that the scheme comes out with the best possible facet set from the first dataset.

3.3.1.2 Selection of Features for Second Approach

The dataset used in this phase was also collected from the University of Wisconsin Hospitals, Madison through kaggle.com. This dataset may be considered as an extension of the dataset used in phase 1. There are 25 more facets that are related to the abnormal lump observed and some parameters are computed from x-rays for each cell nucleus of a breast mass. So, there are a total of 30 facets.

3.3.2 Formation of Feature Vector and Classification

Classification is an important juncture in any machine learning work. Its mission is to discern various categories of data related to a machine learning work using the feature set generated during the facet extraction phase. For classification purposes, Weka [3] was used.

In this work, the facet selection procedure needs to be applied to form the final facet vector. Different standard supervised classifiers will assist the feature selection procedure in this matter. The SFFS technique is used in this work to form the final facet vector. The initial facet vector is formed with the minimum number of facets, termed F_{21}. Then the number of facets is gradually increased to form the final facet set. Classification performance is noted for every facet set and based on that the final facet set is suggested. The differentiating power of the recommended facet set is assessed through the logistic regression, neural network, K-nearest neighbor, and SVM classifiers. In the second dataset, the deep learning concept was applied to the deep neural network.

3.3.2.1 Formation of Feature Vector and Classification for First Approach

Initially, no facets are put into the feature set. This means the formation of the feature set is initiated with a bare feature set as per the rules of the SFFS technique. Then gradually the facets from the dataset are added to the facet vector and its corresponding classification accuracy is monitored. Whenever the classification accuracy falls even after including a new facet in the feature vector, then it can be concluded that the feature vector has reached its optimal length and no further facet accumulation will be profitable. This principle has been implemented in this work to cut down the length of the feature set to avoid computational complexity as well as the curse of dimensionality. There are a total of five facets in the first dataset collected from the University of Wisconsin Hospitals, Madison. These facets are related to the abnormal lump observed and some parameters are computed from an x-ray of that. These facets are mean radius, mean texture, mean perimeter, mean area, and mean smoothness for each cell nucleus of a breast mass. While forming the feature set, the mean radius is first included in the initial feature set and then gradually the other facets are included as per the SFFS technique. These feature sets are denoted by F_{11}, F_{12}, F_{13}, and F_{14}. For classification purposes, the Weka tool [3] was used in this phase also.

But as the prediction of breast cancer is a two-class problem (either benign or malignant), a minimum of two facets (as per Equation 3.1) has to be in the probable feature set as per the convention of machine learning. The convention states

$$Min.no.of\ facets\ in\ feature\ set = \frac{total\ number\ of\ class\ or\ category}{2} + 1 \tag{3.1}$$

This convention is applied to all types of machine learning problems. Equation 3.1 helps to form the probable feature set from the N numbers of facet sets. So, effectively the probable set of facets has been formed considering the mean radius and mean texture (this is denoted by facet set F_{11}) for each cell nucleus of a breast mass. After inclusion of the remaining facets, the classification accuracy of the feature set is calculated for every facet. This is explained in the next section, which describes experimental results. F_{12} is formed by including the mean radius, mean texture, and mean perimeter. F_{13} is formed by including the mean radius, mean texture, and mean perimeter as well as mean area. F_{14} is formed by including the mean radius, mean texture, mean perimeter, mean area, and mean smoothness.

Classifiers are an integral part of any machine learning work because they do the actual classification task with the help of the feature set generated during the feature extraction phase and the facet selection phase. The differentiating powers of all the facet sets formed in all iterations are assessed through logistic regression, neural network, K-nearest neighbor, and SVM. These classifiers are very widespread supervised classifiers.

The dataset contains the biological information of 569 patients. The dataset is divided into two identical groups: one is used for training and the other for testing. The MLP model of the neural network was applied in this work considering the number of neurons in the input echelon equal to the dimensions of the facet set. Hence, for the initial phase, the input echelon consisted of two neurons and then the number of neurons was gradually increased to five in the final phase. There are two neurons in the output stratum, which points to the two categories of predictions of breast cancer: benign and malignant. The output echelon is always made of two neurons irrespective of the different phases where the number of neurons was gradually changed from two to five. In the concealed stratum of this MLP model, the number of neurons was equal to half of the total neurons present in the input phase + 1 for every phase.

A tenfold cross-validation is applied in this work to enforce logistic regression and support vector machine. Here the data is split into ten numbers of unique reduced samples to enhance the classification purpose. Ten was chosen as, through trial and error, it was observed that this value provides the best classification result.

SVM is a very robust classification algorithm. It can be configured as per the requirement. There are different kernel functions for configuring SVM. Through experimental study, the "quadratic" kernel is exercised to obtain the best classification result.

K-nearest neighbor is one of the problem-free supervised classifiers. Also, it is very easy to employ. This classifier was employed with k = 3, as there are only two classes (benign and malignant). As the value of k is set to 3, there is little chance of a tie. Still, if a tie occurs, the random rule and nearest rule are exercised in this classifier to break the tie in order to label the data benign or malignant. The city block distance metric was considered here to quantify the distance between any two sample components.

3.3.2.2 Formation of Feature Vector and Classification for Second Approach

Here the dataset of 569 patients is divided for testing and training by setting apart the complete dataset into two divisions. The MLP model of the neural network was applied in this work considering the number of neurons in the input echelon equal to the dimension of the facet set. There are two neurons in the output stratum which points to the benign or malignant predictions of breast cancer. Logistic regression,

MLP, K-nearest neighbor, and SVM were used with the same configuration as the first approach.

In the second approach, ten facets are considered: radius, texture, perimeter, area, smoothness, compactness, concavity, concave points, symmetry, and fractal dimension. As the SFFS technique has been used for feature selection, the initial facet set, termed F_{21}, was formed with the means of these ten facets, that is, mean radius, mean texture, mean perimeter, mean area, mean smoothness, mean compactness, mean concavity, mean concave points, mean symmetry, and mean fractal dimension. Then, the next set of facets is added to form the facet set F_{22}. In F_{22}, all the standard errors of the aforementioned ten facets are embraced. The worst case values of the ten facets are considered in the final facet set termed F_{23} along with all the facets of F_{22}.

All these facet sets are fed to the classifiers to identify the best facet set. The detailed experimental results are discussed in the next section.

3.4 EXPERIMENTAL RESULTS

The whole experiment was carried out with the freely available datasets collected from the University of Wisconsin Hospitals, Madison through kaggle.com [25]. Both datasets consist of biological facets from the digitized images of the breast mass of 569 patients. These biological facets describe the characteristics of the cell nuclei present in the images.

There are several approaches for feature selection. Feature selection is very important for any machine learning problem solution. In the case of the first dataset, the SFFS technique was applied to find the best feature set. For this, experiments started with an empty feature set, and then gradually the other features were added and hence the feature sets F_{11}, F_{12}, F_{13}, and F_{14} were formed gradually. Similarly, F_{21}, F_{22}, and F_{23} were formed for the second dataset.

For every facet set, half of the files in the dataset were used to train the supervised classifiers used in this work. The rest of the files were used for testing by applying the trained supervised classifiers. After the completion of the discrimination task using the training dataset and testing dataset, the datasets were reversed and the same differentiation task was repeated once more. The average of the two discrimination tasks was considered as the final differentiation conclusion for the prediction of breast cancer for every feature set. For the first dataset, the discrimination results are tabulated in Table 3.1, Table 3.2, Table 3.3, and Table 3.4, respectively for $F_{11,}$ $F_{12,}$ F_{13}, and F_{14}, and for the second dataset the discrimination results are tabulated in Table 3.5, Table 3.6, and Table 3.7, respectively, for $F_{21,}$ F_{22}, and F_{23}.

From the experimental result, it is clear that the feature set comprising all the features mentioned in the first dataset (F_{14}) outperforms the other combination of facets for the first dataset.

The second dataset also contains the biological information of 569 patients. There are 25 more facets available that are related to the irregular lump examined and some parameters are calculated from an x-ray for each cell nucleus of a breast mass. So, there are a total of 30 facets.

TABLE 3.1
Accuracy of Prediction of Breast Cancer (Using F_{11})

Classifier	Discrimination Exactness (in %) Meant for Suggested Feature Set
Logistic regression	89.1037
MLP (multilayer perceptron)	89.2794
K-nearest neighbor	88.4007
SVM (support vector machine)	88.0492

TABLE 3.2
Accuracy of Prediction of Breast Cancer (Using F_{12})

Classifier	Discrimination Exactness (in %) Meant for Suggested Feature Set
Logistic regression	91.3884
MLP (multilayer perceptron)	90.5097
K-nearest neighbor	90.1582
SVM (support vector machine)	88.225

TABLE 3.3
Accuracy of Prediction of Breast Cancer (Using F_{13})

Classifier	Discrimination Exactness (in %) meant for suggested feature set
Logistic regression	91.7399
MLP (multilayer perceptron)	89.9824
K-nearest neighbor	89.8067
SVM (support vector machine)	88.0492

TABLE 3.4
Accuracy of Prediction of Breast Cancer (Using F_{14})

Classifier	Discrimination Exactness (in %) Meant for Suggested Feature Set
Logistic regression	92.6186
MLP (multilayer perceptron)	92.7944
K-nearest neighbor	91.9156
SVM (support vector machine)	92.2671

TABLE 3.5
Accuracy of Prediction of Breast Cancer (Using F_{21})

Classifier	Discrimination Exactness (in %) Meant for Suggested Feature Set
Logistic regression	93.6731
MLP (multilayer perceptron)	93.6731
K-nearest neighbor	91.0369
SVM (support vector machine)	93.8489

TABLE 3.6
Accuracy of Prediction of Breast Cancer (Using F_{22})

Classifier	Discrimination Exactness (in %) Meant for Suggested Feature Set
Logistic regression	94.3761
MLP (multilayer perceptron)	96.1336
K-nearest neighbor	94.3761
SVM (support vector machine)	94.3761

TABLE 3.7
Accuracy of Prediction of Breast Cancer (Using F_{23})

Classifier	Discrimination Exactness (in %) Meant for Suggested Feature Set
Logistic regression	94.2004
MLP (multilayer perceptron)	98.188
K-nearest neighbor	96.1336
SVM (support vector machine)	97.891

From the aforementioned tables it is clear that MLP using F_{23} performs better compared to the others. Facet set F_{23} consists of the mean, standard error, and worst cases of all ten facets, that is, it consists of all the facets of the second dataset. Hence, it is concluded that the second dataset performs better for the prediction of breast cancer using MLP.

3.4.1 Comparative Analysis

The superiority of this work was established through performance comparison of this work with other works. It is observed that the Wisconsin dataset has been used

TABLE 3.8
Comparative Analysis with Existing Work

Approach	Discrimination Exactness (in %)
Bazazeh and Shubair [5] (SVM)	97.0
Proposed approach: MLP (using three hidden layers)	98.188

by many researchers, which this work also employs. Bazazeh and Shubair [5], who also used the Wisconsin dataset, adopted a machine learning approach through random forest, SVM, and Bayesian network classifiers. They obtained their best result by applying SVM. In our proposed scheme, the best accuracy is achieved by applying MLP using all the facets of the second dataset. The best classification performance of the proposed scheme and the scheme proposed by Bazazeh and Shubair was compared. From the comparative result, it is observed that the proposed approach performs better. The comparative classification performance is tabulated in Table 3.8.

3.5 CONCLUSION

This work indicates that the facet set based on the second dataset is able to predict breast cancer with high accuracy. Also, through experiments, it is revealed that breast cancer prediction accuracy will improve if the mean, standard error, and worst cases are considered for the dataset of University of Wisconsin Hospitals, Madison. Also, how inclusion of the facets improves overall breast cancer prediction accuracy is noticed in this work. The dataset used in this work is a benchmark dataset. This work also indicates that future research work may be carried out to find new facets that will improve prediction accuracy. This work yields its novelty in that this scheme is capable of quick and early prediction of breast cancer based on the biological information of 569 patients so that the preliminary steps of treatment can be started and the life of the patient can be saved. The performance of this scheme should be checked for other types of cancer.

REFERENCES

1. Jerez, J. M., Molina, I., García-Laencina, P. J., Alba, E., Ribelles, N., Martín, M., & Franco, L. (2010). Missing data imputation using statistical and machine learning methods in a real breast cancer problem. *Artificial Intelligence in Medicine*, 50(2), 105–115.
2. Ahmad, L. G., Eshlaghy, A. T., Poorebrahimi, A., Ebrahimi, M., & Razavi, A. R. (2013). Using three machine learning techniques for predicting breast cancer recurrence. *Journal of Health and Medical Informatics*, 4(124), 3.
3. Srivastava, S. (2014). Weka: A tool for data preprocessing, classification, ensemble, clustering and association rule mining. *International Journal of Computer Applications*, 88(10): 26–29.

4. Kourou, K., Exarchos, T. P., Exarchos, K. P., Karamouzis, M. V., & Fotiadis, D. I. (2015). Machine learning applications in cancer prognosis and prediction. *Computational and Structural Biotechnology Journal*, 13, 8–17.
5. Bazazeh, D., & Shubair, R. (2016, December). Comparative study of machine learning algorithms for breast cancer detection and diagnosis. In *2016 5th International Conference on Electronic Devices, Systems and Applications (ICEDSA)* (pp. 1–4). IEEE.
6. Parekh, V. S., & Jacobs, M. A. (2017). Integrated radiomic framework for breast cancer and tumor biology using advanced machine learning and multiparametric MRI. *NPJ Breast Cancer*, 3(1), 1–9.
7. Richter, A. N., & Khoshgoftaar, T. M. (2018). A review of statistical and machine learning methods for modeling cancer risk using structured clinical data. *Artificial Intelligence in Medicine*, 90, 1–14.
8. Nindrea, R. D., Aryandono, T., Lazuardi, L., & Dwiprahasto, I. (2018). Diagnostic accuracy of different machine learning algorithms for breast cancer risk calculation: A meta-analysis. *Asian Pacific Journal of Cancer Prevention: APJCP*, 19(7), 1747.
9. Aslan, M. F., Celik, Y., Sabanci, K., & Durdu, A. (2018). Breast cancer diagnosis by different machine learning methods using blood analysis data. *International Journal of Intelligent Systems and Applications in Engineering*, 6(4), 289–293.
10. Yue, W., Wang, Z., Chen, H., Payne, A., & Liu, X. (2018). Machine learning with applications in breast cancer diagnosis and prognosis. *Designs*, 2(2), 13.
11. Wang, D., Li, J. R., Zhang, Y. H., Chen, L., Huang, T., & Cai, Y. D. (2018). Identification of differentially expressed genes between original breast cancer and xenograft using machine learning algorithms. *Genes*, 9(3), 155.
12. Saha, A., Harowicz, M. R., Grimm, L. J., Kim, C. E., Ghate, S. V., Walsh, R., & Mazurowski, M. A. (2018). A machine learning approach to radiogenomics of breast cancer: A study of 922 subjects and 529 DCE-MRI features. *British Journal of Cancer*, 119(4), 508–516.
13. Al Bataineh, A. (2019). A comparative analysis of nonlinear machine learning algorithms for breast cancer detection. *International Journal of Machine Learning and Computing*, 9(3), 248–254.
14. Ferroni, P., Zanzotto, F. M., Riondino, S., Scarpato, N., Guadagni, F., & Roselli, M. (2019). Breast cancer prognosis using a machine learning approach. *Cancers*, 11(3), 328.
15. Rehman, O., Zhuang, H., Muhamed Ali, A., Ibrahim, A., & Li, Z. (2019). Validation of miRNAs as breast cancer biomarkers with a machine learning approach. *Cancers*, 11(3), 431.
16. Ganggayah, M. D., Taib, N. A., Har, Y. C., Lio, P., & Dhillon, S. K. (2019). Predicting factors for survival of breast cancer patients using machine learning techniques. *BMC Medical Informatics and Decision Making*, 19(1), 48.
17. Cain, E. H., Saha, A., Harowicz, M. R., Marks, J. R., Marcom, P. K., & Mazurowski, M. A. (2019). Multivariate machine learning models for prediction of pathologic response to neoadjuvant therapy in breast cancer using MRI features: A study using an independent validation set. *Breast Cancer Research and Treatment*, 173(2), 455–463.
18. Tahmassebi, A., Wengert, G. J., Helbich, T. H., Bago-Horvath, Z., Alaei, S., Bartsch, R., … Morris, E. A. (2019). Impact of machine learning with multiparametric magnetic resonance imaging of the breast for early prediction of response to neoadjuvant chemotherapy and survival outcomes in breast cancer patients. *Investigative Radiology*, 54(2), 110.

19. Wolberg, W., Mangasarian, O., Street, N., and Street, W. (1995). *Breast Cancer Wisconsin (Diagnostic)*. UCI Machine Learning Repository. https://doi.org/10.24432/C5DW2B.
20. Tapak, L., Shirmohammadi-Khorram, N., Amini, P., Alafchi, B., Hamidi, O., & Poorolajal, J. (2019). Prediction of survival and metastasis in breast cancer patients using machine learning classifiers. *Clinical Epidemiology and Global Health*, 7(3), 293–299.
21. Turkki, R., Byckhov, D., Lundin, M., Isola, J., Nordling, S., Kovanen, P. E., … Linder, N. (2019). Breast cancer outcome prediction with tumour tissue images and machine learning. *Breast Cancer Research and Treatment*, 177(1), 41–52.
22. Khan, M. M., Islam, S., Sarkar, S., Ayaz, F. I., Ananda, M. K., Tazin, T., … Almalki, F. A. (2022). Machine learning based comparative analysis for breast cancer prediction. *Journal of Healthcare Engineering*, 2023, 1–15.
23. Balkenende, L., Teuwen, J., & Mann, R. M. (2022, March). Application of deep learning in breast cancer imaging. *Seminars in Nuclear Medicine*, 52(5), 584–596.
24. Nassif, A. B., Talib, M. A., Nasir, Q., Afadar, Y., & Elgendy, O. (2022). Breast cancer detection using artificial intelligence techniques: A systematic literature review. *Artificial Intelligence in Medicine*, 127, 102276.
25. Breast Cancer Prediction Dataset. (2018, September 26). Kaggle. https://www.kaggle.com/merishnasuwal/breast-cancer-prediction-dataset

4 A Survey on the Development of Deep Learning–Based Techniques in the Diagnosis of Parkinson's Disease

B.K. Tripathy, Astha, Anushka Patil, Savvy Gupta and Preeti Kumari

4.1 INTRODUCTION

Healthcare is of paramount importance globally. Various diseases, whether pandemic, epidemic, or common, pose significant threats to human society. Unlike pandemics or epidemics with acute surges, diseases such as Parkinson's disease (PD) and Alzheimer's disease are prevalent and age-related, affecting individuals at some point in their lives. This research focuses on the detection and prediction of PD, examining efforts made by researchers in this field. The Unified Parkinson's Disease Rating Scale (UPDRS) allows assessment of disease progression in patients. Remote patient monitoring systems can detect early-onset disorders, reducing the burden on healthcare workers. Combining images with text, audio, and video data using Machine Learning (ML) techniques enhances assessment accuracy [29].

The UPDRS score assesses the effectiveness of deep brain stimulation (DBS) in surgically treated PD patients and its postoperative neuroprotective and neurorestorative effects, utilizing Deep Learning (DL) algorithms and magnetic resonance imaging (MRI) scan analysis [14].

PD is a neurodegenerative disorder characterized by the loss of specific clusters of brain cells producing neurotransmitters like acetylcholine, dopamine, norepinephrine, and serotonin. These neurotransmitters regulate various physiological and cognitive functions, including movement, mood, and cognition. In PD, neurotransmitter deficiency results in a wide range of kinetic and non-kinetic symptoms. While the degeneration of these brain cells defines the disease, its root causes remain unknown.

DOI: 10.1201/9781003391456-4

Recent research suggests that both genetics and environmental factors play a role in its development [20]. PD affects the nervous system, impacting other body functions controlled by nerves. Early-stage symptoms include a lack of facial expression, reduced arm movement during walking, and speech changes. As PD progresses, it affects walking, writing, speaking, and basic cognitive abilities. Other nerve-related functions deteriorate as dopamine-producing nerves in the brain become damaged or die, leading to severe, progressive symptoms.

Symptoms of PD include limb tremors, particularly in the hands at rest but reduced during movement. Movement becomes slower, causing tasks to take longer. Rising from a chair becomes difficult, and muscle stiffness restricts the range of motion. Balance issues and stooped posture can develop, along with involuntary actions like eye blinking, hand swinging while walking, and unexplained smiling. Changes in speech, such as slowed speech or sudden fast talking, and speech hesitation may occur. Writing difficulties and small handwriting are common. PD is not curable, but medication and brain surgery can manage and sometimes improve symptoms. DL models excel in handling big data, mitigating challenges like feature selection and extraction observed in ML. These models are capable of handling high-dimensional data and mimic the functionality of biological neurons in the human brain.

Incorporating DL techniques into the diagnostic process aims to enhance the accuracy, sensitivity, and specificity of PD diagnosis. DL algorithms excel at extracting intricate patterns and features from diverse data modalities, enabling innovative and noninvasive diagnostic approaches for PD [51]. Early and accurate diagnosis is essential for timely medical intervention, and ML techniques play a vital role in achieving this goal. Recent advancements indicate that DL techniques outperform earlier ML algorithms. This work compiles, categorizes, and suggests approaches for applying DL techniques in early-stage PD prediction and detection. Following an introduction to Deep Neural Networks (DNN) and their applications, we explore the potential impact of PD on various organs through organ risk prediction. Early detection and treatment are primary topics of discussion. Effective treatment hinges on early detection, so we analyze specific behavioral patterns that aid in the diagnostic process. After a comprehensive analysis and survey, we conclude the chapter.

4.2 DEEP NEURAL NETWORKS

Among various models for handling data uncertainty, neural networks (NNs), designed to simulate the human brain, hold a prominent position [1]. NNs consist of processing elements organized in vertical columns called layers, which can include input and output layers. Neurons in each layer are connected to neurons in the following layer, with no connections within a single layer. Some specialized networks incorporate backward connections. The input layer receives and forwards input for further processing. DL operates through hierarchical learning, mirroring the human brain's learning process. DL has become a pivotal component of artificial intelligence (AI), and the fusion of DL concepts with NN architecture is known as DNN [2]. The number of hidden layers is determined by the designer.

DL techniques find extensive application in natural language processing and computer vision. Numerous real-world applications, including drug discovery, self-driving vehicles, medical fields [5], audio signal classification [6], text-based image retrieval [7], computational biology [8], diabetic retinopathy [9], materials development, and finance, are under rigorous study.

Among DNN models, convolutional neural networks (CNNs) [3] excel in classifying image data. Instead of conventional matrix multiplication, the next layer uses a transformation called the convolution operator to process input data. Nonlinear activation functions are commonly employed. Recurrent neural networks (RNNs) represent another popular DNN type, particularly suited for temporal data. The connection structures among nodes can take the form of directed or undirected graphs. Addressing long-term dependencies, long short-term memory (LSTM) is a specialized form of RNN [4]. LSTM's feedback connections enable it to capture intricate temporal relationships. LSTM finds applications in domains involving time-series data, including classification, featurc extraction, and estimation. Notably, CNN and LSTM are among the most accurate models used in distinguishing between fake and real videos.

4.3 DL IN ORGAN RISK PREDICTION

The versatility of DNN in simulating the human brain's functioning positions them as preferred tools for processing and analyzing medical data. DL is employed not only for disease diagnosis but also for tracking disease progression, devising personalized treatment plans, and holistic patient management. PD ranks as the second most common ailment worldwide.

Previous research has primarily focused on the detection and treatment of PD, neglecting the prediction of future organ risks in afflicted individuals. Questions arise: What data provides the best predictions for organ risk, and which organs should PD experts prioritize? To address these issues, low-correlated clinical data were pooled to predict organ risks associated with PD. Initially, the Parkinson's Progression Markers Initiative (PPMI) data was used to recreate clinical records without data. Subsequently, data was employed to identify the disease's primary stages, and health professionals aided in extracting pertinent data elements. Combining low-correlated data led to the development of the organ risk model. It was discovered that the artificial neural network-based multimodal organ risk prediction (ANN-MORP) outperforms other approaches. No prior medical data analysis has contrasted data in this manner.

Upon contrasting feature-based comparisons between the ANN-MORP method and other conventional prediction techniques, the expected precision of this approach reached 76%, surpassing others in terms of speed. The architecture of the algorithm is depicted in Figure 4.1 [10].

Convolutional models have demonstrated superior performance across various generalization frameworks, providing valuable insights for neurological gait classification research. The utilization of multiview visual data–driven DL for predicting Parkinson's stride impairment is discussed further. Remote monitoring systems

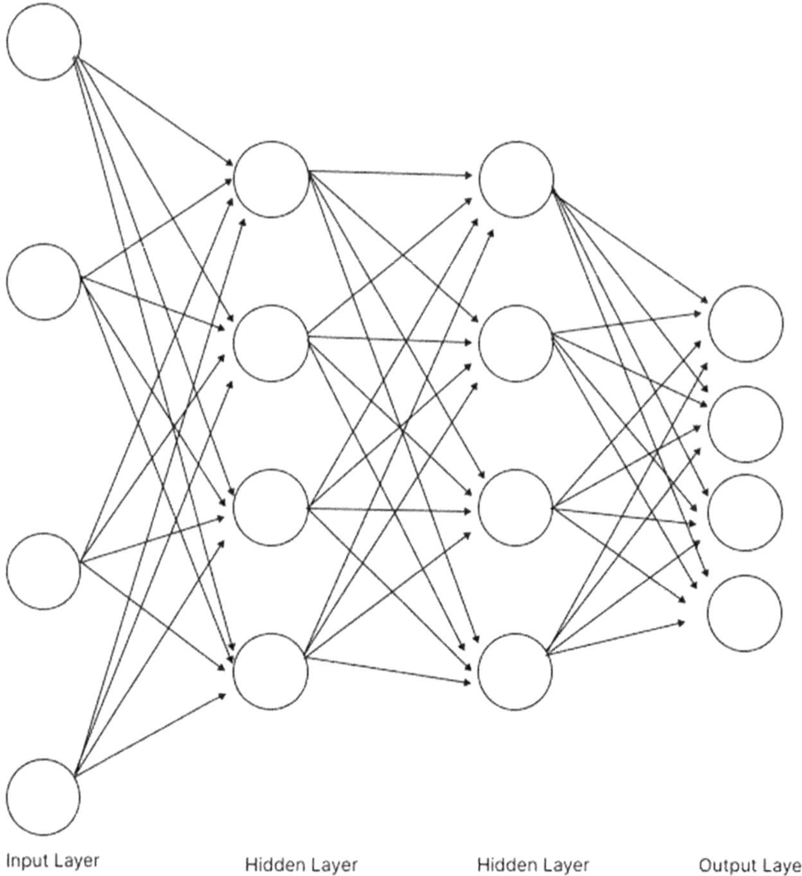

FIGURE 4.1 ANN-MORP algorithm architecture.

facilitate rapid, accurate, and cost-effective neurological gait classification. The contactless architecture simplifies outdoor gait assessments for elderly individuals without the need for licensed practitioners. Convolutional models have consistently outperformed other generalization frameworks. However, no single architecture excels across all features, tasks, and frameworks [11]. These findings suggest that gait research should explore alternative DL architectures to maximize the utilization of input data. Extracting essential physical feature locations in 3D commences with gait extraction, revealing how DL architectures differentiate neurological gait. Furthermore, the generality of this framework is tested across various walking tasks and individuals. Digital camera–based systems have the potential to enhance diagnosis through in-home gait tracking, potentially reducing therapy costs for patients with multiple sclerosis (MS) and PD, while also enabling affordable telemedicine for individuals with MS and PD based on data [12].

PD is a progressive disease that impacts the nervous system over time. As specific brain regions lose dopamine-producing nerves, basic cognitive processes such as verbal expression, writing, and walking become increasingly challenging. As the condition worsens, patients experience progressively severe symptoms. A strategy for predicting PD prevalence is developed using DNN, utilizing the Parkinson's Telemonitoring Speech Data Set from UCI. The Python "TensorFlow" DL module is employed to implement the NN for assessing PD severity. The proposed method is illustrated in Figure 4.2. The process begins with collecting voice recordings from PD patients for analysis. The data is normalized using the min-max method. Subsequently, the input, hidden, and output layers of a DNN are constructed, with the number of neurons in the input layer determined by the number of attributes in the input data. The output layer comprises two neurons, representing "severe" and "non-severe" classifications. The normalized data is then used for training and testing the built DNN [39].

Despite various methods for distinguishing PD using MRI filter images, it remains a significant challenge. This chapter proposes a novel approach for PD detection by combining an AdaBoost classifier with a hybrid particle swarm optimization (PSO) algorithm. AdaBoost outperforms other classifiers in this context. Initially, the finest features of a MRI scan are extracted and identified using curvelet transformation and principal component analysis (PCA). These optimal features are then fed into the AdaBoost classifier. AdaBoost operates in rounds, each involving the training of a new weak learner. An optimization problem is solved in each AdaBoost round to select the best learner that minimizes classification error. Importantly, AdaBoost does not specify how the decision boundary is calculated. To address this, PSO is employed to construct the weak classifier, solving the problem of feature selection and decision boundary determination through an optimization process. An enhanced AdaBoost method using the PSO algorithm accelerates weak classifier development. For initial PSO population parameter calculation, the "CUKOO" algorithm, combined with support vector machine (SVM) and PSO, is employed. Refer to Figure 4.3.

Weak classifiers, represented by decision stumps, replace the PSO-based optimized search for in-depth exploration. Empirical results demonstrate that applying PSO to AdaBoost reduces time consumption. The PD–PCA–PSO–AdaBoost algorithm outperforms other algorithms, surpassing PD–PCA–AdaBoost by 16.47%, PD–PCA–AdaBoost by 12.72%, and PDPSO–SVM–CUKOO–AdaBoost by 5.21%. The hybrid optimization algorithms hold promise for future improvements [34].

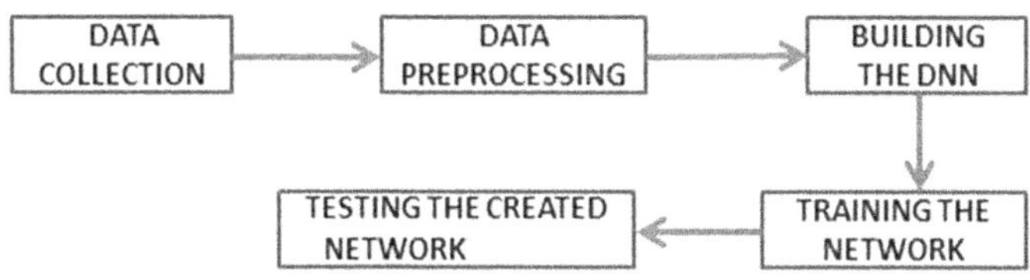

FIGURE 4.2 Deep learning for predicting the severity of PD.

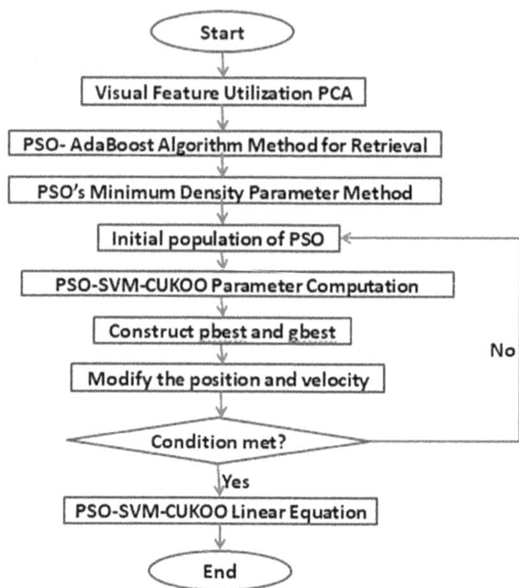

FIGURE 4.3 Flow chart for PSO-based AdaBoost technique.

4.4 EARLY DETECTION OF PD

Developing a PD detection system on a large clinical dataset that incorporates ensemble learning and online learning is a challenging task. However, it can be achieved through the use of deep belief networks (DBNs) and neuro-fuzzy techniques. Expectation–Maximization is employed to cluster large datasets, followed by PCA to address data noise and multicollinearity in PD data. The DBN–adaptive neuro-fuzzy inference system (ANFIS) technique enhances PD data prediction, particularly improving the UPDRS prediction. The general structure of DBN–ANFIS is depicted in Figure 4.4. ANFIS consists of five stages: the product layer, fuzzy layer, de-fuzzy layer, normalized layer, and total output layer.

Figure 4.5 illustrates the utilization of ML for PD detection. The approach addresses missing data and online learning using K-nearest neighbor (KNN) for missing data and interval PCA in conjunction with DBN–ANFIS to enhance incremental learning.

This model employs a dataset with over 5000 records, 16 features, and 2 outputs. Each patient contributes approximately 200 records, resulting in a male-to-female ratio of 1:2. The dataset includes features such as noise-to-harmonics ratio (NHR), multidimensional voice program (MDVP), jitter (Abs), MDVP–shimmer, MDVP–jitter (%), and the total UPDRS and motor UPDRS as the output variables. The model aims to predict these variables and incrementally trains on new data to update prediction models. The refinement of PD dataset attributes enhances UPDRS prediction calculation time and accuracy, reducing time complexity compared to massive

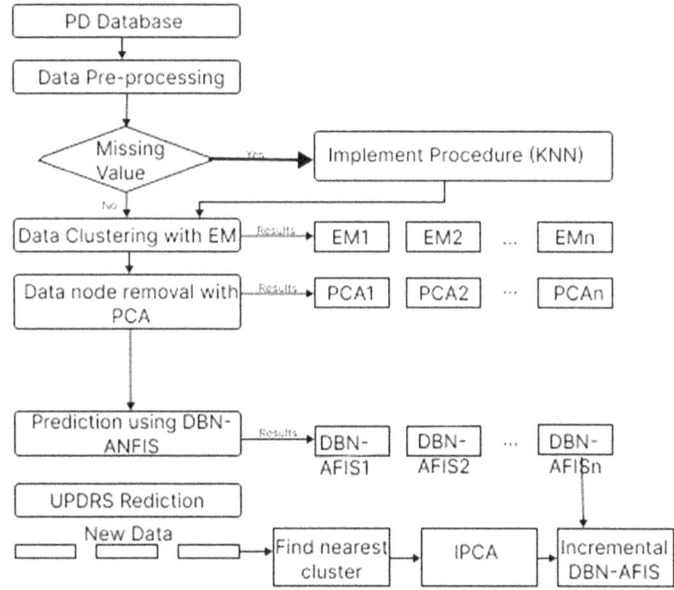

FIGURE 4.4 DBN–ANFIS prediction architecture.

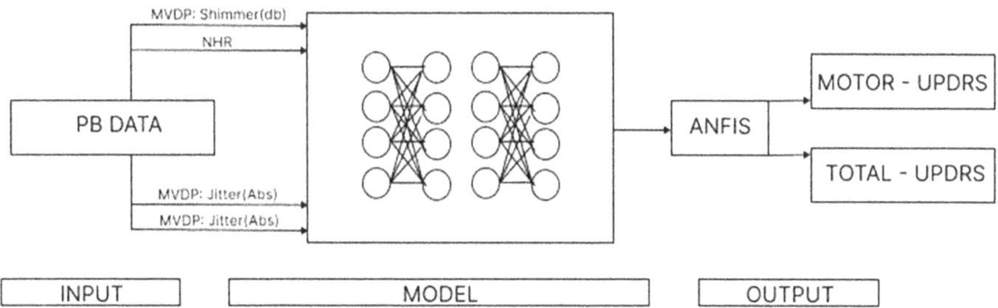

FIGURE 4.5 ML-based PD detection.

input data approaches. Clustering is employed to incrementally improve computing time, and DBN and ANFIS outperform support vector regression and ANFIS in terms of RMSE and modified coefficients of assurance metrics. This research strategy provides an accurate prediction of UPDRS [11].

Research has shown that approximately 90% of PD patients exhibit speech disorders, including dysarthria, monotony, and a low voice. Consequently, these speech characteristics can be used as early indicators of PD. Facial expressions, which offer a noninvasive way to express emotions, are also valuable in identifying PD, particularly when combined with DNN algorithms for analyzing audio recordings. The use of DNN models for classification, as depicted in Figure 4.6, has achieved a detection accuracy of 99.49% [20].

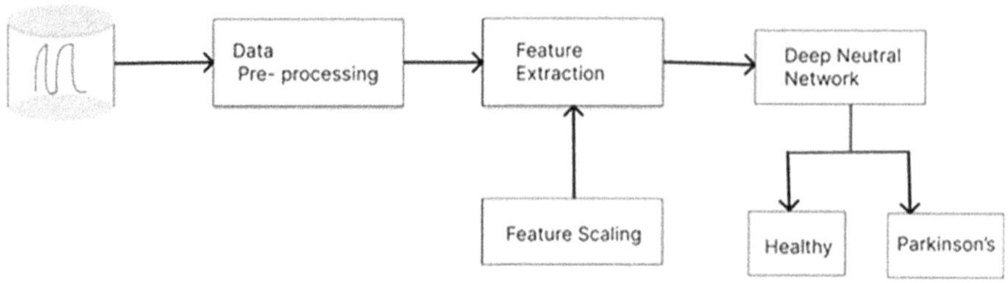

FIGURE 4.6 Workflow diagram for PD detection.

In the early stages of PD, when motor symptoms are absent, the brain's motor coordination channels, such as the thalamus and red nucleus, may compensate for deficiencies. DL models have excelled in brain lesion classification challenges, such as the Multimodal Brain Tumor Image Segmentation Benchmark (BRATS) and ISLES at MICCAI conferences. Autoencoder-based models, including spatial autoencoders, spatial variational autoencoders, and dense variational autoencoders (dVAEs), were tested. Among these, dVAEs exhibited the highest reconstruction errors for subcortical structures. Quantitative MRI data demonstrated that autoencoders could effectively generate anomaly scores for distinguishing de novo PD patients [24].

PD symptoms encompass both motor and non-motor manifestations. Motor symptoms include impaired gait, instability, and stiffness, while non-motor symptoms encompass sleep disturbances, speech difficulties, and loss of smell. A study [25] compared six ML models – Gaussian naive Bayes, decision tree, logistic regression, random forest, SVM, and K-nearest neighbor – using evaluation metrics like accuracy, F1-score, recall, precision, area under the receiver operating characteristic curve (AUC-ROC), and false positive rate. The dataset comprised 188 voice recordings, with 107 from men and 81 from women, spanning ages 37 to 87. Among these, 64 were healthy individuals, while the rest had PD. The results indicated that random forests performed effectively in PD detection. KNN demonstrated the highest accuracy (92.05%) with a k value of 1, and its accuracy decreased as the k value increased. KNN also exhibited the lowest false positive rate (7.97%), outperforming other algorithms in this regard [25].

In India, there are no lab tests or blood tests available for diagnosing PD. Despite this, India has conducted extensive research on the causes and prevalence of PD, surpassing other nations in this regard. The impact of the disease is poised to significantly escalate in the future. Presently, about 300 to 400 individuals out of every 100,000 in the country are grappling with PD. By the year 2030, it is projected that the prevalence of this ailment will double, solidifying its status as one of the most widespread health conditions in the nation. DBS is a surgical procedure that entails the insertion of electrical devices, like electrodes, into the brain to disrupt the signals responsible for PD symptoms. However, the cost associated with this procedure remains prohibitive for many individuals [26].

In India, individuals with PD have access to treatment options such as medication or DBS surgery. In this study, the cross-fold validation method is employed, where the dataset is divided into ten equally sized parts. One part is designated for testing, while the remaining nine parts are used for training the model. The performance of various models is assessed by calculating the average accuracy across ten cross-fold validations. Additionally, NN including DNN, CNN, gated recurrent unit (GRU), LSTM, RNN, and the transfer learning model RESNET50 are evaluated for their performance. Notably, extreme gradient boosting demonstrates superior performance compared to other ML models, both before and after exemplification [26].

Neglecting the first and most prevalent symptom of PD, tremors, can be detrimental to patients. Hand-drawn images and dopamine transporter scan (DaTscan) brain images can be used to predict tremors using models such as VGG 16, ResNet 15, and DenseNet. One model achieved the highest accuracy of 91% for hand-drawn images and 95% for DaTscan images [23]. The PPMI database is utilized to analyze groups of PD patients, aiming to identify biomarkers for improved treatment. The database includes 213 healthy and 441 Parkinson's patient images obtained from the PPMI website, with standardized SPECT images. A decision tree for vocal dataset classification is illustrated in Figure 4.7. VGG 16 proves superior for SPECT images, while DenseNet is more effective for spiral wave representation [14]. Scaling

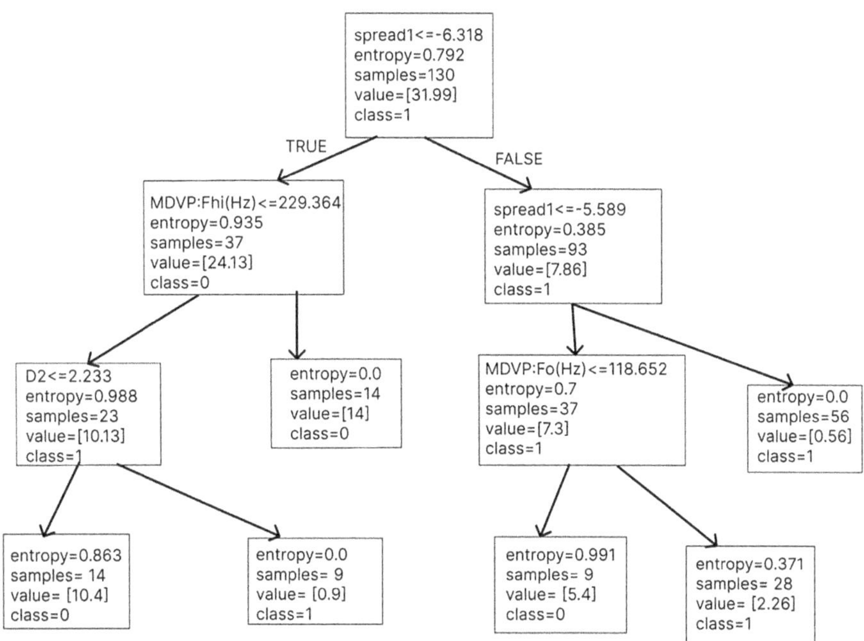

FIGURE 4.7 Decision tree for classification.

all values between 0 and 1 enhances the KNN classifier and artificial neural network (ANN) accuracy to 92% for the voice dataset. DaTscan SPECT images depict smaller dopamine-producing substantia nigra in Parkinson's patients compared to healthy individuals. Spiral and wave drawings classify images as either healthy or Parkinson's-afflicted.

Using a large dataset comprising 5876 records with 22 fields from the UCI ML Repository [22], we evaluated DL and ML methods to determine the optimal pre-diagnosis approach. This dataset includes detailed information about PD patients and healthy individuals. Metrics such as specificity, F1-score, precision, sensitivity, recall, and confusion matrix are used to assess the performance of each method, and the results are visualized in a graph (Figure 4.8) showing training loss and accuracy.

The results indicate that with k = 5, KNN achieves the highest accuracy of 97.43%. It's important to note that the choice of k can influence results. Data-driven methods in ML have revolutionized the extraction and analysis of essential information from metallic element biomarkers. This topic has garnered significant attention in both academic and business spheres for PD diagnosis [22]. ML technologies provide valuable insights for the classification and diagnosis of PD, expediting the decision-making process. The dataset is partitioned into 70/30 train and test sets, each utilized in different models to assess accuracy and classification for each model.

The accuracy of each method is assessed to determine which one is the most effective (Table 4.1). Remarkably, the KNN model achieved the highest accuracy at

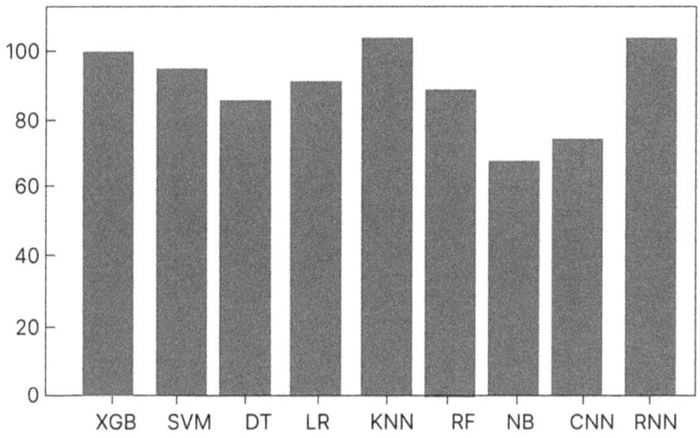

FIGURE 4.8 Bar diagram representation of overall performance for algorithms.

TABLE 4.1
Tabular Description of Results

Algorithm	XGB	SVM	DT	LR	KNN	RF	NB	CNN	RNN
Accuracy (%)	94.87	89.74	87.17	87.17	97.43	92.30	71.79	82.56	96.65

97.43% among all methods examined. These results demonstrate that out of the nine models considered in this study [22], a supervised ML model exhibits the highest accuracy in distinguishing PD patients from healthy individuals.

In ML-based approaches for PD detection, feature selection plays a vital role in stabilizing data dimensions and enhancing model efficiency. Feature selection is also crucial for balancing the risk of overfitting and improving model interpretability. Features selected for detection may encompass clinical assessments, imaging data, and biological markers. Feature selection typically relies on criteria such as statistical significance, correlation with the disease, and clinical relevance.

Tsanas et al. [52] introduced and applied a feature selection technique to patient speech data, alongside data from physically fit individuals, to identify the most relevant acoustic traits that aid in distinguishing between these two groups. The selected features include measures of pitch, jitter, and shimmer, which exhibit high discriminative power in detecting PD. The advantages of feature selection encompass time savings for future data collection, enhanced understanding of disease etiology, reduced computational costs, and improved performance. Combining feature selection with classification algorithms, especially when working with data containing numerous acoustic characteristics, proves highly beneficial.

Through the proposed early diagnosis technique, PD can be accurately identified in its early stages, potentially halting the progression of the disease's symptoms. In comparison to MRI-based techniques, obtaining voice features is simpler and less expensive. Some results suggest that a subset of speech features can efficiently assist researchers in categorizing affected individuals, with feature extraction from candidate PD patients' voice signals requiring less effort. Additionally, classification can be achieved with reduced computational demands.

Pure SVM exhibited the poorest classification performance (79.98%), whereas SVM combined with feature selection performed the best (93.84%) among ANN, SVM, and classification and regression tree (CART). These findings emphasize that selecting the most relevant features significantly enhances categorization performance [37].

$$Accuracy = \frac{TN + TP}{TN + TP + FN + FP} \tag{4.1}$$

The accuracy is determined using Equation 4.1, where TP represents true positives (correctly identified positive instances), TN denotes true negatives (correctly identified negative instances), FP stands for false positives (incorrectly identified negative instances), and FN represents false negatives (incorrectly identified positive instances). The performance of classifiers is also influenced by their settings. Crucial aspects include selecting the optimal parameters for a particular classification algorithm. For SVM, C and gamma parameters must be accurately configured. When employing ANNs for classification, it's essential to carefully choose the network topology, encompassing hidden layers, the number of neurons within each layer, activation functions, learning rate, regularization, and other factors. Each of these parameters necessitates thorough investigation [37].

DL within ML involves training DNNs with multiple layers to extract meaningful patterns from raw data. This approach has gained traction in medical research, particularly in PD identification and assessment. DL's capacity to discern complex patterns and relationships from extensive datasets is one of its strengths. PD is a multifaceted disorder, and DL algorithms have the potential to capture subtle and intricate changes in biological, clinical, and imaging data indicative of the disease's presence. DL techniques can be employed to identify PD based on premotor features such as eye movement speed, sensory loss, subarachnoid space data, and dopamine trait identifiers.

A DL algorithm was developed to differentiate between PD patients and healthy individuals based on brain MRI data, achieving an accuracy of 89%, offering promising results for early PD detection (Figure 4.9). Furthermore, DL techniques can automatically differentiate between healthy individuals and PD patients based on premotor signals, such as rapid eye movement sleep behavior disorder and sensory loss, with a DL model achieving an accuracy of 96.45%. DL algorithms have the remarkable ability to learn both linear and nonlinear features from PD data without the need for manual feature extraction. This study found that DL models outperform 12 other ML models in terms of detection performance, enabling accurate differentiation of individuals with PD from those without.

Notably, DL models demonstrate resilience to network structure, with larger networks, such as DEEP1, exhibiting no signs of both higher accuracy and overfitting in identifying Parkinson's patients. The DEEP EN network, which combines the findings of DEEP1, DEEP2, and DEEP3, significantly enhances the effectiveness of each network. In comparison to any single network, the ensemble network consistently outperforms it in every measure, whether trained for 25 or 50 epochs [29].

The premotor or prodromal phase of PD is now well documented, representing a period of neurodegeneration preceding the emergence of typical clinical motor symptoms. This premotor phase is estimated to last at least 5 years and potentially up to 20 years [12]. During this phase, most symptoms are non-motor in nature, including rapid eye movement sleep behavior disorder and loss of the sense of smell. It's worth noting that none of these symptoms are sensitive enough for screening purposes. However, combining them with potential indicators, such as dopamine

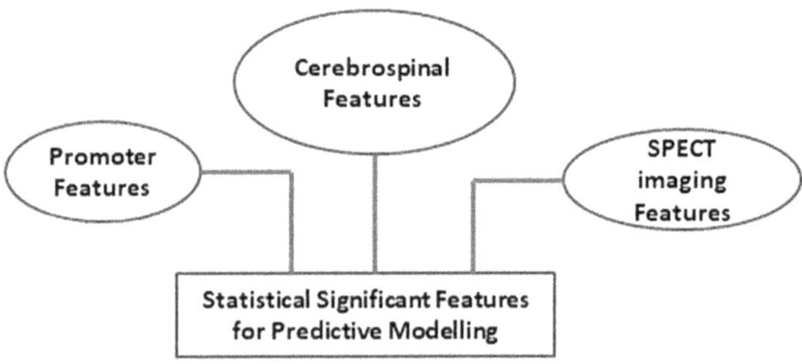

FIGURE 4.9 High-accuracy early PD detection.

transporter (DAT) imaging and cerebrospinal fluid measurements (CSF), can aid in assessing the risk of developing PD.

Early PD can be distinguished from robust normal conditions by utilizing preclinical signs like non-motor aspects of rapid eye movement sleep behavior disorder, sensory loss, CSF metrics, and dopaminergic imaging features. The SVM classifier has demonstrated excellent performance, achieving an accuracy of 96.40%, sensitivity of 97.03%, specificity of 95.01%, and an impressive AUC-ROC of 98.88%. The utilization of non-motor, CSF, and imaging indicators offers a promising approach to preclinical PD diagnosis [41].

The expansion of feature spaces has been observed to enhance the classification accuracy of all PD prediction methods. Classification results obtained with extended features outperform those using the original data features. Logistic regression, which provides the most comprehensive feature space, achieves an accuracy rating of 76.03%. SVM, one of the popular core-based techniques, has been evaluated with various kernels and settings. The linear kernel SVM produces the best outcome with an accuracy of 75.49%. PCA is employed to reduce the dimensionality from 26 features to 5, with these reduced features showing superior distribution. The incorporation of information gain values also proved effective in extending the feature space for gradient boosting and random forest [42].

FP-CIT SPECT (DaTscan) primarily serves to differentiate patients with mild or indeterminate Parkinsonism [46]. Nevertheless, interpreting DAT imaging and categorizing PD can be challenging, leading to a subset of PD patients referred to as scans without evidence of dopaminergic deficit (SWEDD). SWEDD patients, constituting 10%–15% of clinically diagnosed PD cases, exhibit distinct characteristics regarding etiology and prognosis compared to conventional PD. However, DAT imaging's interpretation can sometimes be inconsistent. Visual interpretation of DAT scans offers better exposure (98%) but lower sensitivity (67%) in early PD diagnosis.

A DL-based technique for interpreting FP-CIT SPECT data is developed to enhance PD imaging diagnosis. This method attains excellent accuracy, matching reference quantification performed by experts using SPECT images of affected and healthy individuals as training data. Its high accuracy is further confirmed in an independent sample of PD and non-Parkinsonian tremor patients. The results suggest that this DL-based method can effectively interpret FP-CIT SPECT scans and reduce human judgment variability. It holds the potential to reclassify some individuals with clinical PD diagnoses who exhibit scans without cholinergic deficiency, a distinct subtype of PD. The DL-based approach can offer valuable insights for patients with undetermined Parkinsonism, particularly for SWEDD [34].

Single strategies are often inaccurate, prompting the development of hybrid methods. By combining regression analysis (RA) with an ANN model, the limitations of RA are overcome. In RA, data preparation and probability estimates are carried out, while the second method compares a patient's PD status to a neuron's predetermined threshold value. This approach is compared to established methods such as SVM and KNN classifiers, demonstrating the superiority of the suggested algorithm with an accuracy of 93.46%. This method classifies individuals as having PD or being healthy based on attribute values, leveraging features like reduced pitch period entropy, detrended fluctuation analysis, recurrence period density entropy, elevated pulse rate, and iron accumulation in the substantia nigra. While iron deposition plays a significant role in altering an individual's physical and mental behavior, the current context only calculates iron concentration and does not classify significant changes.

The dataset is initially processed through regression analysis for the hybridized regression analysis and ANN technique for early identification. The ANN is then trained on the regressed dataset to predict the likelihood of exhibiting symptoms. The integrated probability of having PD or being healthy is set to 1. The dataset is employed for identifying PD patients based on speech signals [44].

Researchers have devised a decision-support system that utilizes feature selection to facilitate the prompt identification of PD. This system analyzes voice signal features from both PD patients and healthy individuals, with the primary aim of enhancing model performance and accuracy while reducing computational costs. Feature selection is applied to the 23 voice features to retain only the most informative ones, thus streamlining the analysis. Various feature selection algorithms are employed in conjunction with classification methods such as CART, SVM, and ANN for categorizing affected and healthy individuals. Among these methods, SVM with feature selection (FS) achieves the highest accuracy at 93.84%, while pure SVM performs the poorest at 79.98%. The incorporation of FS methods with classification proves highly beneficial, particularly when dealing with speech signals containing a multitude of phonetic features. The dataset is restructured to include fewer columns for more efficient classification, with CART utilizing seven features, and SVM and ANN utilizing thirteen. Python and its libraries, including scikit-learn, Keras, and TensorFlow, are employed in these experiments. Accuracy is used as a performance metric, with precision reflecting the proportion of correct classifications among total assessments [31].

Several studies have explored PD diagnosis using different classification methods, including SAS based computer programs and predictive modeling techniques. Predictive modeling is a crucial aspect of data mining as it aids in defining population groups. With numerous methods available, comparing results to determine the most effective approach is essential. Max Little of the University of Oxford, in collaboration with the National Centre for Voice and Speech in Denver, Colorado, created a dataset for classification by recording speech signals. The dataset comprises biological voice measurements from 31 individuals, with 23 of them having PD. Each row in the table corresponds to one of these individuals' 195 voice recordings (listed in the "title" column), while each column represents a different voice parameter. The primary objective of the dataset, indicated by the "status" column (set to 0 for healthy and 1 for PD), is to distinguish between healthy and PD individuals.

The input dataset was randomly split into two parts: training and testing. The majority of the input dataset was utilized for training, leaving the remaining portion for testing. Parameters for each classifier were adjusted accordingly. The following modifications were made to the NN classifier: The feed-forward, single-hidden-layer NN employs the backpropagation learning algorithm, and Levenberg–Marquardt (LM) algorithms were utilized for analysis. Both the hidden and output layers employ the logistic sigmoid transfer function, with up to ten neurons used in the hidden layer. Initial weights were randomly determined.

The calculated regression technique was employed in the regression node. Default values for both DMNeural and decision tree nodes were selected. Four distinct classification models were employed, namely DMNeural, NN, regression, and decision tree. Various evaluation metrics were employed to compute the classifiers' performance scores, with special emphasis on the NN classifier, which achieved 92.9% classification accuracy [33].

DL models have demonstrated a high level of accuracy in diagnosing PD. Approximately 57% of DL studies for automatic PD identification have recommended the use of CNN models. CNN models have consistently demonstrated high accuracy rates across a variety of image classification tasks, including handwriting recognition and neuroimaging (SPECT, PET, and MRI). CNN's ability to detect anomalies in one-dimensional signals, such as voice and EEG, has also been observed. In contrast, hybrid models (CNN–LSTM), DNNs, or LSTM models appear to excel when applied to gait analysis. Further research is necessary to determine which model performs best for each specific application. For SPECT and voice analysis, backpropagation NN and genetically optimized NN models, respectively, achieve the highest prediction accuracy. Clinical trials are needed to validate the suitability of the proposed DL model for each modality [45].

Early diagnosis and treatment are pivotal in managing PD symptoms and maintaining patients' independence. However, due to the often ambiguous clinical findings and the scarcity of neurologists specializing in PD diagnosis, there can be delays in diagnosis and suboptimal treatment. Furthermore, the success of cutting-edge treatments like gene therapy, which is currently under investigation, may be heavily influenced by early detection. Introducing computer-aided diagnosis (CAD) tools that rely on DL models could help reduce the workload of neurologists if PD can be diagnosed quickly and accurately. DL methods, particularly the CNN model, have demonstrated a high prediction accuracy for PD and have garnered significant support in studies focusing on image classification. To increase adoption among end users like neurologists and other medical professionals, more information on disease prediction and DL-based CAD tools is needed. Therefore, researchers are encouraged to continue developing DL models that address specific challenges related to disease identification and incorporate visual cues. Moreover, future research may explore more interpretable and explainable approaches in DL-based CAD tools to improve health outcomes for the growing global PD population [45].

4.5 TREATMENT OF PD

Utilizing a DL CNN to assist a patient whose PD primarily manifests as hand tremors. Parameters for DBS were adjusted at six different levels – off as a baseline, 1 mA, 1.75 mA, 2.5 mA, 3.25 mA, and 4 mA – to aid patients with hand tremors due to PD. Researchers employed a DL CNN implemented in TensorFlow and achieved an 85% success rate in distinguishing between different DBS parameter settings for Parkinson's treatment, demonstrating the effectiveness of DL algorithms in this domain. Researchers have also effectively demonstrated the use of BioStamp

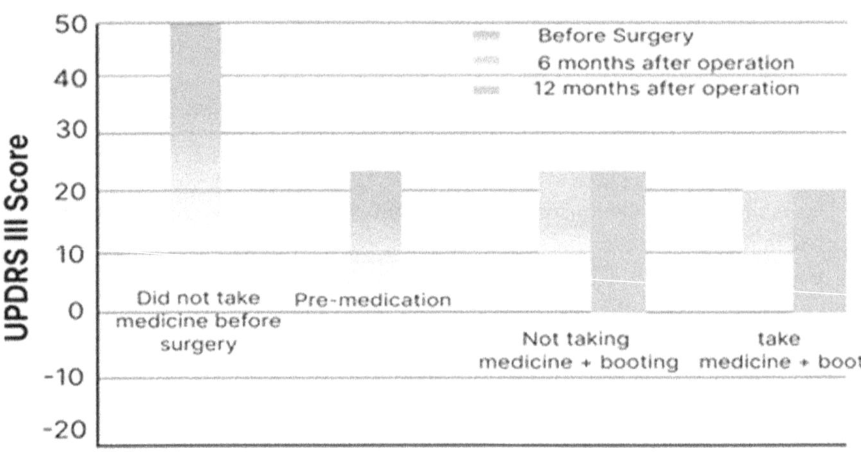

FIGURE 4.10 UPDRS (Unified Parkinson's Disease Rating Scale) score.

nPoint, a similar remote inertial sensor system with remote access to cloud computing resources for storing collected data and analyzing responses to a set of prescribed parameter settings for DBS [13].

In the early stages of its training process, an improved image cropping technique, incorporating new MRI image analysis technologies, is utilized to construct a model, which subsequently diversifies the training process. The data is collected from patients who have undergone bilateral surgical procedures. The square root back-propagation algorithm, also known as RMSProp, is employed to enhance the computational model. This study examines the clinical efficacy of DBS in the surgical treatment of PD and its postoperative neuroprotective and neurorestorative effects. It employs DL algorithms combined with MRI image analysis technology. Moreover, this research enhances the DL technique to make it compatible with clinical imaging, aiming to develop an imaging analysis model corresponding to it. The statistics for the detection rate of the algorithm model when working with extensive data are considered [14] (Figure 4.10 and Table 4.2).

4.6 BEHAVIORAL CHANGES IN A PD PATIENT AND THEIR DETECTION

The voice of an individual with PD undergoes various changes, including instability. Voice analysis, being noninvasive and user-friendly, offers a means to diagnose these changes. NN typically consist of three layers: an input layer, an output layer, and one or more hidden layers. In many cases, the input layer is provided with the data. The Opt–DNN has proven to be more accurate than other ML techniques such as XGBoost, SVM, KNN, and random forest. It achieves an F1-score of 0.9484, an accuracy rate of 95.14%, and a precision of 0.9484. This type of NN with three hidden layers is effective, particularly for small datasets, although it is limited to three hidden layers [21].

TABLE 4.2
Results Obtained Using Various ML Algorithms for PD Detection

ML Algorithm	Precision Score	Recall Score	Cross Val Score In-Sample	Cross Val Score Out-Sample	Accuracy Score
Logistic regression	0.93	0.96	0.91	0.73	0.91
KNN	***0.94***	***0.96***	***0.91***	***0.75***	***0.92***
Decision tree	***0.94***	***0.96***	***0.91***	***0.75***	***0.92***
Random forest	0.88	0.95	0.86	0.7	0.85
AdaBoost	0.82	0.85	0.73	0.73	0.73
Auto_ViML	***0.99***	***0.91***	***0.92***	—	***0.92***

**Note: Rows highlighted and italicized correspond to the algorithms with top 3 accuracy scores.*

Several EEG analysis techniques are applied as a multiclassification approach for monitoring and diagnosing PD. Data is sourced from medical sleep EEG records at Shaanxi People's Hospital. To enhance data accuracy and construct the sample set for experimentation, sleep EEG and related sleep phase information from four groups are utilized. A key comparison is made between rapid eye movement sleep and PD EEG data. Two classification models, TQWT–DRSN (Figure 4.11) and WPT–DRSN (Figure 4.12), are created by combining DL with time-frequency analysis techniques.

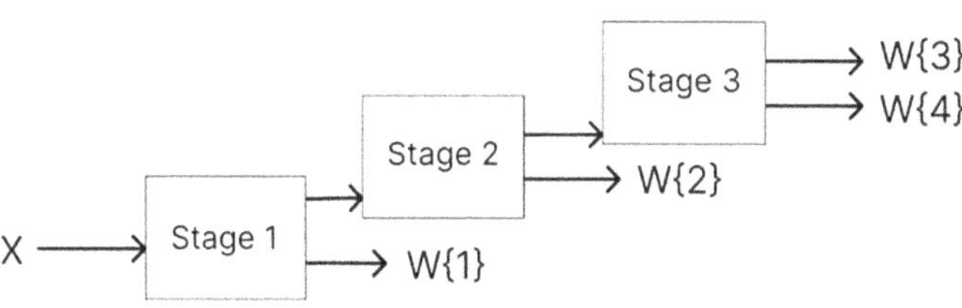

FIGURE 4.11 Tunable Q-factor wavelet transform with J = 3.

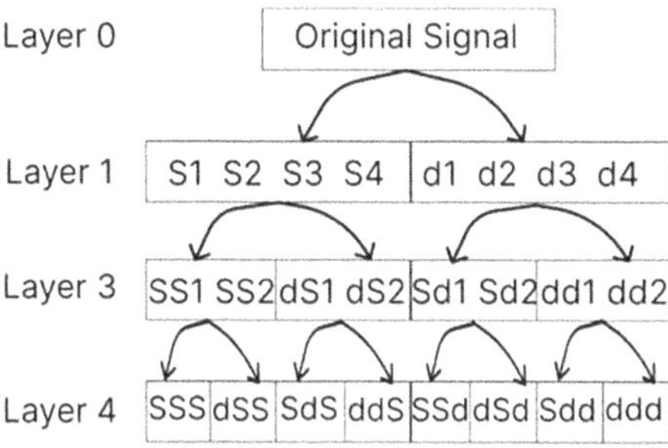

FIGURE 4.12 Three-layer wavelet packets transform.

Disorders related to rapid eye movement sleep in PD are among the conditions classified. The WPT–DRSN (wavelet packet transform–deep residual shrinkage network) achieves remarkable accuracy, with rates of 99.86% in the second class, 97.81% in the third class, and 92.59% in the fourth class, demonstrating its superiority for lower-category classification tasks. This assists doctors in identifying specific neurological disorders in their patients. These proposed methods leverage DL's capabilities in feature learning and representation, incorporating time-frequency data from various sleep stages and EEG channels, distinguishing them from existing methods reliant on artificial feature engineering. These techniques are suitable for early detection, effective management, and prognostic tracking of PD patients, potentially tracking disease progression. While the model excels at classifying data into two groups, its performance may diminish as the number of groups increases [15].

Residual neural networks are employed for real-time detection of freezing of gait (FoG) events, a common but not well understood syndrome in PD patients. FoG detection in real time using residual neural networks represents a significant advancement. The network incorporates LSTM, Moore's algorithm, CNN, and the well-known ResNet-50 model for comparison.

Moore's strategy treats the freeze index as a fundamental indicator for distinguishing FoG from non-FoG. A predefined threshold is set, and FoG events are identified if the freeze index surpasses this threshold. Performance comparisons are made between the proposed deep residual network and a single-layer CNN and a three-layer CNN. LSTM's recurrent connections allow information from previous cell outputs to be used as input for the current cell. The deep residual network design includes 17 convolutional layers across 6 blocks. Although the architectural layers of ResNet-50 are more extensive, the performance of the residual neural network approach is comparable, and in some cases, superior. It excels in detecting short-duration FoG occurrences within limited time frames and can contribute to the detection of these events. The multisensor site study results demonstrate the feasibility of creating a user-friendly system with fewer sensors and employing advanced algorithms for low-latency FoG detection. This approach enhances the quality of life for patients and facilitates the assessment of FoG symptoms [16].

$$SE = \frac{TP}{TP + FN} \times 100\% \tag{4.2}$$

$$SP = \frac{TN}{TN + FP} \times 100\% \tag{4.3}$$

$$GM = \sqrt{SE \times SP} \tag{4.4}$$

Equations 4.2, 4.3, and 4.4 provide formulas for employee sensitivity, specificity, and geometric mean, respectively, to measure performance during the evaluation (Table 4.3). A novel DL architectural paradigm known as DBV (deep neural

TABLE 4.3
Statistical Terms in Binary Classification

	Actual Positive	Actual Negative
Detected positive	True positivity (TP)	False positivity (FP)
Detected negative	False negativity (FN)	True negativity (TN)

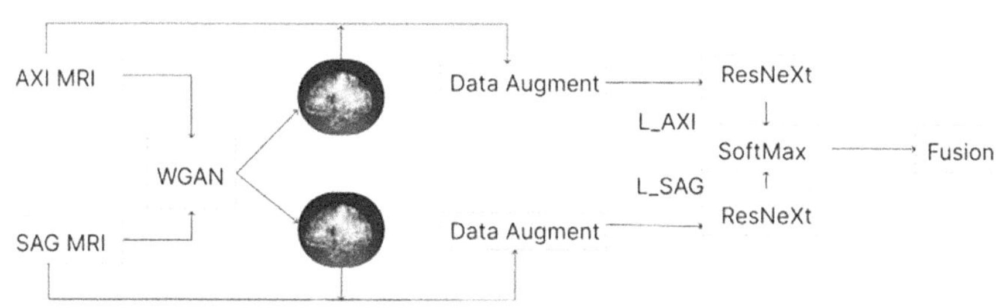

FIGURE 4.13 The DBV framework.

networks with broad views) is introduced. This paradigm utilizes multiview brain MRI data and comprises three phases: training, validation, and testing. DBV builds upon the ResNet architecture and incorporates multimodal learning and layer fusion techniques. Additionally, Keras' WGAN and image data generator are employed for data preprocessing. The DBV model achieves the highest accuracy for PD screening after 20 iterations. The architecture is depicted in Figure 4.13. The results suggest that the DBV model is the preferred choice, as it attains the highest accuracy score and outperforms other powerful existing NN such as LeNet, AlexNet, ResNet, ResNeXt, and DenseNet [18].

Many PD patients exhibit non-motor symptoms that impact various functions. These symptoms encompass disturbances in the sleep–wake cycle, cognitive impairment (including rostral executive dysfunction, episodic memory impairment, Alzheimer's disease, and hallucinosis), anxiety disorders, dyskinesia (primarily orthostatic hypotension), sensory symptoms (hyposmia), and constipation, among others. Some of these signs can manifest years or even decades before the appearance of classic motor symptoms. Diagnosis of PD relies on clinical assessment, considering these signs, medical history, and treatment response. Clinical signs indicative of PD include unilateral resting tremors, bradykinesia, or rigidity. During finger–nose coordination tests, the tested limb's movement diminishes or subsides. Patients may exhibit difficulty with rapid alternating movements during neurological exams. Strength and sensation are typically normal, but reflexes may be challenging to elicit due to stiffness or tremors. In the early stages, PD often affects only one side, making it crucial to pay attention to symptoms that are unilaterally present.

Imaging techniques are valuable for early-stage diagnosis, particularly when clinical findings are inconclusive. A proposed method aims to categorize patients

TABLE 4.4
Confusion Matrices for LSTM, CONV 1D, and CONV 2D

LSTM	Healthy	PD	CONV1D	Healthy	PD	CONV2D	Healthy	PD
Healthy	2381	18	Healthy	2236	163	Healthy	2287	112
PD	120	2196	PD	82	2234	PD	63	2253

TABLE 4.5
Performance Results Network-Wise

Classifier	Accuracy	Precision	Recall	F1-Score
LSTM	0.971	0.992	0.952	0.971
CONV1D	0.948	0.932	0.964	0.948
CONV2D	0.962	0.953	0.973	0.963

as either healthy or having PD based on acoustic tests, as PD often affects voice characteristics. Changes in breathing, speech patterns, and voice volume are common in PD, which can cause voice volume reduction of up to 10 decibels. Therefore, a method based on speech recognition is proposed to aid in diagnosis [27]. The method employs LSTM, 1D, and 2D CNN networks, yielding promising results. The LSTM network achieves an impressive F-score of 97%, indicating its effectiveness. These results suggest that the proposed method could enhance PD diagnosis and reduce the time and effort required.

Table 4.4 presents confusion matrices for the LSTM, CONV1D, and CONV2D NN. In all three cases, patients are predominantly correctly classified. For instance, the LSTM network correctly categorizes 2196 out of 2316 speech samples from patients as positive. The left side of the table, pertaining to the LSTM network, displays the confusion matrix for the expected positive outcomes.

The diagonal elements represent the correct classifications. Specifically, the LSTM network makes only 18 errors when categorizing voice recordings from healthy patients as positive but makes 120 errors when categorizing voice recordings from PD patients as negative. In the other two cases, errors are slightly larger and primarily affect the group of healthy patients. This contrasts with LSTM, where errors are more frequent in the group of patients. Table 4.5 presents the metrics employed to assess classifier performance for all three systems used by Aversano et al. [27], including classifier type, precision, recall, and F-score. Each row demonstrates the performance of a particular classifier.

4.7 PD DETECTION FROM HANDWRITING PATTERNS

PD is a progressive neurological condition that necessitates early detection. However, many clinical diagnostic techniques lack sufficient accuracy. To address this, a CNN and a histogram of oriented gradients (HOG) descriptor are employed to identify PD from handwriting patterns. A dataset comprising 204 photographs of handwritten spiral and wave patterns (102 from healthy individuals and 102 from individuals with PD) is utilized. Given the dataset's limited size, online data augmentation techniques such as rotation, random brightness, and random zooming are applied. The methodology combines a 1D-CNN with the HOG descriptor. The HOG descriptor is based on the idea that objects can be adequately characterized by local intensity gradients and their directions. This is achieved by dividing the input image into "cells" and generating a local 1D histogram of gradient directions for each cell's pixels. The results are aggregated, averaged over a larger spatial region known as a "block," and normalized to enhance lighting invariance. The HOG descriptor features are then input into the 1D-CNN, resulting in an accuracy of approximately 87%. Interestingly, the model performs slightly better on wave patterns than on spiral patterns [28].

4.7.1 PD Detection Using Max Little's Dataset

ML algorithms can aid in early PD detection. Max Little's dataset, recorded at the National Centre for Voice and Speech in Denver, is employed for this purpose. The dataset comprises 195 voice recordings from 31 individuals, including 23 PD patients and 8 healthy individuals, along with 23 features (22 of which are biomedical measures, and 1 binary column denoting "1" for PD and "0" for healthy individuals). The comparison steps are illustrated in Figure 4.14. The stacking model surpasses other utilized models in terms of accuracy and F1 scoring, according to a detailed analysis. Stacking combines predictions from the best two or more base ML

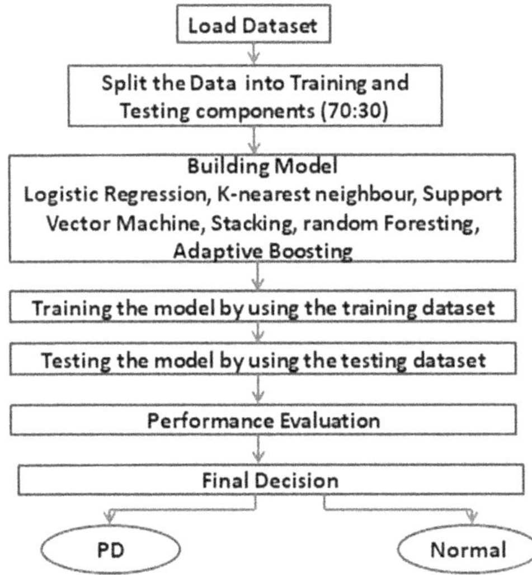

FIGURE 4.14 Flowchart of the comparative analysis of models.

algorithms to create a new meta-learning algorithm. Its advantage lies in harnessing the capabilities of multiple high-performing methods to produce predictions that outperform any single model. The stacking model boasts an impressive accuracy of 93%, a standard deviation of 5%, and an average F1-score of 94%, based on the analysis results [29].

4.8 VOICE ANALYSIS–BASED PD DETECTION

Another proposed method for PD detection relies on motor symptoms associated with voice. Voice analysis begins with two vocal tasks: vowel voicing and sentence articulation, both representing phonation and speech tasks. The classifiers' performance is evaluated using audio data recorded by AC (acoustic cardioid) and SP (smartphone) microphones. The audio speech data is divided into voiced and voiceless segments using the Praat Computer Program Toolkit. Feature extraction is then employed to generate additional records for each feature set and modality, resulting in a total of 144 extraction records. The method utilizes a hold-out strategy to evaluate the database with four classifiers: KNN, MLP, optimum-path forest, and SVM. Default hyper-parameter settings are used for KNN, MLP, and SVM training. The study examines 18 feature sets and 14 classifiers on a voice dataset, evaluating results in terms of error and accuracy. Statistical analysis of the results using N-way ANOVA and the Nemenyi test indicates no statistically significant difference between the AC and SP microphones. This supports the notion that PD can be detected using a smartphone. Notably, the phonation task yields the most promising results, with AC achieving an accuracy of 94.55%, AUC of 87.84%, and EER (equal error rate) of 19.01%, while SP achieves an accuracy of 92.94%, AUC of 92.40%, and EER of 14.15%. The method produces various results, all demonstrating relatively superior performance. In terms of accuracy, both AC and SP modalities are found to be consistent, rendering the phonation task suitable and efficient for application [30].

4.9 SPATIOTEMPORAL PEN TRACE ANALYSIS

PD is one of the most common movement disorders, characterized by a loss of dopaminergic function in the substantia nigra pars compacta. Diagnostic criteria are primarily based on clinical features, which can lack sensitivity and specificity, occasionally leading to misdiagnosis. This method focuses on recording the pen position on a tablet and calculating a vector of measurements to characterize the pen trace spatiotemporally. This includes metrics such as normalized velocity variability, velocity's standard deviation and mean, and signal entropy. These metrics aim to detect subtle features like speed variability and "jumps" from the horizontal plane, which may be more pronounced in individuals with movement disorders compared to healthy subjects [31].

Velocity profiles that deviate from constant-speed lines do not appear natural. The effects of PD are most noticeable at rest or during steady movements. To ensure consistency, participants were instructed to maintain a constant drawing speed. All subjects underwent a practice phase in which they drew several lines to familiarize themselves with the procedure. Participants drew with their wrist fixed in relation to the forearm, while the hand moved away from the body. The forearm was unsupported by either the table or the pad, and the pen was the only point of contact with the pad's surface. The dataset is used to compute mean horizontal velocity (MV), normalized velocity variability (NVV) in units of one second, standard deviation of horizontal velocity (SDV), and entropies (ETP) of the horizontal and vertical components of the signal using histograms of the x-component (x_hist) and y-component (y_hist). Equations 4.5 to 4.9 define the aforementioned variables:

$$MV = \frac{1}{N}\sum_{i=1}^{N} v_i \tag{4.5}$$

$$NVV = \frac{1}{T\,|\,MV\,|}\sum_{i=1}^{N-1} |\, v_{i-1} - v_i \,| \tag{4.6}$$

$$SDV = \sqrt{\frac{1}{N-1}\sum_{i=1}^{N} |v_i - MV|^2} \tag{4.7}$$

$$ETP_x = \sum_{i=1}^{N} P(x_i)\log(P(x_i)) \tag{4.8}$$

$$ETP_Y = \sum_{i=1}^{N} P(y_i)\log(P(y_i)) \tag{4.9}$$

The score vectors for each subject are averaged to compute the components of different metrics' score vectors. This is done in six different ways: ALL (mean over all efforts of a subject), HH (mean of the scores of the highest-scoring hand), LH (mean of the scores of the lowest-scoring hand), HLH (difference between HH and LH), and LD (difference between the highest-scoring and lowest-scoring movement direction). ALL is used when no specific component is mentioned. A comparison of NVV values between the H (healthy) and PD groups reveals that the PD group does not exhibit a normal distribution across all six components, while the H group does.

Correlation tests were conducted between the H and Y variables of the patients, UPDRS component III summation, UPDRS upper limb tremor component summation scores, and score vectors for the entire PD population. It was observed that none of the metrics and UPDRS scores had any significant correlation. Subsequently, low Pearson product–moment correlation coefficients with high p-values were combined. NVV, a novel metric, was computed and compared with four metrics of each subject's digitized line. NVV quantifies the horizontal pen speed during line drawing, regardless of the average speed of line drawing. An accuracy of 91% was achieved by applying a novel ML algorithm to unlabeled PD and H data. A score vector represents each subject, and the resulting model outperformed existing algorithms in the literature using handwriting markers for PD classification. It is noteworthy that these tasks used by other algorithms are time-consuming and more complex. NVV emerged as the most crucial feature in a rigorous experiment with a tenfold, 20-cross-validation framework. Its performance remained consistent across all 200 random folds. The newly developed ML models, in conjunction with NVV, were employed in medical practices. This facilitated the quantification of PD manifestation characteristics using touch-sensitive tablets or pen-tablet digitizers, allowing for the creation of patient profiles to aid physicians in remote monitoring. This noninvasive quantification of subjective disease symptoms supports further research and understanding of PD by the scientific community [32].

4.10 DIFFERENTIATING PD AND PROGRESSIVE SUPRANUCLEAR PALSY (PSP) THROUGH GAIT ANALYSIS

Progressive supranuclear palsy (PSP) is a type of Parkinsonism that shares similarities with PD in its initial stages. PD is recognized as the second most prevalent neurodegenerative condition globally. As gait dysfunctions are a significant motor symptom in both conditions, analyzing gait can provide healthcare professionals with subclinical data that indicates nuanced distinctions between these illnesses. The study involved gathering gait analysis data from 46 individuals categorized into three groups: individuals with PD at different stages and patients with PSP. Spatial and temporal parameters were analyzed. An imbalanced minority artificial dataset was balanced through oversampling, and cross-validation was employed to generate distinct training and testing sets. Random forests and gradient boosted trees were utilized for analysis.

The slicing approach was applied to balance the unbalanced dataset, resulting in 81 records. A total of 33 spatial and temporal features were initially available, but the number was reduced to 16 by calculating the average of computed values for the right and left sides. A fivefold cross-validation was chosen due to limited records. When categorizing PSP patients, random forests showed the highest overall accuracy (86.4%) and specificity (96.3%), while gradient boosted trees exhibited high accuracy (84.0%) and the best sensitivity (96.3%). Compared to all patients, the PSP group demonstrated the highest sensitivity and specificity, exceeding 90% and 95% cut-offs. The de novo PD group had sensitivity and specificity ratings close to 90%. The stable PD group exhibited the highest specificity (around 90%) but the lowest sensitivity (between 65% and 70%). This indicates the capacity to accurately classify the tested group but not the others. This study applied a data mining approach to gait analysis spatial and temporal metrics to differentiate individuals with typical (PD) and atypical Parkinsonism (PSP) based on gait patterns. This tool may assist clinicians in identifying PSP from PD, especially in the early stages when differential diagnosis is challenging [35].

The proposed method utilizes a hybrid approach that combines PCA with linear discriminant analysis (LDA) to identify specific gait patterns associated with PD. Figure 4.15 depicts the gait footage of both PD patients and healthy participants used for system evaluation. The effectiveness of feature extraction using PCA and LDA coefficients was also compared. The computer vision–based gait analysis system

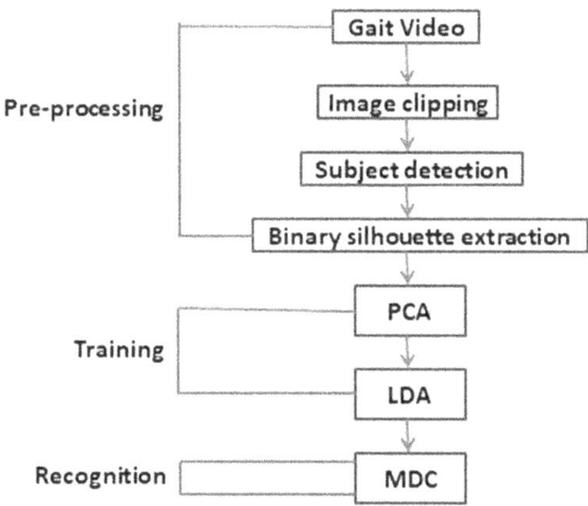

FIGURE 4.15 Workflow of architectural diagram for processing steps.

comprises three components: preprocessing, training, and recognition. Videos of subjects, including seven people with PD and seven healthy individuals, walking from left to right and back, were recorded using a SONY HDR-HC3 camcorder. These video recordings were then converted into image snippets sampled at a rate of 15 frames per second. To enable feature extraction using PCA and LDA, each subject was encoded as a vector. An MDC (multi-dimensional classifier) was employed to assess the classification performance of the proposed method. This approach focuses on identifying and categorizing PD gait patterns by extracting inherent information from image sequences of walking human silhouettes. During training, both PCA and LDA achieved a classification rate of 100%. According to the experiment, LDA–MDC outperformed PCA–MDC by 18.31%. LDA–MDC improved the detection rate in both normal and PD participants. PCA, mainly used as a preprocessing step in LDA–MDC for data dimensionality reduction, did not effectively separate different groups of silhouette vectors [36].

Brain scans and neurological examinations, such as the UPDRS, are commonly used for diagnosis but are costly and require specialized expertise. Therefore, a reliable software system is needed to aid in PD diagnosis. The advent of digitization tools has made it feasible to record measurements from handwritten activities using tablet and pen devices. ML methods, including DL, have been employed to classify signals and images, such as audio signals and handwritten text lines. DL, including CNN and CNN–LSTM models, has enabled PD detection through automatic classification of online handwriting. CNN uses chain and spectral analysis methods to encode time series into images, while CNN–LSTM uses raw time sequences directly. Both models account for local short-term information before normalization. Concatenation algorithms standardize the time sequence into a fixed dimension visual representation without retaining this local data, resulting in worse performance. Furthermore, enhancing the CNN–bidirectional LSTM model's understanding of the dynamics of temporal feature activation improves its performance [31].

4.11 CONCLUSIONS

The application of DL has the potential to revolutionize the diagnosis and treatment of PD. DL algorithms can handle vast amounts of input rapidly and accurately, aiding in the identification of patterns and correlations that may not be apparent to human specialists. This could lead to more precise and dependable diagnoses, shorter treatment durations, and improved outcomes for patients. Additionally, individualized treatment plans generated through DL algorithms may result in more effective therapies and improved outcomes for individuals with PD. In this work, we presented the developments carried out so far in the detection of PD using DL techniques. The future of DL in the diagnosis and treatment of PD looks promising, and it is expected to become an increasingly vital tool for medical professionals in the years ahead.

4.12 FUTURE SCOPE

DL could accelerate and enhance the accuracy of PD diagnosis. By rapidly analyzing large datasets, these algorithms may shorten diagnosis times, particularly in remote or resource-limited areas. Furthermore, one can analyze wearable devices and other data sources to detect PD early, enabling timely interventions. Improved diagnostic precision is possible with DL algorithms examining extensive datasets for patterns that elude human specialists. This leads to accurate diagnosis of PD in its early stages. DL algorithms can also analyze wearable devices and other data sources for disease monitoring and evaluation of treatment effectiveness. Targeted and efficient approaches to PD treatment can be framed. New algorithms based on DL can be developed to create personalized treatment programs based on a patient's unique symptoms and medical history, potentially leading to improved therapies and longer life expectancies for millions of individuals affected by the disease.

REFERENCES

1. Tripathy, B.K. and Anuradha, J. (2015). *Soft Computing-Advances and Applications.* Cengage Learning Publishers, New Delhi.
2. Bhattacharyya, S., Snasel, V., Hassanian, A. E., Saha, S. and Tripathy, B. K. (2020). *Deep Learning Research with Engineering Applications.* De Gruyter Publications. DOI: 10.1515/9783110670905
3. Maheswari, K., Shaha, A., Arya, D., Rajkumar, R. and Tripathy, B. K. (2020). Convolutional neural networks: A bottom-up approach. In Bhattacharyya, S., Hassanian, A. E., Saha, S. and Tripathy, B.K. (Eds) *Deep Learning Research with Engineering Applications.* De Gruyter Publications, pp. 21–50. DOI: 10.1515/9783110670905-002
4. Adate, A. and Tripathy, B.K. (2019). S-LSTM-GAN: Shared recurrent neural networks with adversarial training. In Kulkarni, A., Satapathy, S., Kang, T. and Kashan, A. (Eds) *Proceedings of the 2nd International Conference on Data Engineering and Communication Technology.* Advances in Intelligent Systems and Computing, Vol. 828, Springer, Singapore, pp. 107–115.

5. Kaul, D., Raju, H. and Tripathy, B.K. (2022). Deep learning in healthcare. In Acharjya, D.P., Mitra, A. and Zaman, N. (Eds) *Deep Learning in Data Analytics- Recent Techniques, Practices and Applications)*, Studies in Big Data, Vol. 91. Springer, Cham, pp. 97–115. DOI: 10.1007/978-3-030-75855-4_6
6. Bose, A. and Tripathy, B.K. (2020). Deep learning for audio signal classification. In Bhattacharyya, S., Hassanian, A. E., Saha, S. and Tripathy, B.K. (Eds) *Deep Learning Research and Applications*, De Gruyter Publications, pp. 105–136. DOI: 10.1515/9783110670905-00660
7. Singhania, U. and Tripathy, B.K. (2021). *Text-Based Image Retrieval Using Deep Learning, Encyclopaedia of Information Science and Technology*, Fifth Edition, pages 11. DOI: 10.4018/978-1-7998-3479-3.ch007
8. Bhardwaj, P., Guhan, T. and Tripathy, B.K. (2021). Computational biology in the lens of CNN. In Roy, S.S. and Taguchi, Y.H. (Eds) *Handbook of Machine Learning Applications for Genomics, Studies in Big Data*, Vol. 103, Springer, Singapore. DOI: 10.1007/978-981-16-9158-4_5
9. Prabhavathy, P., Tripathy, B.K., Venkatesan, M. (2022). Analysis of diabetic retinopathy detection techniques using CNN models. In Mishra, S., Tripathy, H.K., Mallick, P. and Shaalan, K. (Eds) *Augmented Intelligence in Healthcare: A Pragmatic and Integrated Analysis*. Studies in Computational Intelligence, Vol. 1024, Springer, Singapore. DOI: 10.1007/978-981-19-1076-0_6
10. Raizada, S., Verma, Y., Mala, S., Shankar, A. and Thakur, S. (2021). Organ risk prediction for Parkinson's disease using deep learning techniques. *11th International Conference on Cloud Computing, Data Science & Engineering (Confluence)*, Noida, pp. 978–983. DOI: 10.1109/Confluence51648.2021.9377174
11. Nilashi, M., Abumalloh, R.A., Yusuf, S.Y.M., Thi, H.H., Alsulami, M., Abosaq, H., Alyami, S. and Alghamdi, A. (2023). Early diagnosis of Parkinson's disease: A combined method using deep learning and neuro-fuzzy techniques. *Computational Biology and Chemistry*, 102, 107788. DOI: 10.1016/j.compbiolchem.2022.107788
12. Kaur, R., Motl, R.W., Sowers, R. and Hernandez, M.E. (2023). A vision-based framework for predicting multiple sclerosis and Parkinson's disease gait dysfunctions—A deep learning approach. *IEEE Journal of Biomedical and Health Informatics*, 27(1), 190–201. DOI: 10.1109/JBHI.2022.3208077
13. LeMoyne, R. Mastroianni, T. Whiting, D. and Tomycz, N. (2020). Application of deep learning to distinguish multiple deep brain stimulation parameter configurations for the treatment of Parkinson's disease. *19th IEEE International Conference on Machine Learning and Applications (ICMLA)*, Miami, FL, pp. 1106–1111. DOI: 10.1109/ICMLA51294.2020.00178
14. Zhang, J., Zhou, C., Xiao, X., Chen, W., Jiang, Y., Zhu, R. and Xin, T. (2022). Magnetic resonance imaging image analysis of the therapeutic effect and neuroprotective effect of deep brain stimulation in Parkinson's disease based on a deep learning algorithm. *International Journal for Numerical Methods in Biomedical Engineering*, 38(11), e3642. DOI: 10.1002/cnm.3642
15. Zhang, R., Jia, J. and Zhang, R. (2022). EEG analysis of Parkinson's disease using time–frequency analysis and deep learning. *Biomedical Signal Processing and Control*, 78. DOI: 10.1016/j.bspc.2022.103883
16. Miao, R., Shokur, S., De Lima Pardini, A.C., Boari, D. and Bouri, M. (2021). Detecting freezing of gait in Parkinson's disease patient via deep residual network. *2021 20th IEEE International Conference on Machine Learning and Applications (ICMLA), Machine Learning and Applications (ICMLA)*, 320–325. DOI: 10.1109/ICMLA52953.2021.00056

17. Dixit, S., Gaikwad, A., Vyas, V., Shindikar, M. and Kamble, K. (2022). United neurological study of disorders: Alzheimer's disease, Parkinson's disease detection, Anxiety detection, and Stress detection using various machine learning algorithms. *2022 International Conference on Signal and Information Processing (IConSIP), Signal and Information Processing (IConSIP)*, 1–6. DOI: 10.1109/ICoNSIP49665.2022.10007434
18. Zhang, X., Yang, Y., Wang, H., Ning, S. and Wang, H. (2019). Deep neural networks with broad views for Parkinson's disease screening. *2019 IEEE International Conference on Bioinformatics and Biomedicine (BIBM), Bioinformatics and Biomedicine (BIBM)*, 1018–1022. DOI: 10.1109/BIBM47256.2019.8983000
19. Deepa, P. and Khilar, R. (2022). Parkinson's disease classification from speech signal parameters using deep neural network. *2022 IEEE 4th International Conference on Cybernetics, Cognition and Machine Learning Applications (ICCCMLA)*, Goa, pp. 44–48. DOI: 10.1109/ICCCMLA56841.2022.9989106.
20. Nissar, I., Mir, W.A., Izharuddin and Shaikh, T.A. (2021). Machine learning approaches for detection and diagnosis of Parkinson's disease - a review. *2021 7th International Conference on Advanced Computing and Communication Systems (ICACCS)*, Coimbatore, pp. 898–905. DOI: 10.1109/ICACCS51430.2021.9441885.
21. Anila, M. and Pradeepini, G. (2021). Diagnosis of Parkinson's disease using deep neural network model. *2021 International Conference on Smart Generation Computing, Communication and Networking(SMARTGENCON)*, Pune, pp. 1–7. DOI: 10.1109/SMARTGENCON51891
22. Mounika, P. and Rao, S.G. (2021). Machine learning and deep learning models for diagnosis of Parkinson's disease: A performance analysis. *2021 Fifth International Conference on I-SMAC (IoT in Social, Mobile, Analytics and Cloud) (I-SMAC)*, Palladam, pp. 381–388. DOI: 10.1109/I-SMAC52330.2021.9640632
23. Manimegalai, R., Ramya, A., Swedha, S.U., Pruthvi, M. and Lokesh, S. (2022). Deep learning based approach for identification of Parkinson's syndrome. *2022 International Conference on Intelligent Innovations in Engineering and Technology (ICIIET)*, Coimbatore, pp. 335–341. DOI: 10.1109/ICIIET55458.2022.9967676
24. Ramírez, V.M., Kmetzsch, V., Forbes, F. and Dojat, M. (2020). Deep learning models to study the early stages of Parkinson's disease. *2020 IEEE 17th International Symposium on Biomedical Imaging (ISBI)*, Iowa City, IA, pp. 1534–1537. DOI: 10.1109/ISBI45749.2020.9098529
25. Yadav, D. and Jain, I. (2022). Comparative analysis of machine learning algorithms for Parkinson's disease prediction. *2022 6th International Conference on Intelligent Computing and Control Systems (ICICCS)*, Madurai, pp. 1334–1339. DOI: 10.1109/ICICCS5 3718.2022.9788354
26. Varalakshmi, P., Priya, B.T., Rithiga, B.A., Bhuvaneaswari, R. (2021). Parkinson disease detection based on speech using various machine learning models and deep learning models. *2021 International Conference on System, Computation, Automation and Networking (ICSCAN)*, Puducherry, pp. 1–6. DOI: 10.1109/ICSCAN53069.2021.9526372
27. Aversano, L., Bernardi, M.L. Cimitile, M. Iammarino, M., Montano, D. and Verdone, C. (2022). A machine learning approach for early detection of Parkinson's disease using acoustic traces. *2022 IEEE International Conference on Evolving and Adaptive Intelligent Systems (EAIS)*, Larnaca, Cyprus, pp. 1–8. DOI: 10.1109/EAIS51927.2022.9787728
28. Aghzal, M. and Mourhir, A. (2020). Early diagnosis of Parkinson's disease based on handwritten patterns using deep learning. *2020 Fourth International Conference on Intelligent Computing in Data Sciences (ICDS)*, Fez, Morocco, pp. 1–6. DOI: 10.1109/ICDS50568.2020.9268738

29. Hussain, A. and Sharma, A. (2022). Machine learning techniques for voice-based early detection of Parkinson's disease. *2022 2nd International Conference on Advance Computing and Innovative Technologies in Engineering (ICACITE)*, Greater Noida, pp. 1436–1439. DOI: 10.1109/ICACITE53722.2022.9823467
30. Almeida, J.S., Rebouças Filho, P.P., Carneiro, T., Wei, W., Damaševičius, R., Maskeliūnas, R. and de Albuquerque, V.H.C. (2019). Detecting Parkinson's disease with sustained phonation and speech signals using machine learning techniques. *Pattern Recognition Letters*, 125, 55–62.
31. Senturk, Z.K. (2020). Early diagnosis of Parkinson's disease using machine learning algorithms. *Medical Hypotheses*, 138, 109603.
32. Kotsavasiloglou, C., Kostikis, N., Hristu-Varsakelis, D. and Arnaoutoglou, M. (2017). Machine learning-based classification of simple drawing movements in Parkinson's disease. *Biomedical Signal Processing and Control*, 31, 174–180.
33. Das, R. (2010). A comparison of multiple classification methods for diagnosis of Parkinson disease. *Expert Systems with Applications*, 37(2), 1568–1572.
34. Sanjay, V. and Swarnalatha, P. (2022, December). Machine learning techniques for Parkinson's disease detection. *2022 Smart Technologies, Communication and Robotics (STCR)* (pp. 1–6). IEEE.
35. Ricciardi, C., Amboni, M., De Santis, C., Improta, G., Volpe, G., Iuppariello, L., ... Biomedical Engineering Unit (2019). Using gait analysis' parameters to classify Parkinsonism: A data mining approach. *Computer Methods and Programs in Biomedicine*, 180, 105033.
36. Cho, C.W., Chao, W.H., Lin, S.H. and Chen, Y.Y. (2009). A vision-based analysis system for gait recognition in patients with Parkinson's disease. *Expert Systems with Applications*, 36(3), 7033–7039.
37. Senturk, Z.K. (2020). Early diagnosis of Parkinson's disease using machine learning algorithms. *Medical Hypotheses*, 138. DOI: 10.1016/j.mehy.2020.109603
38. Wang, W., Lee, J. Harrou, F. and Sun, Y. (2020). Early detection of Parkinson's disease using deep learning and machine learning. *IEEE Access*, 8, 147635–147646. DOI: 10.1109/ACCESS.2020.3016062
39. Grover, S., Saloni Bhartia, A., Abhilasha Yadav, S.K.R. (2018). Predicting severity of Parkinson's disease using deep learning. *Procedia Computer Science*, 132, 1788–1794. DOI: 10.1016/j.procs.2018.05.154
40. Taleb, C., Likforman-Sulem, L., Mokbel, C. et al. (2020). Detection of Parkinson's disease from handwriting using deep learning: A comparative study. *Evolutionary Intelligence*. DOI: 10.1007/s12065-020-00470-0
41. Prashanth, R., Roy, S.D., Mandal, P.K., Ghosh, S. (2016). High-accuracy detection of early Parkinson's disease through multimodal features and machine learning. *International Journal of Medical Informatics*, 90, 13–21. DOI: 10.1016/j.ijmedinf.2016.03.001
42. Celik, E. and Omurca, S.I. (2019). Improving Parkinson's disease diagnosis with machine learning methods. *2019 Scientific Meeting on Electrical-Electronics & Biomedical Engineering and Computer Science (EBBT)*, Istanbul, Turkey, pp. 1–4. DOI: 10.1109/EBBT.2019.8742057
43. Choi, H. Ha, S., Im, H.J. Ha Paek, S. and Lee, D.S. (2017). Refining diagnosis of Parkinson's disease with deep learning-based interpretation of dopamine transporter imaging. *NeuroImage: Clinical*, 16, 586–594. DOI: 10.1016/j.nicl.2017.09.010
44. Sahu, L., Sharma, R., Sahu, I., Das, M., Sahu, B. and Kumar, R. (2021, August 16). Efficient detection of Parkinson's disease using deep learning techniques over medical data. DOI: 10.1111/exsy.12787

45. Loh, H.W., Hong, W., Ooi, C.P., Chakraborty, S., Barua, P.D., Deo, R.C., Soar, J., Palmer, E.E. and Acharya, U.R. (2021). Application of deep learning models for automated identification of Parkinson's disease: A review (2011–2021). *Sensors*, 21(21):7034. DOI: 10.3390/s21217034
46. Marshall, V. and Grosset, D. (2003, December). Role of dopamine transporter imaging in routine clinical practice. *Movement Disorders*, 18(12):1415–23. DOI: 10.1002/mds.10592
47. Marshall, V. and Grosset, D. (2003). Role of dopamine transporter imaging in routine clinical practice. *Movement Disorders: Official Journal of the Movement Disorder Society*, 18(12), 1415–1423.
48. Marek, K., Seibyl, J., Eberly, S., Oakes, D., Shoulson, I., Lang, A.E., … Parkinson Study Group PRECEPT Investigators. (2014). Longitudinal follow-up of SWEDD subjects in the PRECEPT study. *Neurology*, 82(20), 1791–1797.
49. Parkinson Study Group. (2000). A randomized controlled trial comparing pramipexole with levodopa in early Parkinson's disease: Design and methods of the CALM-PD study. *Clinical Neuropharmacology*, 23(1), 34–44.
50. Schwingenschuh, P., Ruge, D., Edwards, M.J., Terranova, C., Katschnig, P., Carrillo, F., … Bhatia, K.P. (2010). Distinguishing SWEDDs patients with asymmetric resting tremor from Parkinson's disease: A clinical and electrophysiological study. *Movement Disorders*, 25(5), 560–569.
51. Kwon, D.H., Kim, J.S., Shin, H.J. and Kim, S. (2021). Deep learning-based Parkinson's disease detection using handwriting analysis. *IEEE Access*, 9, 25632–25641. DOI: 10.1109/ACCESS.2021.3053040
52. Tsanas, A., Little, M.A., McSharry, P.E., Spielman, J. and Ramig, L.O. (2012). Novel speech signal processing algorithms for high-accuracy classification of Parkinson's disease. *IEEE Transactions on Biomedical Engineering*, 59(5), 1264–1271.

5 A Deep Learning-based Approach for Detecting Diabetic Retinopathy in Retina Images

Sahana Das, Asifuzzaman Lasker, Mridul Ghosh, Sk Md Obaidullah and Kaushik Roy

5.1 INTRODUCTION

Diabetic Retinopathy (DR) is a widespread epidemic worldwide, particularly prevalent in Indian society, leading to an excessive number of cases that result in complications like DR. Therefore, it is essential to design a diagnostic framework to assist ophthalmologists and reduce patient morbidity. The global diabetic population has reached 422 million, with India being countries with a high prevalence of diabetes zone in the globe.

Within the span of years, the count of cases escalated from 108 million to a substantial 422 million, with approximately half of the afflicted individuals living in a handful of countries [1]. In the preceding two decades, there's been a significant upsurge in the prevalence of diabetes, affecting a shocking number of people globally. Around 500 million individuals, regardless of their age, suffer from this disease 5, and this figure is projected to exceed 700 million in the next 22 years, representing a considerable healthcare challenge. Diabetes can induce a plethora of complications, including the impairment of vision. This paper emphasizes Diabetic Retinopathy, which can lead to blindness. DR arises due to the augmentation of blood glucose that adversely affects the minute vessels in the retina. Consequently, an abundance of fluid amasses in the retina, leading to the thickening and swelling of the macula [2].

Screening for diabetic retinopathy requires specialized clinical expertise, experience, and a considerable amount of time for ophthalmologists to make a diagnosis. Typically, ophthalmologists conduct an eye test to analyze the retina image captured by specialized equipment to determine the DR. This process can be time-consuming, and there is a shortage of professional ophthalmologists to meet the demand for diagnoses. Consequently, the development of an automatic classification algorithm [8] for assessing the severity of DR is crucial in enhancing the efficiency and accuracy of DR diagnosis. Retinal fundus imaging can serve as a valuable input for this

DOI: 10.1201/9781003391456-5

algorithm [7]. The advancement of deep learning has enabled the efficient detection and segmentation [10] of infected parts of the retina, allowing for high-performance diagnosis and grading. Machine learning methods are extensively employed for the classification and grading of Diabetic Retinopathy [9,11]. Researchers in the medical field, having successfully integrated the CAD system, are now exploring new technologies such as deep learning, a type of AI system. In medical informatics, the application of deep learning [12] has significantly increased as it is able to efficiently analyze humongous amounts of data. In terms of speed and experimentation.

Attia et al. [18] executed a study exploring a variety of deep learning-focused methods for the classification of DR. A critical evaluation of machine learning-based techniques was carried out by Gupta and Chhikara [19], shedding light on the limitations of existing approaches. Li et al. [24] developed a quartet of CNN-based frameworks capable of handling high-resolution images with multiscale inputs. Examining the complexity of the VGG network, Hajabdollahi et al. [25] constructed a modified variant of VGG16-Net [26] using an innovative pruning strategy. Upon testing on the Messidor database, it was revealed that trimming down 35% of the feature maps of VGG16-Net led to a slight decrease of 1.89% in accuracy. An alternative CNN-based framework was proposed by Kazakh-British et al. [34], incorporating both original and anisotropic diffusion filter images. The recent development in deep learning-based work witnessed the proposition of diverse lightweight convolutional neural networks [13,14]. Akram et al. suggested a composite classification approach [33] to enhance the performance of retinal lesion detection. They expanded the scope of m-Mediods-based modeling by fusing it with a Gaussian Mixture Model, developing a hybrid classifier that boosted the accuracy of classification.

Winder et al. [27] concentrated on the development of algorithms aimed at automatically identifying retinopathy within digital color retinal images. The algorithms were structured into five distinct phases, including the segmentation of the optic disk and retinal vasculature. Mookiah et al. [30] carried out a comparative analysis of multiple techniques used for detecting diabetic retinopathy (DR) in images. Their work presents a comprehensive investigation into a variety of approaches employed for DR image recognition, along with a precise tabulation of potential methods and their corresponding accuracy results. Rakshitha et al. [31] illuminated the use of innovative imaging transformation methods, such as contourlet transform, curvelet transform, and wavelet transform, for the enhancement of retinal images. They provided a comparison between these three imaging transformations in their paper.

The primary accomplishment of this study, as presented by the authors, involves the formulation of a streamlined convolutional neural network framework. The framework is trained employing a stratified cross-validation method, enhancing the precision in identifying and detecting diabetic retinopathy (DR) within retinal images. We adapted our network utilizing four publicly accessible datasets that comprise varying quantities of images, from relatively few to a large number. Leveraging the capabilities of CNNs [15,16,17], our intent was to amplify the efficacy and precision of DR diagnosis via automated retinal image analysis.

The structure of this chapter unfolds as follows: Section 2 elucidates the materials involved, whereas Section 2.2 explores the methodologies incorporated. Section 3 offers a detailed discussion on the experimental outcomes, and ultimately, Section 4 puts forth the derived conclusions of the article.

5.2 Materials and Methods

The dataset has found extensive use among researchers and practitioners for the design and evaluation of machine learning mechanisms and deep learning models, aiming at the automated diagnosis of diabetic retinopathy. The clinical observations are illustrated in figure 5.3.

DRD [20]: This dataset encompasses 23,207 high-resolution RGB retina images that have been classified into five classes (0-4) by skilled professionals based on the DR severity. The dataset's distribution is notably imbalanced, with Class-0 (no diabetic retinopathy) being the most represented and Class-4 (proliferative diabetic retinopathy) being the least. Among the other datasets, this one houses the maximum number of images, making it a precious asset for training machine-learning models in the detection of diabetic retinopathy.

Messidor-2 Dataset [21]: This dataset incorporates 1,739 retina images that have been assessed by ophthalmologists on a scale from 0 to 4, according to the severity of DR. This dataset is substantially smaller compared to the others, and the class distribution is greatly imbalanced, with Class-0 being the most frequent and Class-4 the least.

IDRiD [22]: This dataset includes 363 retinal images of diabetic patients, categorized into five classes (0-4) by ophthalmologists. Similar to the other datasets, the class distribution in IDRiD is imbalanced, with Class-0 being the most frequent and Class-3 the least. The dataset's relatively small size might restrict its utility in training machine learning models.

RFMiD [23]: This dataset houses 1,920 retinal images of patients suffering from various ocular conditions, including diabetic retinopathy, glaucoma, age-related macular degeneration, and more. The images have been labeled by ophthalmologists based on the diseases present. The class distribution in this dataset is also skewed, with Class-0 being the most common and Class-4 the least. Nonetheless, when compared to the Messidor-2 and Indian Diabetic Retinopathy datasets, RFMiD is considerably larger.

Figure 5.1, represent the datasets that vary in terms of size, class distribution, and the number of classes they contain. The Diabetic Retinopathy dataset is the largest and has the highest number of classes, while the IDRiD dataset is the smallest and has the lowest number of classes. All datasets suffer from class imbalance, which can affect the performance of machine learning models trained on these datasets. Therefore, it is important to take into account the characteristics of each dataset when selecting them for training and testing machine learning models. So, in this context, the authors used stratified k-fold cross-validation with 12 folds to overcome the data imbalance problem.

Training framework

In this study, a framework based on convolutional neural networks (CNN) has been developed for the classification of diabetic retinopathy (DR) using retinal images.

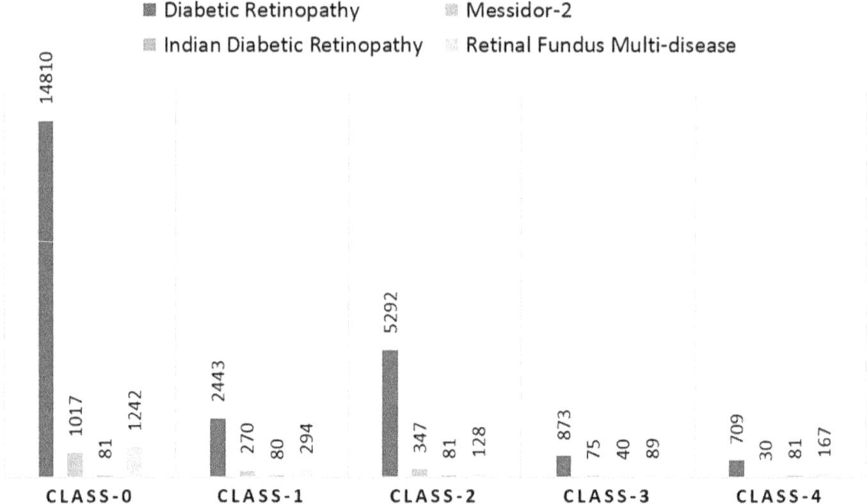

FIGURE 5.1 Overview of four datasets with five classes.

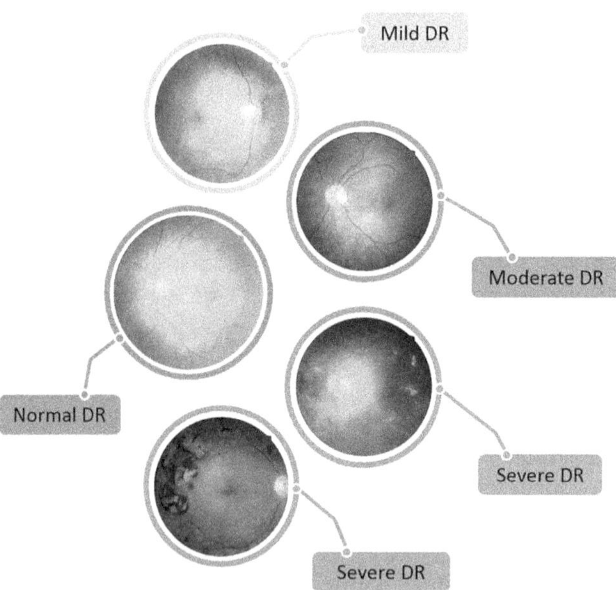

FIGURE 5.2 Colour notation of severity with green representing a normal DR and red representing a severe33 DR.

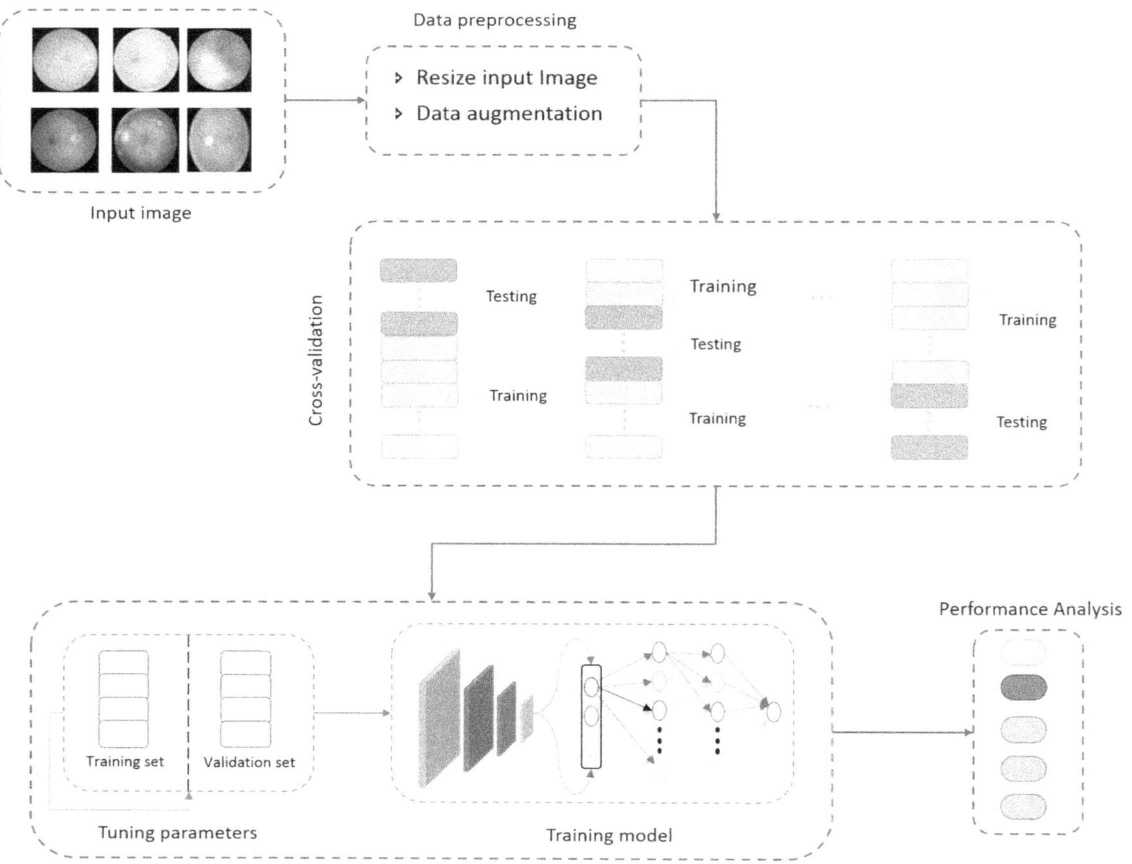

FIGURE 5.3 Proposed classification framework for diabetic retinopathy.

The dataset, which was subjected to preprocessing and resized to dimensions of 256x256 pixels, comprised retinal images of varying quality, captured using diverse cameras and exhibiting different DR severity levels. In terms of evaluation, a stratified k-fold cross-validation method was employed. This approach is often used to assess the performance of machine learning models when dealing with datasets that have imbalanced class distribution, such as the dataset in this study. Figure 5.3 depicts the entire workflow of the proposed framework, comprising pairs of convolution and pooling layers, followed by two dense layers. The first convolution layer features 16 filters of size 5x5, and the second one comprises 32 filters of size 3x3. The first pooling layer is 3x3 in size, and the second is 2x2. The first and second dense layers have dimensions of 128 and 256, respectively. The 'relu' activation function was employed between the convolution and pooling layers. A dropout of 0.4 was introduced between the first and second dense layers. Lastly, the softmax function was utilized for class prediction across five classes. Training incorporated consideration of epochs from 50 to 250, with intervals of 50 epochs, and a batch size of 32. Performance evaluation was conducted using standard metrics including accuracy, precision, recall, and F1 score.

Performance measurement parameters

Accuracy serves as the foremost metric when evaluating the performance of any deep learning model, as indicated in Equation 1. Mathematically, it is characterized by the proportion of accurate predictions to all predictions made.

$$Acc = \frac{Number\ of\ Correct\ \Pr edictions}{Total\ Number\ of\ \Pr edictions} = \frac{1}{i^n} \sum\nolimits_n I(y_i = \hat{y}_i) \qquad (1)$$

This is the count of instances where the model's prediction y^i matches the actual value yi. The indicator functions I(condition): This is a function that outputs 1 if the condition inside is true and 0 otherwise. In this case, the condition is yi = y^i, which checks if the predicted value equals the actual value.

Since only accuracy does not justify the performance of the system, precision τ, sensitivity ε, and f-measure ω were also applied using this equation 2, which described as follows:

$$\tau = \frac{\gamma}{\gamma + \omega}, \varphi = \frac{\delta}{\delta + \varepsilon}, \mu = 2 * \frac{\delta * \varphi}{\delta + \varphi} \qquad (2)$$

Where γ, ω and ε denote true-positive, false-positive, and, false-negative rate, respectively.

Receiver Operating Characteristic Curve (ROC Curve): At different classification thresholds, the ROC curve is a graphical representation of the performance of a binary classification model. Various threshold settings are plotted against the true positive rate (TPR). We can visualize the accuracy of the model in detecting diseases using the ROC curve by comparing it to other models.

TABLE 5.1
Metrics for detecting diabetic retinopathy based on the number of images, sorted in ascending order.

Dataset Name	Precision	Recall	F1-score	Accuracy
RFMiD	90.72	84.47	88.6	89.10
IDRiD	96.64	95.47	95.32	96.74
Messidor-2	94.02	93.64	92.20	94.75
DBD	78.68	77.61	79.25	79.96

5.3 RESULT

From the results which are tabulated in Table 5.1, we can see that the Indian Diabetic Retinopathy dataset achieved the highest accuracy of 96.46%, followed by Messidor-2 with 94.68% accuracy, Diabetic Retinopathy with 79.89% accuracy, and Retinal Fundus Multi-disease with 88.76% accuracy. In terms of precision, the Messidor-2 dataset had the highest precision score of 0.9662, followed by the Indian Diabetic Retinopathy dataset with a precision score of 0.9386. The lowest precision score was observed in the Retinal Fundus Multi-disease dataset with a score of 0.6878. Regarding recall, the Indian Diabetic Retinopathy dataset achieved the highest score of 0.9187, followed by Messidor-2 with a score of 0.9568. The lowest recall score was observed in the Retinal Fundus Multi-disease dataset with a score of 0.6462.

In terms of F1-score, the Indian Diabetic Retinopathy dataset achieved the highest score of 0.9265, followed by Messidor-2 with a score of 0.9612. The lowest F1-score was observed in the Retinal Fundus Multi-disease dataset with a score of 0.6641. Overall, the results suggest that the Indian Diabetic Retinopathy dataset performed the best across all metrics, followed closely by Messidor-2.

However, it's important to note that the performance of each dataset may be influenced by factors such as the size and quality of the dataset, as well as the specific characteristics of the images included in the dataset. The ROC curve in figure 5.4 is a graphical representation of the true positive rate against the false positive rate. It is useful for evaluating the performance of a model across various thresholds.

The result of our method has been compared with the recent techniques which is shown in Table 5.2. The results reveal significant improvements in precision compared to previous studies ([35], [36], [37], and [38]). Specifically, our method showcases enhancements of 7.06% (Messidor-2), 6.68% (DBD), 24.1%, and 6.04% when compared to [35], [36], [37], and [38] respectively, as evident from Tables 5.1 and 5.2.

5.4 CONCLUSION

In conclusion, diabetic retinopathy is a significant global health challenge with an increasing prevalence, particularly in India. Early detection and consistent screening

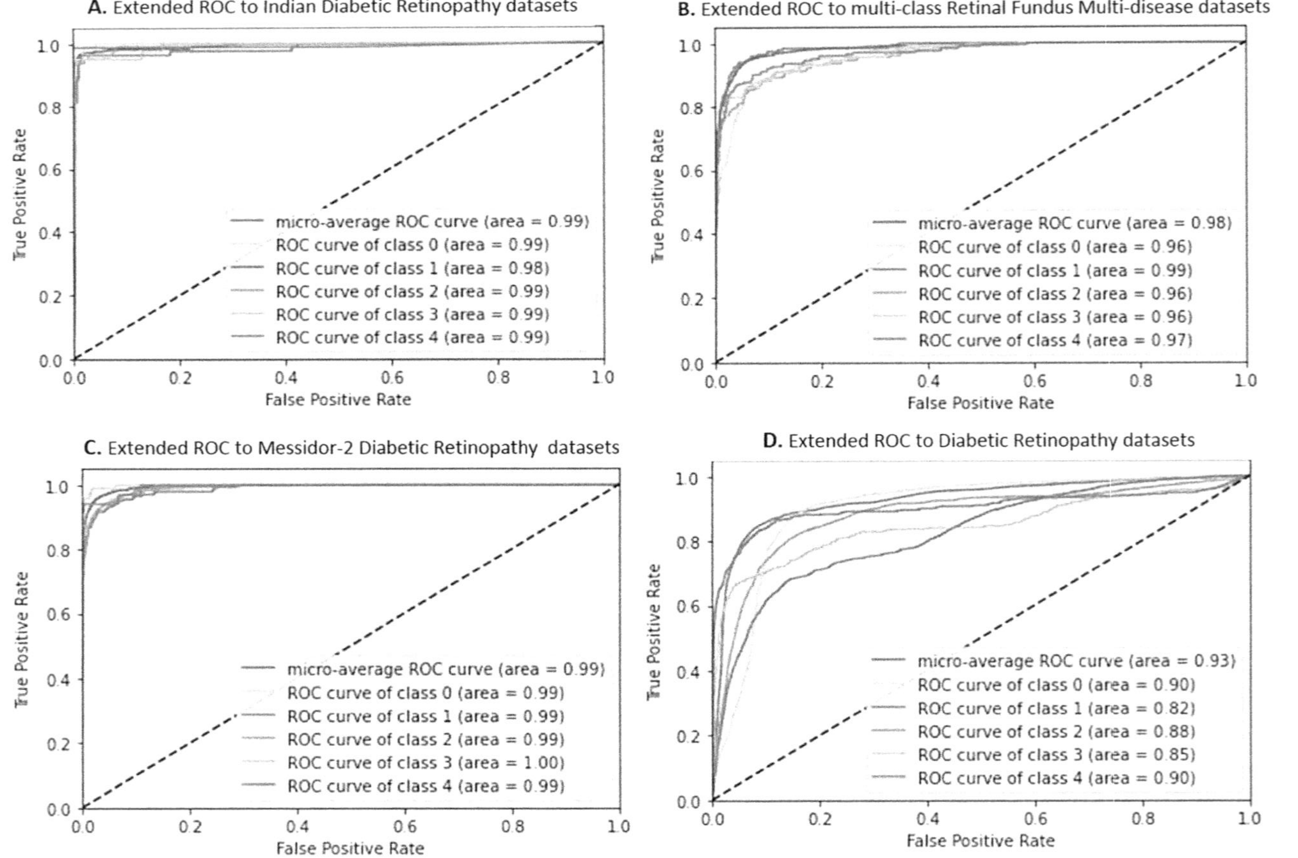

FIGURE 5.4 ROC curve of four distinct datasets e.g. A. Diabetic Retinopathy in Indians, B. Retinal Fundus Multi-disease, C. Messidor-2 Diabetic Retinopathy and D. Diabetic Retinopathy of cross-validation training with a deep learning framework

TABLE 5.2
Comparison between our work with state-of-the-art framework.

Dataset Name	Precision	Recall	AUC	Accuracy (%)
Gabriel et al. [35] (Messidor-2)	87.00	90.00	94.40	94.40
Rakhlin et al. [36] (DBD)	72.00	92.00	92.00	-
Voting Inception ((RFMiD) [37]	66.62	68.76	67.18	74.44
CANet (IDRiD) [38]	90.6	92.0	96.3	92.6

are crucial to managing the disease and preventing further complications, and retinal fundus imaging is an effective tool for detecting DR. However, manual screening is time-consuming, and there is a shortage of professional ophthalmologists to meet the demand for diagnoses. This paper highlights the importance of developing an automated diagnostic model to assist ophthalmologists and reduce patient morbidity. The advancement of AI techniques, specifically machine learning and deep learning, has enabled the efficient detection

REFERENCES

1. Smolen, J. S., Burmester, G. R., & Combeet, B. (2016). NCD risk factor collaboration (NCD-RisC). Worldwide trends in diabetes since 1980: A pooled analysis of 751 population-based studies with 4·4 million participants. *Lancet*, 387, 1513–1530—In this Article, Catherine Pelletier.
2. Vo, H. H., & Verma, A. (2016, September). Discriminant color texture descriptors for diabetic retinopathy recognition. In *2016 IEEE 12th International Conference on Intelligent Computer Communication and Processing (ICCP)* (pp. 309–315). IEEE.
3. Prasad, D. K., Vibha, L., & Venugopal, K. R. (2015, December). Early detection of diabetic retinopathy from digital retinal fundus images. In *2015 IEEE Recent Advances in Intelligent Computational Systems (RAICS)* (pp. 240–245). IEEE.
4. Patil, P., Shettar, P., Narayankar, P., & Patil, M. (2016, September). An efficient method of detecting exudates in diabetic retinopathy: Using texture edge features. In *2016 International Conference on Advances in Computing, Communications and Informatics (ICACCI)* (pp. 1188–1191). IEEE.
5. Winder, R. J., Morrow, P. J., McRitchie, I. N., Bailie, J. R., & Hart, P. M. (2009). Algorithms for digital image processing in diabetic retinopathy. *Computerized medical Imaging and Graphics*, 33(8), 608–622.
6. Williams, R., Airey, M., Baxter, H., Forrester, J. K. M., Kennedy-Martin, T., & Girach, A. (2004). Epidemiology of diabetic retinopathy and macular oedema: A systematic review. *Eye*, 18(10), 963–983.
7. Yavuz, Z., & K¨ose, C. (2017). Blood vessel extraction in color retinal fundus images with enhancement filtering and unsupervised classification. *Journal of Healthcare Engineering*, 4897258.

8. Lasker, A., Obaidullah, S. M., Chakraborty, C., & Roy, K. (2022). Application of machine learning and deep learning techniques for COVID-19 screening using radiological imaging: A comprehensive review. *SN Computer Science*, 4(1), 65.
9. Narasimha-Iyer, H., Can, A., Roysam, B., Stewart, V., Tanenbaum, H. L., Majerovics, A., & Singh, H. (2006). Robust detection and classification of longitudinal changes in color retinal fundus images for monitoring diabetic retinopathy. *IEEE Transactions on Biomedical Engineering*, 53(6), 1084–1098.
10. Lasker, A., Ghosh, M., Obaidullah, S. M., Chakraborty, C., Goncalves, T., & Roy, K. (2022, November). Ensemble stack architecture for lungs segmentation from X-ray images. In *Intelligent Data Engineering and Automated Learning–IDEAL 2022: 23rd International Conference*, IDEAL 2022, Manchester, November 24–26, 2022, Proceedings (pp. 3–11). Springer International Publishing.
11. Narasimha-Iyer, H., Can, A., Roysam, B., Stewart, V., Tanenbaum, H. L., Majerovics, A., & Singh, H. (2006). Robust detection and classification of longitudinal changes in color retinal fundus images for monitoring diabetic retinopathy. *IEEE Transactions on Biomedical Engineering*, 53(6), 1084–1098.
12. Ghosh, M., Obaidullah, S. M., Gherardini, F., & Zdimalova, M. (2021). Classification of geometric forms in mosaics using deep neural network. *Journal of Imaging*, 7(8), 149.
13. Ghosh, M., Roy, S. S., Mukherjee, H., Obaidullah, S. M., Gao, X. Z., & Roy, K. (2021). Movie title extraction and script separation using shallow convolution neural network. *IEEE Access*, 9, 125184–125201.
14. Ghosh, M., Baidya, G., Mukherjee, H., Obaidullah, S. M., & Roy, K. (2022). A deep learning-based approach to single/mixed script-type identification. *Advanced Computing and Systems for Security*, 13, 121–132.
15. Lasker, A., Ghosh, M., Obaidullah, S. M., Chakraborty, C., & Roy, K. (2023). LWSNet-a novel deep-learning architecture to segregate Covid-19 and pneumonia from x-ray imagery. *Multimedia Tools and Applications*, 82(14), 21801–21823.
16. Ghosh, M., Mukherjee, H., Obaidullah, S. M., Santosh, K. C., Das, N., & Roy, K. (2021). LWSINet: A deep learning-based approach towards video script identification. *Multimedia Tools and Applications*, 80(19), 29095–29128.
17. Lasker, A., Ghosh, M., Obaidullah, S. M., Chakraborty, C., & Roy, K. (2023). A deep learning-based framework for COVID-19 identification using chest X-ray images. In *Advancement of Deep Learning and its Applications in Object Detection and Recognition* (pp. 23–46). River Publishers.
18. Attia, A., Akhtar, Z., Akhrouf, S., & Maza, S. (2020). A survey on machine and deep learning for detection of diabetic retinopathy. *ICTACT Journal on Image and Video Processing*, 11(2), 2337–2344.
19. Gupta, A., & Chhikara, R. (2018). Diabetic retinopathy: Present and past. *Procedia Computer Science*, 132, 1432–1440.
20. Kaggle Dataset [Online]. https://kaggle.com/c/diabetic-retinopathy detection
21. Laboratoire de Traitement de l'Information M´edicale (LaTIM - INSERM U650). Messidor-2 dataset (M´ethodes d'Evaluation de Syst`emes de Segmentation et d'Indexation D´edi´ees a′ l'Ophtalmologie R´etinienne). (2011). http://latim.univ-brest.fr/indexfce0.html. Accessed March 19, 2023.
22. Porwal, P., Pachade, S., Kamble, R., Kokare, M., Deshmukh, G., Sahasrabuddhe, V. & Meriaudeau, F. (2018). Indian diabetic retinopathy image dataset (IDRiD): A database for diabetic retinopathy screening research. *Data*, 3(3), 25.
23. Pachade, S., Porwal, P., Thulkar, D., Kokare, M., Deshmukh, G., Sahasrabuddhe, V., & Mériaudeau, F. (2021). Retinal fundus multi-disease image dataset (RFMiD): A dataset for multi-disease detection research. *Data*, 6(2), 14.

24. Li, F., Yuan, D., Zhang, M., Liang, C., Zhou, X., & Zhang, H. (2019, July). Multi-scale stepwise training strategy of convolutional neural networks for diabetic retinopathy severity assessment. In *2019 International Joint Conference on Neural Networks (IJCNN)* (pp. 1–5). IEEE.
25. Hajabdollahi, M., Esfandiarpoor, R., Najarian, K., Karimi, N., Samavi, S., & Soroushmehr, S. R. (2019, July). Hierarchical pruning for simplification of convolutional neural networks in diabetic retinopathy classification. In *2019 41st Annual International Conference of the IEEE Engineering in Medicine and Biology Society (EMBC)* (pp. 970–973). IEEE.
26. Simonyan, K., & Zisserman, A. (2014). Very deep convolutional networks for large scale image recognition. arXiv preprint arXiv:1409.1556.
27. Winder, R. J., Morrow, P. J., McRitchie, I. N., Bailie, J. R., & Hart, P. M. (2009). Algorithms for digital image processing in diabetic retinopathy. *Computerized Medical Imaging and Graphics*, 33(8), 608–622.
28. Haleem, M. S., Han, L., Van Hemert, J., & Li, B. (2013). Automatic extraction of retinal features from colour retinal images for glaucoma diagnosis: A review. *Computerized Medical Imaging and Graphics*, 37(7–8), 581–596.
29. Roychowdhury, S., Koozekanani, D. D., & Parhi, K. K. (2013). DREAM: Diabetic retinopathy analysis using machine learning. *IEEE Journal of Biomedical and Health Informatics*, 18(5), 1717–1728.
30. Mookiah, M. R. K., Acharya, U. R., Chua, C. K., Lim, C. M., Ng, E. Y. K., & Laude, A. (2013). Computer-aided diagnosis of diabetic retinopathy: A review. *Computers in Biology and Medicine*, 43(12), 2136–2155.
31. Rakshitha, T. R., Devaraj, D., & Kumar, S. P. (2016, May). Comparative study of imaging transforms on diabetic retinopathy images. In *2016 IEEE International Conference on Recent Trends in Electronics, Information & Communication Technology (RTEICT)* (pp. 118–122). IEEE.
32. Vo, H. H., & Verma, A. (2016, September). Discriminant color texture descriptors for diabetic retinopathy recognition. In *2016 IEEE 12th International Conference on Intelligent Computer Communication and Processing (ICCP)* (pp. 309–315). IEEE.
33. Akram, M. U., Khalid, S., Tariq, A., Khan, S. A., & Azam, F. (2014). Detection and classification of retinal lesions for grading of diabetic retinopathy. *Computers in Biology and Medicine*, 45, 161–171.
34. Kazakh-British, N. P., Pak, A. A., & Abdullina, D. (2018, October). Automatic detection of blood vessels and classification in retinal images for diabetic retinopathy diagnosis with application of convolution neural network. In *Proceedings of the 2018 International Conference on Sensors, Signal and Image Processing* (pp. 60–63).
35. Zago, G. T., Andreao, R. V., Dorizzi, B., & Salles, E. O. T. (2020). Diabetic retinopathy detection using red lesion localization and convolutional neural networks. *Computers in Biology and Medicine*, 116, 103537.
36. Rakhlin, A. (2017). Diabetic retinopathy detection through integration of deep learning classification framework. *BioRxiv*, 225508.
37. He, X., Deng, Y., Fang, L., & Peng, Q. (2021). Multi-modal retinal image classification with modality-specific attention network. *IEEE Transactions on Medical Imaging*, 40(6), 1591–1602.
38. Li, X., Hu, X., Yu, L., Zhu, L., Fu, C. W., & Heng, P. A. (2019). CANet: Cross-disease attention network for joint diabetic retinopathy and diabetic macular edema grading. *IEEE Transactions on Medical Imaging*, 39(5), 1483–1493.

6 Optimization of CNN for Content-Based Image Retrieval in Healthcare

Arnab Gain

6.1 INTRODUCTION

Healthcare is an integral part of life. With the increasing rate of various diseases and patients, better healthcare services have become a very important concern. The healthcare system must be very efficient to handle a large amount of patient data, including medical images, to improve patient outcomes, increase efficiency, and reduce costs. Due to this reason, the healthcare system has been united with artificial intelligence (AI), Internet of Things (IoT), machine learning (ML), blockchain, and other advanced technologies. The important concern of this chapter is the application of IoT in the area of healthcare. Healthcare 4.0 is most relevant to this approach because it involves the integration of advanced technologies and data analytics to transform the delivery of healthcare. IoT is a network where objects like buildings, vehicles, devices, and other items are embedded with connectivity, software, and sensors. IoT enables real-time data collection and transmission for these objects, allowing them to be monitored, analyzed, and optimized for better performance, efficiency, and productivity.

The Internet of Medical Things (IoMT) is IoT for medical devices and applications. In IoMT, these medical devices and applications are linked to the internet, enabling data collection, data transmission, and data analysis in real time. IoMT includes a wide range of medical devices, such as wearables, remote monitoring devices, implantable devices, and smart sensors. These devices are used for various healthcare applications, including patient monitoring, remote patient care, chronic disease management, and medication adherence. Figure 6.1 depicts the relationship among IoT, IoMT, and Healthcare 4.0.

In IoMT, content-based image retrieval (CBIR) is essential because it makes it possible to retrieve medical images accurately and quickly, permitting quick diagnosis, well-informed treatment choices, and aiding medical research while maximizing efficiency, costs, and patient outcomes. By enabling seamless access to a variety of image databases and encouraging collaboration and information exchange among healthcare professionals, it also improves remote consultations, telemedicine, and medical education.

 DOI: 10.1201/9781003391456-6

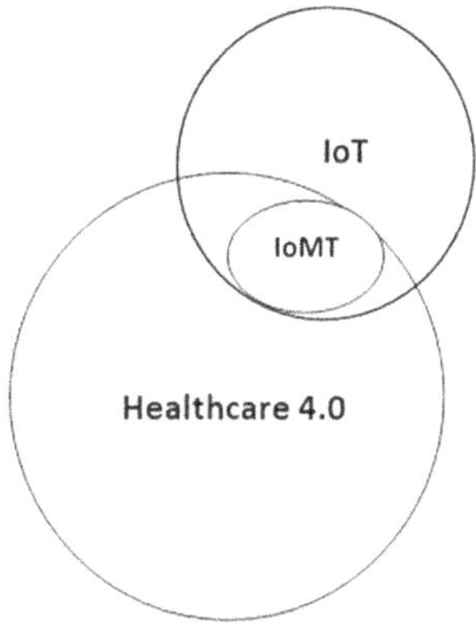

FIGURE 6.1 Relationship among Healthcare 4.0, IoT, and IoMT.

Medical image processing plays a vital role in CBIR when applied in the area of IoMT. Many researchers are applying ML to the CBIR technique to process medical images. This approach has improved the accuracy of diagnoses, medical image analysis, and patient outcomes. Hence, the focus of this proposed work is ML, which enables a machine to learn and make predictions or decisions based on data without being programmed explicitly to do so, and it can create intelligent systems that can improve their performance or accuracy over time by continuously learning from new data and adapting to changing environments.

ML can revolutionize the area of medicine as it has enabled more accurate and personalized diagnosis, treatment, and prevention of diseases. This chapter proposes an ML algorithm consisting of a set of convolutional neural network (CNN) models. For an image dataset given as input, this proposed algorithm generates an optimized neural network that can perform on that dataset with high accuracy. There are many CNN models for solving problems, including medical imaging problems. Hence, for a particular image dataset, only one or some of the neural network (NN) models perform with more accuracy, precision, recall, and F1 score. Due to this reason, many researchers have been applying optimization algorithms for NN models [20–33].

Differential evolution (DE) is a well-known optimization algorithm that is considered for solving ML applications [30]. The proposed work applied a modified version of the DE technique to search the best CNN architecture. In the mutation step of the differential evolution, the trial solution is created by adding the target vector with the weighted difference of two randomly selected population vectors. This approach may result in an optimization challenge of inefficient exploration. In the modified version of DE, the mutation step has been updated to alleviate this challenge and improve the convergence of DE. Furthermore, this proposed work has designed a CBIR framework, and with the help of the proposed optimized neural network model, the framework efficiently recognized medical images. To verify the improvement in performance of the proposed work, a simulation-based experiment was done with three publicly accessible medical image sets: Brain Tumor Classification (MRI) dataset [9], Breast Cancer Patients MRI's dataset [36], and Covid-19 Radiography Database [10]. The proposed approach is superior according to the simulation results.

This book chapter is further divided into the following sections: the preliminaries are discussed in Section 6.2; Section 6.3 presents a literature review regarding related works; the methodology is given in Section 6.4. Section 6.5 contains the experimental analysis, and the last section, i.e., Section 6.6, contains a conclusion and suggestions for future scope.

6.2 PRELIMINARIES

6.2.1 Content-Based Image Retrieval (CBIR)

CBIR is a technique used to search images based on the visual content of those images. CBIR algorithms analyze the visual features of images, which include color, texture, and shape, and use these features to search for those images in a database that are similar to them.

While CBIR and IoMT are two distinct technologies, they can be used in conjunction to enable more effective healthcare applications. For example, CBIR algorithms could be used to analyze medical images and help identify potential health issues. IoMT devices could be used to monitor patient health and track the effectiveness of treatments. The combination of these technologies has helped to improve patient outcomes and reduce healthcare costs by enabling more efficient and accurate diagnosis and treatment.

6.2.2 Machine Learning (ML)

ML involves developing algorithms to improve the performance of computer systems on a particular task by learning from a set of data. ML utilizes NN models for the learning process, which is involved in analyzing and identifying patterns in data. These models use these patterns to make predictions and decisions about new data. A subfield of ML is deep learning (DL), which involves building deep neural networks (DNNs) that can learn from large datasets.

6.2.2.1 Transfer Learning (TL)

Transfer learning (TL) is an ML technique in which a pretrained model is used for solving related problems. Training is done on a pretrained model to do a specific task regarding a large dataset. After it has learned features that are useful to the new task

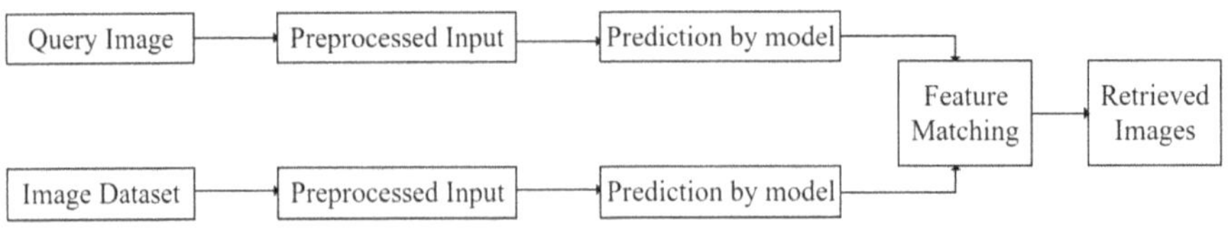

FIGURE 6.2 CBIR framework designed for the proposed work.

with a smaller dataset, TL can help improve accuracy, reduce the need for labeled data, and accelerate the training process. It has been successful in many applications, including computer vision. However, careful consideration of factors such as the similarity between tasks and the choice of a pretrained model is necessary for effective TL.

6.2.2.2 Ensemble Learning

Another ML technique is ensemble learning. It combines multiple models to improve the overall predictive model performance. Instead of relying on a single model, ensemble learning uses a group of models to make predictions, with the idea that the combined predictions will be more accurate than any individual model.

There are several different methods for ensemble learning, but some common approaches include:

- Bagging: This method is involved in training multiple models on different subsets of training data and averaging each model's predictions.
- Boosting: In this method, models are trained sequentially, with each new model attempting to correct the errors of the previous model.
- Stacking: This approach involves training multiple models and then using their predictions as inputs to a metamodel that makes the final prediction after that.

Ensemble learning can be used with various ML algorithms, such as decision trees, NNs, and support vector machines. It is a very popular technique because it can often improve the accuracy of predictive models without requiring significant additional computational resources.

6.2.2.3 Convolutional Neural Networks (CNNs)

CNNs are one type of deep neural network used mainly in tasks regarding the area of computer vision. They are designed to automatically detect and extract meaningful features from input images, making them a powerful tool for tasks including the classification of images, which plays an important role in CBIR.

The key feature of CNNs is the utilization of convolutional layers (CLs); these layers create an output feature map set by applying a set of learned filters to the images taken as input. These filters are designed to detect specific input image features, such as edges or textures, and can be learned through the training process.

CNNs also typically include pooling layers (PLs). These layers not only reduce the spatial dimensions of feature maps but also downsample the output of the CLs. This approach helps to reduce the number of parameters in the model and prevents overfitting.

In addition to CLs and PLs, CNNs often include fully connected layers. They take the flattened output of previous layers to classify the input image. During training, the weights of all layers are updated using backpropagation, which adjusts the model parameters to minimize the difference between the predicted labels and actual labels of the training data.

Input Image (224 x 224 x 3)	Conv1 + Relu (96 filters, 11 x 11)	MaxPooling (3 x 3)	Conv2 + Relu (256 filters, 5 x 5)	MaxPooling (3 x 3)	Conv3 + Relu (384 filters, 3 x 3)	Conv4 + Relu (384 filters, 3 x 3)	Conv5 + Relu (256 filters, 3 x 3)	MaxPooling (3 x 3)	FC1 (4096 units)	FC2 (4096 units)	FC3 (1000 units, output)	Output (1000 classes)

FIGURE 6.3 Architecture of AlexNet.

6.2.2.3.1 AlexNet

Alex et al. developed a deep CNN architecture (Figure 6.3) named AlexNet [3]. It has eight layers: five are CLs and three are fully connected layers, with over 60 million trainable parameters. AlexNet was the first DL architecture. It won the ImageNet Large Scale Visual Recognition Challenge (ILSVRC) in 2012. It has achieved state-of-the-art results in classifying images with a significant margin over the second-place entry. AlexNet is known for using techniques such as data augmentation, dropout, and rectified linear unit (ReLU) activation functions. These have helped to improve the performance of CNNs.

The details of the layers in AlexNet are as follows:

1. Convolutional layer 1: This layer has 96 filters of size 11 × 11 × 3. This layer has a stride of 4 and a 0-padding. It takes the input image and convolves it with these filters to produce 96 output feature maps.
2. Max pooling layer 1: This layer has a kernel of size 3 × 3 and a stride of 2. It downsamples feature maps from the previous layer by taking the maximum value in each 3 × 3 region.
3. Convolutional layer 2: This layer has 256 filters of size 5 × 5 × 48 (the number of output feature maps from the previous layer is 48), having a stride of 1 and 2-padding.
4. Max pooling layer 2: This layer has the same configuration as max pooling layer 1, except that it operates on the feature maps from convolutional layer 2.
5. Convolutional layer 3: This layer has 384 filters having the size of 3 × 3 × 256, with stride of 1 and 1-padding.
6. Convolutional layer 4: It has 384 filters of size 3 × 3 × 192 (the number of output feature maps from the previous layer is 192), having a stride of 1 and 1-padding.
7. Convolutional layer 5: The number of filters in this layer is 256 where each filter is of size 3 × 3 × 192, having a stride of one and 1-padding.

8. Max pooling layer 3: It has the same configuration as max pooling layer 1 and 2, except that it operates on the feature maps from convolutional layer 5.
9. Fully connected layer 1: It has 4096 neurons. This layer is connected with all neurons in max pooling layer 3.
10. Fully connected layer 2: Like fully connected layer 1, this layer also has 4096 neurons and it is connected with all the neurons in the previous layer (i.e., fully connected layer 1).
11. Fully connected layer 3: This layer is next to fully connected layer 2. The number of neurons in this layer is 1000 (corresponding to the number of classes in the ImageNet classification challenge) and is connected with all the neurons in the previous layer.

Each of the convolutional layers uses the ReLU activation function. In the fully connected layers, the hyperbolic tangent (tanh) is used as an activation function. After the first two fully connected layers, dropout regularization is used to reduce overfitting.

6.2.2.3.2 VGG19

At the University of Oxford, the Visual Geometry Group developed a deep CNN architecture (Figure 6.4) and named it VGG19 [1]. It contains 19 layers, of which 16 layers are CLs and 3 are fully connected layers. It has over 143 million trainable parameters. VGG19 is known for its simplicity and is utilized as a benchmark for image classification. It has achieved state-of-the-art results on various image recognition benchmarks, which include the ILSVRC in 2014. VGG19 is trained on large datasets of images and can recognize a wide range of visual features.

Specifically, the network contains 16 CLs. A ReLU activation function follows each of them. The CLs use a small filter size of 3 × 3, having a stride of 1 pixel. The network consists of three fully connected layers. A ReLU activation function follows each of them. Each of the first two fully connected layers contains 4096 units, while

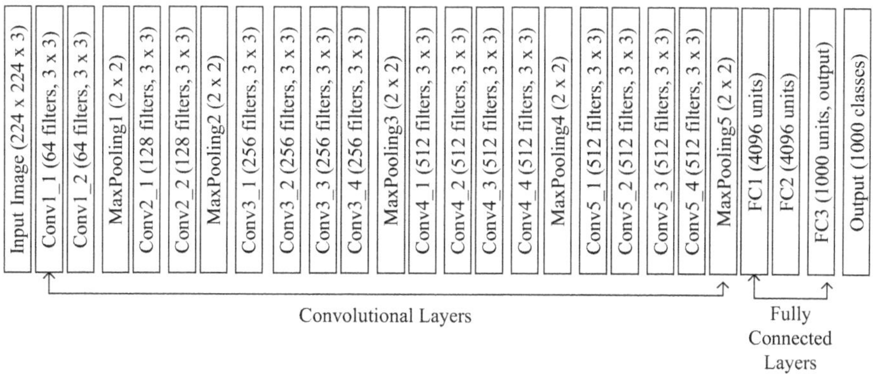

FIGURE 6.4 Architecture of VGG19.

TABLE 6.1
Architecture of InceptionV3

Size of Kernel	Type (Size of Input)
3 × 3/2	Convolution (299 × 299 × 3)
3 × 3/1	Convolution (149 × 149 × 32)
3 × 3/1	Convolution (147 × 147 × 32)
3 × 3/2	Pooling (147 × 147 × 64)
3 × 3/1	Convolution (73 × 73 × 64)
3 × 3/2	Convolution (71 × 71 × 80)
3 × 3/1	Convolution (35 × 35 × 192)
3 modules	Inception module (35 × 35 × 288)
5 modules	Inception module (17 × 17 × 768)
2 modules	Inception module (8 × 8 × 1280)
8 × 8	Pooling (8 × 8 × 2048)
Logits	Linear (1 × 1 × 2048)
Output	Softmax (1 × 1 × 1000)

the last one contains 1000 units, which corresponds to the number of classes in the ImageNet dataset.

6.2.2.3.3 *InceptionV3*

Another deep CNN architecture (Table 6.1) that Google researchers developed is InceptionV3 [2]. It contains 48 layers, including multiple Inception modules, and has over 23 million trainable parameters. Inception modules use multiple convolutional filters of different sizes and types for extracting input image features at different scales. It helps network for learning features that are more robust and discriminative. InceptionV3 is used for classifying images. This model has been successfully applied to various image recognition benchmarks, which include the ILSVRC in 2015. InceptionV3 is capable of recognizing a wide range of visual features with high accuracy.

6.2.2.3.4 *ResNet*

He et al. from Microsoft Research introduced a CNN architecture in 2015 named ResNet [5]. ResNet stands for "Residual Network" and is designed to solve the vanishing gradient problem in CNNs. An important innovation of ResNet is the introduction of "residual connections" or "skip connections", which enable information to bypass one or more layers in the network. It allows the network to learn residual mappings instead of full mappings, which can be easier to optimize. Residual connections also make it possible to train CNNs, up to hundreds of layers, without encountering the vanishing gradient problem.

The ResNet architecture (Figure 6.6) comprises "residual blocks" containing convolutional layers and identity mappings. A residual block takes an input feature map

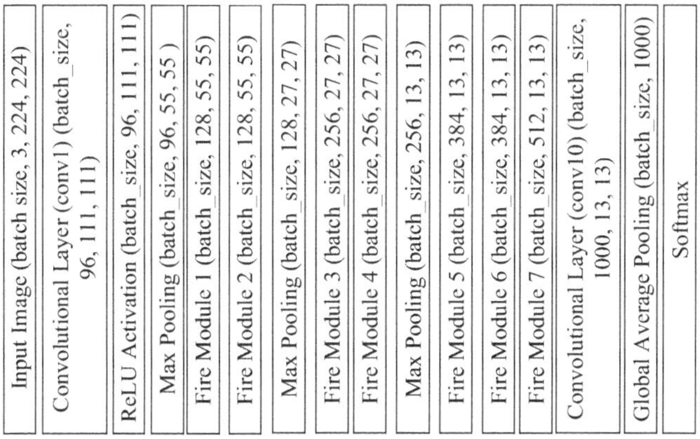

Input Image (batch size, 3, 224, 224)
Convolutional Layer (conv1) (batch_size, 96, 111, 111)
ReLU Activation (batch_size, 96, 111, 111)
Max Pooling (batch_size, 96, 55, 55)
Fire Module 1 (batch_size, 128, 55, 55)
Fire Module 2 (batch_size, 128, 55, 55)
Max Pooling (batch_size, 128, 27, 27)
Fire Module 3 (batch_size, 256, 27, 27)
Fire Module 4 (batch_size, 256, 27, 27)
Max Pooling (batch_size, 256, 13, 13)
Fire Module 5 (batch_size, 384, 13, 13)
Fire Module 6 (batch_size, 384, 13, 13)
Fire Module 7 (batch_size, 512, 13, 13)
Convolutional Layer (conv10) (batch_size, 1000, 13, 13)
Global Average Pooling (batch_size, 1000)
Softmax

FIGURE 6.5 Architecture of SqueezeNet.

and then passes through a series of CLs, followed by application of the residual connection. The residual block output is then added to the original input, which creates a shortcut path for the gradient. In this proposed work, ResNet-50 has been used.

6.2.2.3.5 SqueezeNet

SqueezeNet [8] is used to classify images with high accuracy and low computational complexity. It was introduced in a research paper published in 2016 and is known for achieving very high accuracy with very few parameters and a smaller model.

The main idea behind SqueezeNet is to use 1 × 1 convolutional filters in convolutional layers. This idea decreases the number of parameters and computational complexity while maintaining expressive power. This architecture (shown in Figure 6.5) also introduces "Fire Module", which combines 1 × 1 and 3 × 3 convolutional layers to extract features efficiently.

6.2.2.3.6 InceptionResNetV2

Google introduced InceptionResNetV2 [6] in 2016 as an improvement over the original Inception and InceptionV3 models. InceptionResNetV2 is a deep CNN architecture that combines the Inception architecture with residual connections, similar to the ResNet architecture. It uses a combination of CLs, PLs, and Inception modules for extracting features from input images. This architecture (Table 6.2) introduces residual connection, which solves the vanishing gradient problem by providing a direct path for gradients to flow during backpropagation and improves training of deep networks. InceptionResNetV2 has successfully been applied in computer vision applications. It has a total of 164 layers and over 55 million parameters.

6.2.2.3.7 MobileNet

Google introduced MobileNet [4] in 2017 to reduce the space and time complexity while working with CNNs, but the accuracy is not sacrificed. The MobileNet architecture is shown in detail in Figure 6.7. There is a global average pooling layer. The mean of the feature map is computed over the spatial dimension in this layer. After

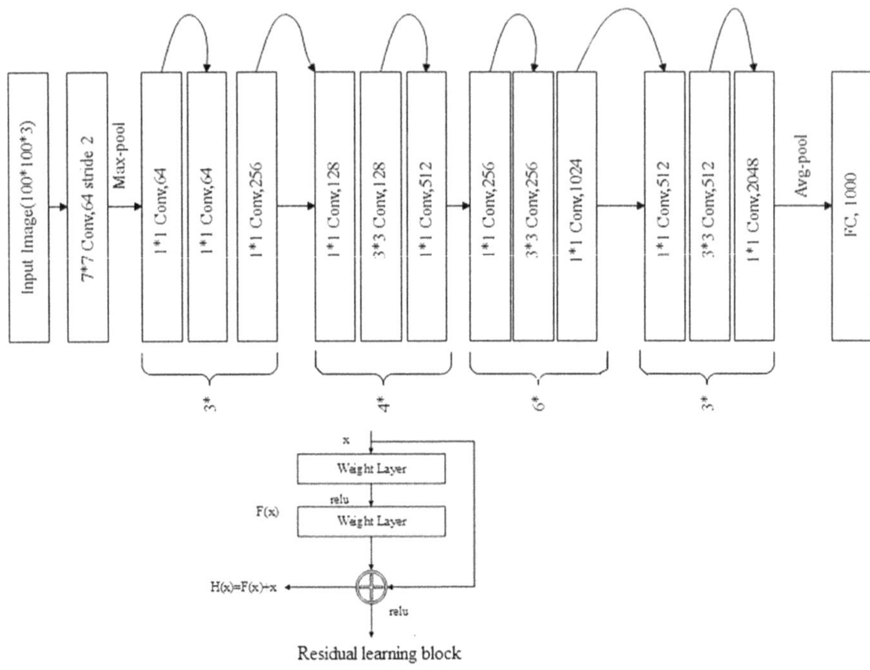

FIGURE 6.6 Architecture of ResNet.

TABLE 6.2
Architecture of InceptionResNetV2

Name of the Layer	Shape of Output
Input	299 × 299 × 3
Stem	35 × 35 × 256
Inception-ResNet-A	35 × 35 × 256
Reduction-A	17 × 17 × 896
Inception-ResNet-B	17 × 17 × 896
Reduction-B	8 × 8 × 1792
Inception-ResNet-C	8 × 8 × 1792
Average Pooling	1 × 1 × 1792
Dropout	1 × 1 × 1792
Output	1 × 1 × 1000

that, there is a fully connected layer and a softmax function. MobileNet also uses linear bottlenecks, which reduce the number of channels in the intermediate layers. It helps to further reduce the computational requirements and model size, while still preserving accuracy. Here is a brief overview of the layers in MobileNet:

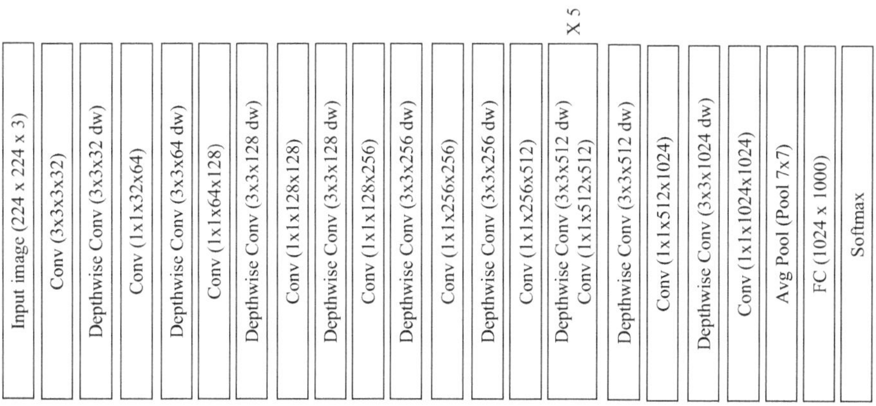

Input image (224 x 224 x 3)
Conv (3x3x3x32)
Depthwise Conv (3x3x32 dw)
Conv (1x1x32x64)
Depthwise Conv (3x3x64 dw)
Conv (1x1x64x128)
Depthwise Conv (3x3x128 dw)
Conv (1x1x128x128)
Depthwise Conv (3x3x128 dw)
Conv (1x1x128x256)
Depthwise Conv (3x3x256 dw)
Conv (1x1x256x256)
Depthwise Conv (3x3x256 dw)
Conv (1x1x256x512)
X 5
Depthwise Conv (3x3x512 dw)
Conv (1x1x512x512)
Depthwise Conv (3x3x512 dw)
Conv (1x1x512x1024)
Depthwise Conv (3x3x1024 dw)
Conv (1x1x1024x1024)
Avg Pool (Pool 7x7)
FC (1024 x 1000)
Softmax

FIGURE 6.7 Architecture of MobileNet.

1. Input layer: This layer takes as input an image of the size specified by the user.
2. Convolutional layer: It executes a standard convolution operation with a specified number of filters, kernel size, and stride. Then, the output is passed through one batch normalization layer and one ReLU function.
3. Depthwise separable convolutional layer: A depthwise convolution (DC) operation is executed in this layer, which is followed by a pointwise convolution (PC) operation. The DC uses one filter separately for each input channel, while the PC uses 1×1 convolutions for combining the outputs of DC. The output is then passed through one batch normalization layer and one ReLU function.
4. Max pooling layer: It performs a max pooling operation with specified kernel size and stride.
5. Linear bottleneck layer: This layer reduces the number of channels in intermediate feature maps using 1×1 convolutions, applies a depthwise separable convolution, and then expands the number of channels back to the original number using another 1×1 convolution. The output is then passed through one batch normalization layer and one linear activation function.
6. Fully connected layer: This layer takes the output of the last convolution layer and applies the global average pooling operation to produce a feature vector of a fixed length. That feature vector is then moved across one fully connected layer with a defined number of neurons and one softmax function to produce the final classification output.

MobileNet typically consists of multiple convolutional layers and depthwise separable CLs, with varying parameters such as number of filters, kernel sizes, and strides. The number and size of these layers can be adjusted to tradeoff model size, accuracy, and computational efficiency.

6.2.2.3.8 DenseNet

In 2017, Huang et al. proposed a CNN architecture called Densely Connected Convolutional Networks or DenseNet [7]. DenseNet introduced direct connections between all layers to solve problems regarding vanishing gradients. In DenseNet, input to every layer is the feature maps of all preceding layers, which allows it to use all the previous layers' feature maps in its computations. This connectivity pattern helps improve feature reuse, reduce parameters, and improve the flow of gradients during backpropagation. In Figure 6.8, the architecture of a dense block is given.

In this proposed work, DenseNet-201 was used (Figure 6.9). The architecture consists of three dense blocks; a transition layer follows each. The first dense block takes as input a 224 × 224 RGB image and outputs 256 feature maps. The subsequent dense blocks expand the number of feature maps to 896 and 1792, respectively. Each transition layer reduces the spatial dimension of feature maps by half and reduces the number of feature maps by utilizing a combination of 1 × 1 CLs and average pooling.

The feature maps are passed through a global average pooling layer at the end of the last dense block. This global average pooling layer averages feature maps over their spatial dimensions, resulting in a 1792-dimensional feature vector. Then, this feature vector is passed across a fully connected layer for producing final output probabilities over the 1000 classes of the ImageNet dataset.

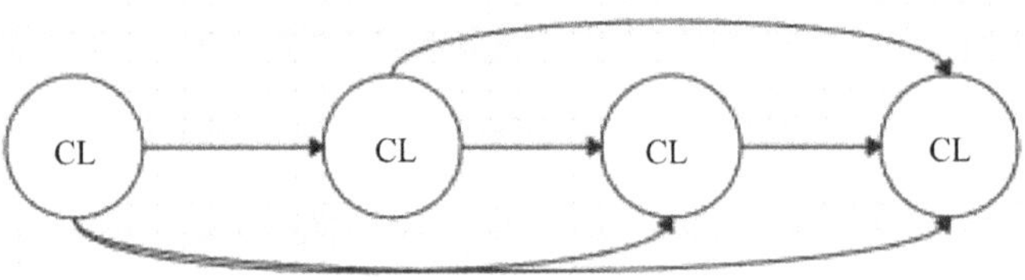

FIGURE 6.8 Dense block.

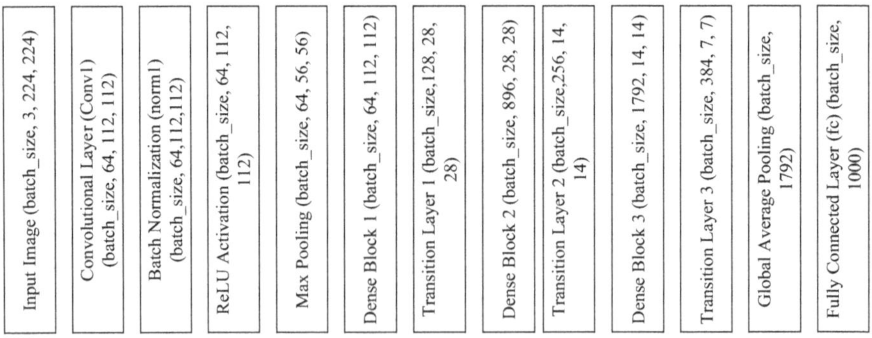

Input Image (batch_size, 3, 224, 224)
Convolutional Layer (Conv1) (batch_size, 64, 112, 112)
Batch Normalization (norm1) (batch_size, 64,112,112)
ReLU Activation (batch_size, 64, 112, 112)
Max Pooling (batch_size, 64, 56, 56)
Dense Block 1 (batch_size, 64, 112, 112)
Transition Layer 1 (batch_size,128, 28, 28)
Dense Block 2 (batch_size, 896, 28, 28)
Transition Layer 2 (batch_size,256, 14, 14)
Dense Block 3 (batch_size, 1792, 14, 14)
Transition Layer 3 (batch_size, 384, 7, 7)
Global Average Pooling (batch_size, 1792)
Fully Connected Layer (fc) (batch_size, 1000)

FIGURE 6.9 Architecture of DenseNet-201.

6.2.2.4 Differential Evolution (DE)

A specific stochastic and population-based optimization algorithm is differential evolution. It was developed to solve nonlinear optimization problems. DE maintains a population of candidate solutions and iteratively generates new solutions by creating solutions using mutation operation and combining them with the existing solutions through the process of crossover. Then the evaluation of new candidate solutions is done, and the best ones are selected to form the next generation of the population.

Optimization algorithms typically involve:

- Searching through a large space of possible solutions.
- Evaluating each potential solution based on the objective function and constraints.
- Refining the search until the best solution is found or a stopping criterion is met.

Different optimization techniques may be more suitable for different types of problems, depending on the structure and complexity of the objective function and constraints.

6.3 LITERATURE SURVEY

In recent eras, IoMT played a vital role in smart healthcare systems, because it not only allows remote monitoring of patients but also allows for telemedicine. Efficient management of an enormous amount of data is extremely challenging in contemporary times. Researchers have applied various ML approaches to meet this challenge. Egala et al. [37] proposed the random forest support vector machine, where a random forest algorithm is utilized for optimal feature selection of patient-related information, and an SVM is used for decision-making. It is also a formidable challenge to retrieve relevant medical images from a very large amount of patient-related information. Li et al. [11] conducted a survey on the CBIR technique and proposed applying deep learning to the CBIR technique, which can mitigate this challenge.

Senthilkumar and Somasundaram [12] have proposed a CBIR system by utilizing DL techniques for feature extraction and similarity measurement. Their proposed system has retrieved medical images from large databases based on their content that can be used in various Healthcare 4.0 applications such as disease diagnosis, treatment planning, and medical education. Shamna et al. [13] introduced a topic and location model-based automated CBIR system for medical images. The guided latent Dirichlet allocation method was used to create the topic information. A unique location model was developed to incorporate the geographical data of visual words. They also presented position-weighted precision for ranking the retrieved images. Tortorella et al. [14] surveyed 109 healthcare professionals. Based on their survey, they discovered that four Healthcare 4.0 technologies have a significant impact on the monitoring, predicting, responding, and learning abilities of a resilient system.

These four technologies are “digital platform for collaborative sharing of patient data”, “interconnected medical emergency support”, “remote consultation and development of the plan and care in real-time”, and “digital non-invasive care”. Sisodia and Jindal conducted a comprehensive literature analysis on Industry 4.0 in the healthcare business [15]. They have conducted meta-analyses of prior literature using several criteria. The study’s most important conclusion is that the likelihood of the health environment increases if some efficient security procedures are employed by pairing with better big data handling techniques. A unique architecture for safe and quick image retrieval in a cloud setting was put out by Noor et al. [16]. They performed scaling on images to various dimensions and developed encryption–decryption for safe storage. After that, they included iBuck, which is a middleware, to retrieve images quickly and easily. Maji and Bose [17] used pretrained CNN models to extract features from a large image dataset and proposed a database preclustering method based on those extracted features. They analyzed the time required for CBIR and their cases were shorter in time. The paper by Al-Qahtani et al. [18] provided a comprehensive review of CBIR techniques in the Healthcare 4.0 context. In the paper, the challenges and opportunities of CBIR in healthcare were discussed, such as the large and complex nature of medical images and the potential benefits of using CBIR for improving medical diagnosis and treatment. The paper provided a detailed overview of various CBIR techniques, including feature extraction, similarity measures, and relevance feedback, and discussed their application in medical image retrieval. The authors also identified current research trends and future directions for CBIR in healthcare, such as the integration of deep learning and cloud computing technologies. Shakarami and Tarrah [19] utilized CNN for CBIR. They used an improved AlexNet combined with oriented gradients and local binary patterns. After that, they used principle component analysis to reduce the number of dimensions. They proved superiority of their approach experimentally.

Optimization is a very important approach in ML because it involves finding the best solution to a problem. Due to this reason, it is leading to improve the performance of various ML techniques to solve various tasks [34, 35]. Kingman and Ba [20] introduced the Adam optimization algorithm, which is popular in DL for its ability to converge quickly and achieve better performance. The algorithm combined the benefits of both momentum-based optimization and RMSProp and has been extensively tested on several benchmark datasets. LeCun, Bottou, Bengio, and Haffner [21] introduced CNNs and provided a comprehensive analysis of their effectiveness in recognizing handwritten digits, laying the foundation for the development of CNNs as a fundamental tool for various ML tasks. LeCun, Bottou, Orr, and Müller [22] provided a comprehensive review of various backpropagation optimization techniques and proposed several modifications for the improvement of convergence and algorithm speed. Smith [23] proposed the use of cyclical learning rates as a technique for the improvement of DNN performance. The paper showed that using cyclical learning rates can result in more rapid convergence and improved generalization performance than traditional learning rate schedules. Zhang et al. [24] proposed a new optimization algorithm that can make the convergence speed and generalization performance of DNNs better. The proposed algorithm incorporated an auxiliary optimizer to search the weight space and help the main optimizer escape from local minima. Luo et al. [25] presented a new family of optimization algorithms that dynamically adjust the learning rate based on the gradient information. The proposed algorithms can effectively prevent the optimizer from diverging or oscillating while allowing for aggressive updates in flat regions. Liu et al. [26] proposed a modification to the Adam optimizer that addresses its susceptibility to noisy gradients as well as make the robustness and generalization performance of DNNs better. The authors of [27] introduced a novel optimizer that adapts the learning rate and momentum based on the belief in observed gradients, achieving the latest performance on various benchmarks. Akoury et al. [28] introduced diffGrad, a novel optimizer for deep neural networks, which adjusts step sizes for each parameter based on the difference between present and past gradients. It has shown its effectiveness across CIFAR10 and CIFAR100 datasets in terms of convergence and performance on synthetic nonconvex functions and image categorization tasks. Feurer et al. [31] proposed a concept called AutoML, which includes a wide range of methods and tools to optimize both the hyperparameters and the architecture of NNs. Han et al. enhanced the performance of the single-hidden-layer feedforward neural network by using particle swarm optimization (PSO) [32]. The artificial fish swarm optimization (AFSO) method and an artificial neural network based on adaptive optimization were proposed by Manjula et al. [33] for the classification of speech stuttering. Tiwari and Pant [29] introduced a brownfield IoMT network for image data. Further, they developed a framework for CBMIR. It used DenseNet-201 architecture to generate image descriptors. After that, to classify the data, they configured a DNN model through DE. They trained and validated their model [9, 10, 36] and experimentally showed that their performance is better than DenseNet-201, ResNet50, InceptionResnetV2, Resnet101V2, InceptionNetV3, and VGG19. One of the problems that has to be faced during optimization is premature convergence. Aon et al. [38] have proposed an intelligent multiobjective genetic algorithm using a self-organizing map (IMOGA/SOM) as a solution to this problem. According to their approach, MOGA-generated solutions train the SOM. The trained SOM leads to better convergence.

In some cases, more than one optimization algorithm is applied to solve a particular problem. Mukherjee et al. [39] applied five multiobjective evolutionary algorithms for optimizing cutting parameters of glass fiber reinforced plastic. These algorithms were the (1) non-dominated sorting genetic algorithm II, (2) archive-based steady-state micro genetic algorithm, (3) archive-based hybrid scatter search, (4) generalized differential evolution 3, and (5) multiobjective particle swarm optimization.

6.3.1 Shortcomings of the Previous Works

Although the aforementioned works are well-designed and robust, there are some shortcomings:

- Inappropriate for large datasets: Shakarami and Tarrah [19] applied their work on smaller datasets, but in the case of CBIR regarding IoMT, there is a large amount of data. Hence, this type of approach is not appropriate in that case.

- Local optima: Most of the previous work, except [38], suffers from premature convergence. Although there exists a global optimum solution, the optimization algorithm gets trapped in local optima. As a result, that algorithm cannot find out the global optima that is better than the local optima.
- Computational complexity: Sometimes the number of objectives is more than one [38]. Due to this reason, the growing computational cost and search space dimensionality are exponential with the increasing complexity of the problem, which makes the computation times longer.

6.4 PROPOSED METHODOLOGY

Figure 6.10 shows the overall flow of the proposed work. The approaches taken by the proposed work have been classified into four parts: image preprocessing, model optimization, classification, and image retrieval. In the following steps, the overall flow is described:

Step 1: Preprocessing is performed on the images taken from the dataset. This step is done to generate image descriptors of the images in the input image dataset.

Step 2: In the subsequent step, a collection of CNN models is optimized by applying the differential evolution algorithm, leveraging the extracted image descriptors as the basis for optimization.

Step 3: Subsequently the optimal CNN model is trained using image descriptors extracted from those input images.

Step 4: Classification of all input images is done using the selected CNN model, and thereafter their labels are determined based on the results of this classification process.

Step 5: When a client submits a query image, the incoming image undergoes preprocessing. Subsequently, the optimized CNN model is employed to classify the query image.

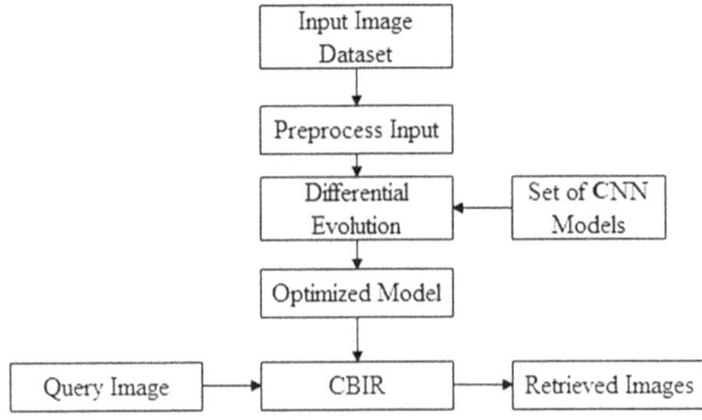

FIGURE 6.10 Overall flow of the proposed work.

Step 6: Similarity is evaluated between every image from the input dataset and the image passed as a query. The image having the most similarity with the query image will get the highest rank (first). This proposed CBIR framework retrieves the first three ranked images.

Algorithm 6.1 DE-Based NN Optimization for CBIR(Image Dataset,Query Image)

```
Input:    ID = Set of input images taken from
            image dataset
          QR = Query image given by client
Output:   RI1 = Rank no 1 retrieved image
          RI2 = Rank no 2 retrieved image
          RI3 = Rank no 3 retrieved image
Begin     I1 = PreprocessInput(ID)
          Q1 = PreprocessInput(QR)
          DE (Set_of_CNNs)          /*Set of CNNs are optimized using
                                      Differential Evolution*/
          OptimizedCNN (I1)         /* The optimized CNN is applied to I1*/

          CBIR(I1,Q1)
End       RetrievedImages
```

Overall details of the proposed work are shown by Algorithm 6.1. A detailed description of the process of the CBIR technique is explained in Section 6.4.4 and Figure 6.2 shows the CBIR framework for this proposed work.

6.4.1 Preprocess Input

The proposed work performs three operations on an image to preprocess it:

1. Gaussian blur operation
2. Morphological operation
3. Contrast limited adaptive histogram equalization (CLAHE) operation

6.4.1.1 Gaussian Blur

In this proposed work, the Gaussian blur operation is done for four reasons:

1. It prevents overfitting by reducing the impact of small variations in the input data.
2. It helps in data augmentation, by artificially generating new training data with varying degrees of blur.
3. It reduces the impact of noise on the input images, which improves overall network performance.
4. It reduces the impact of high-frequency components, such as edges, which makes the network more robust to variations in image quality.

The equation for Gaussian blur for this proposed work is

$$I * G(x, y) \tag{6.1}$$

where I represents the input image, and G(x, y) represents the Gaussian kernel, which is a trainable parameter in the convolutional layer.

$$G(x,y) = \frac{1}{2\pi\sigma^2} e^{\frac{-(x^2+y^2)}{2\sigma^2}} \tag{6.2}$$

where x and y represent the spatial distances from the center of the kernel, and σ denotes the standard deviation of the Gaussian function. The Gaussian kernel used in this proposed work is of size (5,5).

6.4.1.2 Morphological Operation

The morphological operation has been applied after Gaussian blur in this proposed work to improve the quality of the image and enhance the important features of this work. The Gaussian blur operation has been used to reduce noise and smooth the image, after that morphological operation has been used to extract features and reduce noise even further. By applying morphological operation after Gaussian blur, the network has better identified and classified important objects in those images. Furthermore, morphological operations have removed small objects and filled in small gaps that have been introduced by the Gaussian blur operation, and thus morphological operations have improved the overall quality of the image. In this work, the size of the structuring element that will be generated is (3,3) and is of rectangular shape.

The equation for the opening operation is

$$g(x,y) = \text{Dilation}(B)(\text{Erosion}(B)(f(x,y))) \tag{6.3}$$

The equation for the closing operation is

$$g(x,y) = \text{Erosion}(B)(\text{Dilation}(B)(f(x,y))) \tag{6.4}$$

The equation for the morphological dilation operation is

$$g(x,y) = \text{maximum}\{f(x+i,y+j) : (i,j) \in B\} \tag{6.5}$$

The equation for the morphological erosion operation is

$$g(x,y) = \text{minimum}\{f(x+i,y+j) : (i,j) \in B\} \tag{6.6}$$

where f(x,y) represents the input image from the dataset, g(x,y) denotes the output of the morphological operation, and B is the structuring element.

6.4.1.3 Contrast Limited Adaptive Histogram Equalization (CLAHE)

To enhance the contrast of an image while maintaining its local features, CLAHE has been applied in this proposed work. The local features that were preserved by the morphological operations can be further enhanced and made more visible by this operation. In this proposed work, the limiting factor that limits the amplification of contrast in the image is 2.0. The size of the tiles on which the histogram equalization has been applied is taken as (8,8) for this proposed work.

6.4.2 Differential Evolution–Based Optimization

In this proposed work, DE has been exploited as an optimization technique to systematically search the CNN models, ultimately identifying the optimal CNN architecture adaptive to the characteristics of a given input dataset. Subsequently, this optimized CNN model has been applied for the task of classification, leveraging its enhanced performance to achieve superior results in the context of the given dataset. The flowchart for optimization of the model using the differential evolution algorithm is shown in Figure 6.11.

6.4.2.1 Population Initialization

In the population initialization phase, a random population of size n is generated as per Equation 6.7. The value of Pri in Equation 6.8 is a randomly generated fractional number. The selection of a specific CNN model is determined based on this randomly generated fractional number, which is sampled from a uniform distribution within the range [0.0, 2.0). This proposed work considers eight CNN models: InceptionResNetV2, AlexNet, MobileNet, SqueezeNet, InceptionV3, ResNet-50, DenseNet-201, and VGG19. For each individual in the study, one of the CNN models is randomly selected for fitness evaluation using this randomly generated number.

The equation for a population set in a generation is

$$\text{Pop\_gen} = (\text{Pr1}, \text{Pr2}, \ldots \text{Prn}) \tag{6.7}$$

$$\text{Pri} = \text{uniform\_distribution}([0.0, 2.0)) \tag{6.8}$$

where Pop_gen is the entire set of populations and the parameter for each individual is represented as pop1. The population size is represented by n. Here, each individual in the population has been denoted by Pri, where i is an integer value and $\text{i} \in \{1, 2, \ldots n\}$.

6.4.2.2 Fitness Evaluation

In this chapter, an individual represents a CNN model, and the fitness value of each individual is assessed using the validation loss metric. Sparse categorical cross entropy has been used to measure validation loss in this proposed work. Equation 6.9 is considered as fitness function for this proposed work.

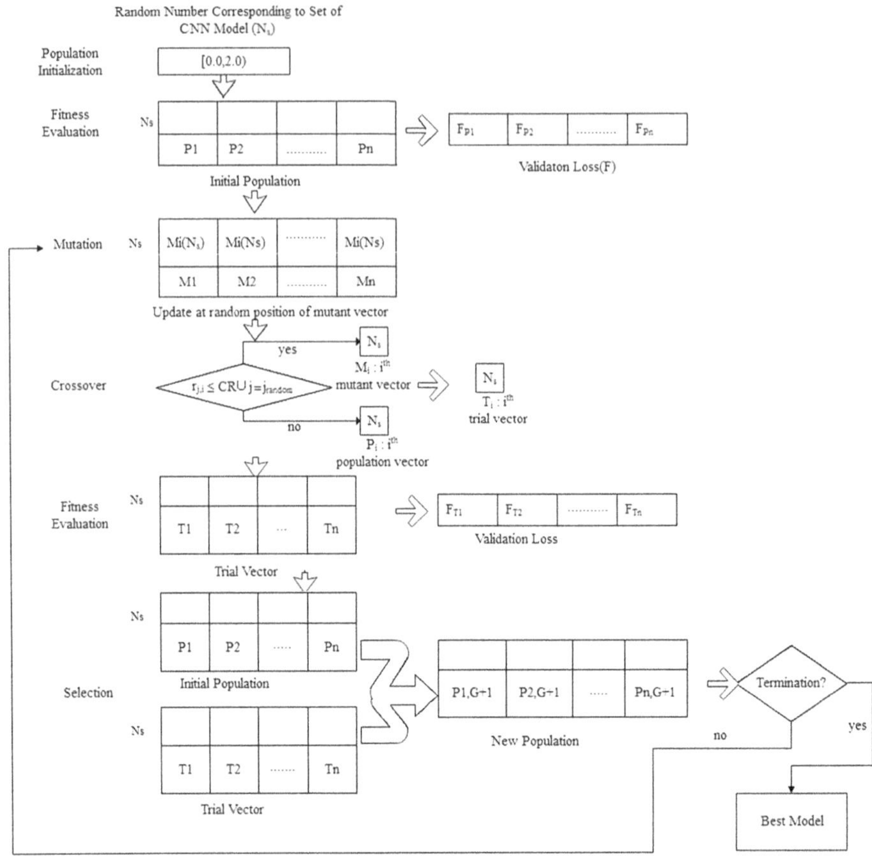

FIGURE 6.11 Flowchart for optimization of the model using a differential evolution algorithm.

$$CrossEntropyLoss(F) = -\sum_{i=1}^{n} y_i \log(\hat{y}_i) \tag{6.9}$$

where the true class label is denoted as y_i, $\hat{y}_i$ represents the predicted probability, and n is quantity of classes.

For evaluating the fitness of an individual, this proposed work has trained the CNN model of the individual by considering the number of epochs as 24 and batch size as 256 and calculated validation accuracy and loss. In this proposed work, 10% of the total images in each image dataset is allocated to the validation set.

6.4.2.3 Mutation

In order to expand the search space, a mutation operation is performed. Here Mui is the mutant vector, which is generated corresponding to each individual Pi. In this proposed work, the mutation operation is updated. This approach is done to expand the search space more than a traditional differential evolution approach. Here according to this proposed work, the equation for generating the mutant vector Muj = (mu1, j, ... md, j) is

$$Muj = \begin{cases} best\ of\ the\ followings \\ P1 + F*(\mathrm{P2} - \mathrm{P3}) \\ P1 + F*(\mathrm{P2} + \mathrm{P3}) \\ P1 - F*(\mathrm{P2} - \mathrm{P3}) \\ P1 - F*(P2 + P3) \end{cases} \tag{6.10}$$

here Muj represents the mutant vector; $P1$, $P2$, and $P3$ are the original population vectors; and F is the scaling factor and $F \in (0.2, 0.9)$.

Among the following, as given in Equation 6.10, either the maximum of those four values or the minimum of those four values is to be considered as the best one and is assigned as the value of the mutant vector. In order to do this, between the maximum and the minimum, which one will be considered is decided at random. It is done to expand the search space further and overcome the inefficient exploration problem. Among the set of mutant vectors, one particular mutant vector will be replaced by the mutant vector generated by using Equation 6.10.

6.4.2.4 Crossover

In differential evolution, the crossover operation is used to generate a new candidate solution for a given problem after mutation. This operation is done to increase the diversity of the population and it creates a manifold of the optimized models by improving the overall quality of the solutions. The crossover operation is performed between the original population vectors or population set and their corresponding mutant vectors. Specifically, for each vector of the population, a trial vector is formed by combining elements of the original vector and the corresponding mutant vector using a crossover operation. The crossover operation is typically performed at a random index, called the "crossover point", and a new vector is created that is a combination of the original population vector and the mutant vector up to the crossover point, followed by the remaining elements from the original vector.

As a result of crossover, the trial vector Ti = ($t_{1,i}, t_{2,i}, \ldots t_{d,i}$) is generated, as shown in Equation 6.11

$$t_{j,i} = \begin{cases} M_{j,i}, if\ r_{j,i} \leq CoR \cup j = j_{random} \\ P_{j,i} \qquad\qquad\qquad Otherwise \end{cases} \tag{6.11}$$

where CoR represents the crossover rate and $CoR \in [0,1]$, $r \in [0,1]$ represents a random number. j and j_{random} is a random integer number, where $j \in [1, 2, \ldots, d]$ and $j_{random} \in [1, 2, \ldots, d]$. Here, $M_{j,i}$ represents the mutant vector, and $P_{j,i}$ is the original population vector.

6.4.2.5 Selection

The selection operation is the last operation carried out in a particular iteration of differential evolution. This operation is performed between the original population vectors and trial vectors. The selection operation is done to select those individuals with better fitness values by comparing each vector from the original population set and trial vectors. This operation is done according to Equation 6.12:

$$P_{i,G+1} = \begin{cases} t_{i,G}, & \text{if } F\left(t_{i,G}\right) \le F\left(P_{i,G}\right) \\ P_{i,G}, & \text{otherwise} \end{cases} \tag{6.12}$$

where $F(.)$ is the fitness function, and $P_{i,G+1}$ is the population set for the next generation.

This process will iterate until it meets the termination criteria. In this proposed work, the number of generations (G) is the termination criterion. After the completion of this process, the optimized CNN is configured for the task of classification. The learning rate is kept at 0.001 during the training.

6.4.3 Classification Using Best Model

The subsequent operation of this proposed work is classification by applying the CNN model optimized by DE. CNN models are employed in the content-based image retrieval framework for learning complex patterns and features in images. Then those models performed similarity matching between query and database images.

6.4.4 Image Retrieval

In this proposed work, image retrieval is done to provide an efficient and effective way to search and retrieve images on the basis of their visual contents. After classification is done, each image of the dataset is labeled by its corresponding class labels. When a client sends an image as a query, that query image arrives at the system. Then the query image is preprocessed. Then the preprocessed query image passes to the same CNN model that has been used to classify the images of the input dataset. After that, the predicted output is generated and it is compared with each of the images of the dataset, which also have been predicted by the model. This is done by measuring the similarity score. In Algorithm 6.2, a detailed description of this section is given, as well as what is done in the method CBIR(I1,Q1) of Algorithm 6.1.

Algorithm 6.2 CBIR (I1,Q1)

Input: I1 = Result after images from input dataset are preprocessed
Q1= Result after query image are preprocessed

Output: RI1 = Rank no 1 retrieved image
RI2 = Rank no 2 retrieved image
RI3 = Rank no 3 retrieved image

```
Begin   PI = PredictByModel (I1)
        PQ = PredictByModel (Q1)
        SimScr = ED (PI,PQ)      /* Calculate similarity score based on Euclidean distance
                                    between each image in input image dataset and the
                                    image sent as a query*/
        SrtSmImg()               /* Sort images according to similarity score between the
                                    image sent as a query and each image in input image
                                    dataset */
        DspImg()                 /* Display images according to sorting performed based
End                                 on similarity score*/
```

6.5 EXPERIMENTAL ANALYSIS

6.5.1 Experimental Setup

The proposed work has been experimented with JupyterLab version 3.3.2 with Python 3.9.16 on Anaconda platform version 2.3.2 on an Intel® Core™ i3-6006U CPU @ 2.00GHz processor with 64-bit operating system, x64-based processor, 8.00 GB RAM, and Windows 10 Operating System. In this study, three publicly available datasets have been used: Brain Tumor Classification (MRI) dataset [9], Covid-19 Radiography Database [10], and Breast Cancer Patients MRI's dataset [36]. [9] includes a dataset of 3554 images, with 926 belonging to the "glioma tumor" category, 937 to the "meningioma tumor" category, 901 to the "pituitary tumor" category, and 895 categorized as "no tumor". Reference [10] includes a dataset consisting of a total of 21,173 images. Within this dataset, there are 3616 images categorized as "Covid", 6012 images categorized as "lung opacity", 10,200 images categorized as "normal", and 1345 images categorized as "viral pneumonia". Reference [36] consists of a dataset comprising 1480 images, of which 700 belong to the healthy class and 700 belong to the sick class.

The datasets have been split into two categories: "train set" and "test set". This splitting is done at a 70:30 ratio. Additionally, the train set is divided into two categories at a ratio of 90:10: "training set" and "validation set". This approach is taken because providing the model with an entire set of training data might end up overfitting. For each class, if there are not sufficient records in a dataset to train a model, splitting it into three sets will significantly decrease the number of records. Moreover, during training, classes with more records may outnumber those classes that have fewer records. A dataset must have a sufficient number of records for each class, which is balanced in order to resolve this issue and overcome the problem regarding overfitting and underfitting. In order to improve the number of labeled records available, the dataset having imbalanced classes needs to be transformed at random. Zooming, sample-wise centering, shearing, sample-wise standard normalization, and rotation are used in this proposed work to perform the data augmentation. The tenfold cross-validation technique has been applied here.

TABLE 6.3
Parameters Used and Their Values

Parameter	Value
Generation (G)	5
Population (n)	6
Scaling factor (F)	0.5
Crossover rate (CR)	0.5
Learning rate	0.001
Batch size	32
Number of epochs	24

TABLE 6.4
Confusion Matrix

	Predicted Class 1	Predicted Class 2
Actual class 1	TP	FN
Actual class 2	FP	TN

In this chapter, seven parameters were used. Those parameters have been shown along with their values in Table 6.3. Based on the confusion matrix, this study utilized standard metrics for evaluating the system's performance. Standard metrics used in this proposed work are precision, recall, accuracy, and F1 score. The confusion matrix is shown in Table 6.4, where TP is true positive cases, i.e., those images having brain tumor or Covid-19 or breast cancer are correctly classified. FP represents false positive, where an ordinary tissue is wrongly classified. FN is false negative, which denotes that actual brain tumor or Covid-19 or breast cancer images are wrongly classified as non-tumor or normal or healthy. TN represents true negative, where ordinary tissues are correctly predicted as such. For this proposed work, the similarity score in CBIR is measured with the help of Euclidean distance.

6.5.2 Experimental Results

The work proposed in this chapter has two purposes. One is to optimize some pretrained CNN models to explore which one is best for a given input image dataset. After the best CNN model is explored, it is applied for classification. Another purpose is to form a CBIR framework where the explored model is utilized. Here we have done a comparison of our work with six existing well-known and mostly used CNN models. They are DenseNet-201 [7], ResNet50 [5], InceptionResNetV2 [6], ResNet101V2 [40], InceptionNetV3 [2], and VGG19 [1]. This comparison is done for

TABLE 6.5
Performance Evaluation Based on Validation Accuracy

Technique	Validation Accuracy		
	Covid-19 Radiography Database	Brain Tumor Classification (MRI) Dataset	Breast Cancer Patients MRI's Dataset
ResNet50	0.93	0.61	0.89
DenseNet-201	0.95	0.93	0.93
InceptionResNetV2	0.94	0.91	0.91
ResNet101V2	0.95	0.92	0.94
InceptionNetV3	0.95	0.92	0.87
VGG19	0.92	0.95	0.94
Proposed work	**1.00**	**0.99**	**0.98**

three publicly available image sets: Brain Tumor Classification (MRI) dataset [9], Breast Cancer Patients MRI's dataset [36], and Covid-19 Radiography Database [10]. Experimental results have been compared based on validation accuracy, validation loss, accuracy, precision, recall, F1 score, and time efficiency.

Tables 6.5–6.10 represent the validation accuracy, validation loss, accuracy, precision, recall, and F1 score, respectively. The best performance is shown in the boldfaced entry of each table.

Table 6.11 shows performance evaluation based on time efficiency. Here boldfaced entries in the table show the best performance. Table 6.11 demonstrates that the performance of InceptionNetV3 is better than all the other techniques in the case the of Covid-19 Radiography Database and Brain Tumor Classification (MRI)

TABLE 6.6
Performance Evaluation Based on Validation Loss

Technique	Validation Loss		
	Covid-19 Radiography Database	Brain Tumor Classification (MRI) Dataset	Breast Cancer Patients MRI's Dataset
ResNet50	0.32	1.00	0.28
DenseNet-201	0.21	0.21	0.20
InceptionResNetV2	0.22	0.26	0.29
ResNet101V2	0.22	0.27	0.19
InceptionNetV3	0.22	0.23	0.45
VGG19	0.20	0.20	0.16
Proposed work	**2.9769e-09**	**0.03**	**0.04**

TABLE 6.7
Performance Evaluation Based on Accuracy

Technique	Accuracy		
	Covid-19 Radiography Database	**Brain Tumor Classification (MRI) Dataset**	**Breast Cancer Patients MRI's Dataset**
ResNet50	0.95	0.94	0.71
DenseNet-201	0.94	0.61	0.70
InceptionResNetV2	0.91	0.91	0.63
ResNet101V2	0.91	0.92	0.71
InceptionNetV3	0.91	0.92	0.63
VGG19	0.92	0.94	0.52
Proposed work	**1.00**	**0.97**	**0.98**

TABLE 6.8
Performance Evaluation Based on Precision

Technique	Precision		
	Covid-19 Radiography Database	**Brain Tumor Classification (MRI) Dataset**	**Breast Cancer Patients MRI's Dataset**
ResNet50	0.95	0.80	0.71
DenseNet-201	0.94	0.63	0.75
InceptionResNetV2	0.95	0.77	0.78
ResNet101V2	0.95	0.79	0.72
InceptionNetV3	0.95	0.63	0.63
VGG19	0.95	0.78	0.75
Proposed work	**1.00**	**0.97**	**0.98**

TABLE 6.9
Performance Evaluation Based on Recall

Technique	Recall		
	Covid-19 Radiography Database	**Brain Tumor Classification (MRI) Dataset**	**Breast Cancer Patients MRI's Dataset**
ResNet50	0.95	0.80	0.71
DenseNet-201	0.94	0.63	0.75
InceptionResNetV2	0.95	0.77	0.78
ResNet101V2	0.95	0.79	0.72
InceptionNetV3	0.95	0.63	0.63
VGG19	0.95	0.78	0.75
Proposed work	**1.00**	**0.97**	**0.98**

TABLE 6.10
Performance Evaluation Based on F1 Score

Technique	F1 Score		
	Covid-19 Radiography Database	Brain Tumor Classification (MRI) Dataset	Breast Cancer Patients MRI's Dataset
ResNet50	0.95	0.72	0.71
DenseNet-201	0.94	0.47	0.68
InceptionResNetV2	0.95	0.71	0.58
ResNet101V2	0.95	0.71	0.70
InceptionNetV3	0.95	0.47	0.63
VGG19	0.95	0.69	0.38
Proposed work	**1.00**	**0.97**	**0.98**

TABLE 6.11
Performance Evaluation Based on Time Efficiency

Technique	Time Efficiency		
	Covid-19 Radiography Database	Brain Tumor Classification (MRI) Dataset	Breast Cancer Patients MRI's Dataset
ResNet50	2583 seconds	1936 seconds	1892 seconds
DenseNet-201	3100 seconds	2023 seconds	1928 seconds
InceptionResNetV2	2111 seconds	1226 seconds	**1049 seconds**
ResNet101V2	3932 seconds	2519 seconds	1911 seconds
InceptionNetV3	**2026 seconds**	**1132 seconds**	1099 seconds
VGG19	11062 seconds	10002 seconds	9632 seconds
Proposed work	3221 seconds	2147 seconds	2015 seconds

dataset, but in the case of the Breast Cancer Patients MRI's dataset, performance of InceptionResNetV2 is better than all the other techniques.

6.5.3 Experimental Results for CBIR

The second approach of this proposed work is described in detail in this section. We have designed a CBIR framework. Three images have been considered as query images for this framework. In Table 6.12, the details about how our proposed CBIR technique experimentally works are given. As shown in Table 6.12, these three images belong to glioma tumor, Covid, and sick, and the corresponding input image datasets are the Brain Tumor Classification (MRI) dataset, Covid-19 Radiography

TABLE 6.12
Images Retrieved from CBIR Framework Based on Rank and Similarity Score

Dataset Name	Class	Queried Image	Retrieved Images Rank-1	Retrieved Images Rank-2	Retrieved Images Rank-3
Brain Tumor Classification (MRI)	Glioma tumor	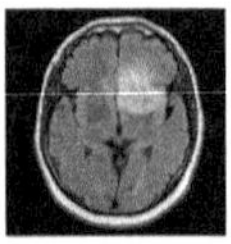	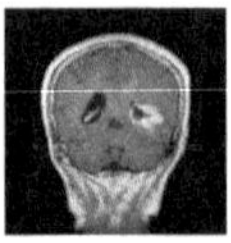	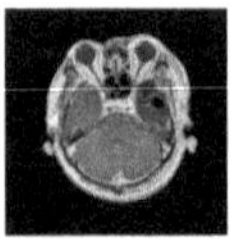	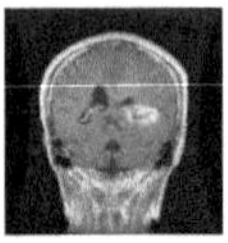
			Similarity score 1.19	Similarity score 1.19	Similarity score 1.19
Covid-19 Radiography	Covid	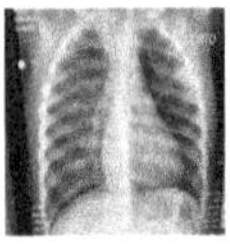	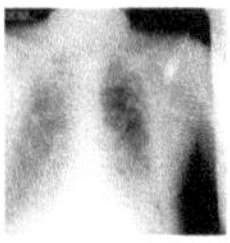	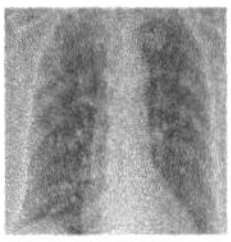	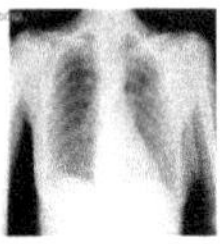
			Similarity score 0.49	Similarity score 0.49	Similarity score 0.49
Breast Cancer Patients MRI's	Sick	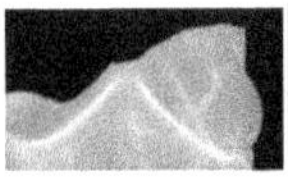	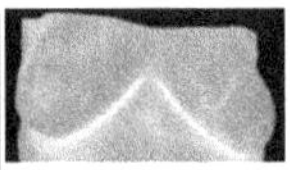	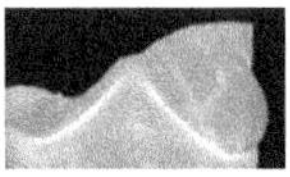	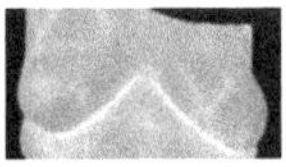
			Similarity score 1.32	Similarity score 1.32	Similarity score 1.31

Database, and Breast Cancer Patients MRI's dataset, respectively. If any of the three input images passes as a query, the proposed CBIR technique retrieves three images from the corresponding image dataset. The model explored by the proposed work is utilized to predict features of the query image and images from the corresponding input image dataset. On the basis of those features, the top three images are retrieved by the CBIR framework from the input image dataset. Those images are ranked according to similarity with the query image. The similarity score is measured by using the Euclidean distance between the query image and each of those images. According to the experimental results shown in Table 6.12, the top three retrieved images belong to the same class of the query image.

6.6 CONCLUSION AND FUTURE SCOPE

This proposed work has modified DE to efficiently explore the optimized CNN model that is suitable for a given dataset. This optimized CNN model has performed effectively for the task of classification as well as CBIR. The proposed work achieved 100% accuracy in the case of the Covid-19 Radiography Database, 98% accuracy in the case of the Breast Cancer Patients MRI's dataset, and 97% accuracy in the case of the Brain Tumor Classification (MRI) dataset. This work can be further enhanced by exploring non-imaging datasets and including additional metadata for the CBIR framework connected to the IoMT network. As a future scope, a combined approach for more than one optimization algorithm can be considered.

REFERENCES

1. Simonyan, K., & Zisserman, A. (2014). Very deep convolutional networks for large-scale image recognition. arXiv preprint arXiv:1409.1556.
2. Szegedy, C., Vanhoucke, V., Ioffe, S., Shlens, J., & Wojna, Z. (2016). Rethinking the inception architecture for computer vision. In *Proceedings of the IEEE Conference on Computer Vision and Pattern Recognition* (pp. 2818–2826).
3. Krizhevsky, A., Sutskever, I., & Hinton, G. E. (2017). Imagenet classification with deep convolutional neural networks. *Communications of the ACM*, 60(6), 84–90.
4. Howard, A. G., Zhu, M., Chen, B., Kalenichenko, D., Wang, W., Weyand, T., ... Adam, H. (2017). MobileNets: Efficient convolutional neural networks for mobile vision applications. arXiv preprint arXiv:1704.04861.
5. He, K., Zhang, X., Ren, S., & Sun, J. (2016). Deep residual learning for image recognition. In *Proceedings of the IEEE Conference on Computer Vision and Pattern Recognition* (pp. 770–778).
6. Szegedy, C., Ioffe, S., Vanhoucke, V., & Alemi, A. (2017, February). Inception-v4, inception-ResNet and the impact of residual connections on learning. In *Proceedings of the AAAI conference on Artificial Intelligence* (Vol. 31, No. 1), 4278–4284.
7. Huang, G., Liu, Z., Van Der Maaten, L., & Weinberger, K. Q. (2017). Densely connected convolutional networks. In *Proceedings of the IEEE Conference on Computer Vision and Pattern Recognition* (pp. 4700–4708).
8. Iandola, F. N., Han, S., Moskewicz, M. W., Ashraf, K., Dally, W. J., & Keutzer, K. (2016). SqueezeNet: Alexnet-level accuracy with 50x fewer parameters and <0.5 MB model size. arXiv preprint arXiv:1602.07360.
9. Bhuvaji, S., Kadam, A., Bhumkar, P., Dedge, S., & Kanchan, S. (2020). Brain tumor classification (MRI) [Dataset]. Kaggle. https://doi.org/10.34740/KAGGLE/DSV/1183165.
10. COVID-19 Radiography Database Kaggle. https://www.kaggle.com/tawsifurrahman/covid19-radiography-database (accessed November 27, 2021).
11. Li, X., Yang, J., & Ma, J. (2021). Recent developments of content-based image retrieval (CBIR). *Neurocomputing*, 452, 675–689.
12. Senthilkumar, S., & Somasundaram, S. (2019). Content-based medical image retrieval using deep learning for healthcare 4.0. In *Advances in Signal Processing and Intelligent Recognition Systems* (pp. 524–532). Springer. https://doi.org/10.1007/978-981-13-8297-9_46.
13. Shamna, P., Govindan, V. K., & Nazeer, K. A. (2019). Content based medical image retrieval using topic and location model. *Journal of Biomedical Informatics*, 91, 103112.
14. Tortorella, G. L., Saurin, T. A., Fogliatto, F. S., Rosa, V. M., Tonetto, L. M., & Magrabi, F. (2021). Impacts of Healthcare 4.0 digital technologies on the resilience of hospitals. *Technological Forecasting and Social Change*, 166, 120666.
15. Sisodia, A., & Jindal, R. (2021). A meta-analysis of industry 4.0 design principles applied in the health sector. *Engineering Applications of Artificial Intelligence*, 104, 104377.
16. Noor, J., Salim, S. I., & Al Islam, A. A. (2021). Strategizing secured image storing and efficient image retrieval through a new cloud framework. *Journal of Network and Computer Applications*, 192, 103167.

17. Maji, S., & Bose, S. (2021). CBIR using features derived by deep learning. *ACM/IMS Transactions on Data Science (TDS)*, 2(3), 1–24.
18. Al-Qahtani, S. M., Alghamdi, M. A., Al-Mogren, M., Al-Khalifa, H. S., Al-Ali, A. R., & Alsaleem, S. A. (2020). A review of content-based image retrieval in healthcare 4.0. *Journal of Healthcare Engineering*, 1–12. https://doi.org/10.1155/2020/1732426.
19. Shakarami, A., & Tarrah, H. (2020). An efficient image descriptor for image classification and CBIR. *Optik*, 214, 164833.
20. Kingma, D. P., & Ba, J. (2015). Adam: A method for stochastic optimization. In *Proceedings of the 3rd International Conference on Learning Representations (ICLR).* (pp. 1–15). https://doi.org/10.48550/arXiv.1412.6980
21. LeCun, Y., Bottou, L., Bengio, Y., & Haffner, P. (1998). Gradient-based learning applied to document recognition. *Proceedings of the IEEE*, 86(11), 2278–2324.
22. LeCun, Y., Bottou, L., Orr, G. B., & Müller, K. R. (1998). Efficient backprop. In G. Montavon (ed.), *Neural Networks: Tricks of the Trade* (pp. 9–50). Springer.
23. Smith, L. N. (2017). Cyclical learning rates for training neural networks. In *2017 IEEE Winter Conference on Applications of Computer Vision (WACV)* (pp. 464–472). IEEE.
24. Zhang, M. R., Lucas, J., Hinton, G., & Ba, J. (2019). Lookahead optimizer: k steps forward, 1 step back. In *Advances in Neural Information Processing Systems* (pp. 9598–9608).
25. Luo, L., Xiong, Y., & Liu, Y. (2019). Adaptive gradient methods with dynamic bound of learning rate. In *Proceedings of the AAAI Conference on Artificial Intelligence* (Vol. 33, pp. 3552–3559).
26. Liu, L., Jiang, H., He, P., Chen, W., Liu, X., & Gao, J. (2019). Rectified Adam: A method for robust optimization of deep neural networks. In *Proceedings of the AAAI Conference on Artificial Intelligence* (Vol. 33, pp. 7241–7248).
27. Zhuang, J., Tang, T., Ding, Y., Tatikonda, S. C., Dvornek, N., Papademetris, X., & Duncan, J. (2020). Adabelief optimizer: Adapting stepsizes by the belief in observed gradients. *Advances in neural information processing systems*, 33, 18795–18806.
28. Dubey, S. R., Chakraborty, S., Roy, S. K.,, Mukherjee, S., Singh, S. K., & Chaudhuri, B. B. (2019). diffGrad: an optimization method for convolutional neural networks. IEEE transactions on neural networks and learning systems, 31(11), 4500–4511.
29. Tiwari, A., & Pant, M. (2022). Optimized deep-neural network for content-based medical image retrieval in a brownfield IoMT network. *ACM Transactions on Multimedia Computing, Communications, and Applications (TOMM)*, 18(2s), 1–26.
30. Baioletti, M., Di Bari, G., Milani, A., & Poggioni, V. (2020). Differential evolution for neural networks optimization. *Mathematics*, 8(1), 69.
31. Feurer, M., & Hutter, F. (2019). Hyperparameter optimization. In Frank Hutter, Lars Kotthoff and Joaquin Vanschoren (eds.), *Automated Machine Learning: Methods, Systems, Challenges* (pp. 3–33). Springer Cham.
32. Han, F., Zhao, M. R., Zhang, J. M., & Ling, Q. H. (2017). An improved incremental constructive single-hidden-layer feedforward networks for extreme learning machine based on particle swarm optimization. *Neurocomputing*, 228, 133–142.
33. Manjula, G., Shivakumar, M., & Geetha, Y. V. (2019, January). Adaptive optimization based neural network for classification of stuttered speech. In *Proceedings of the 3rd International Conference on Cryptography, Security and Privacy* (pp. 93–98).
34. Gain, A., & Dey, P. (2020). Adaptive position–based crossover in the genetic algorithm for data clustering. In Sourav De, Sandip Dey, Siddhartha Bhattacharyya (eds.), *Recent Advances in Hybrid Metaheuristics for Data Clustering* (pp. 39–59).
35. Dey, P., & Gain, A. (2023). A survey on energy-efficient routing in wireless sensor networks using machine learning algorithms. *Novel Research and Development Approaches in Heterogeneous Systems and Algorithms* (pp. 272–291).

36. Breast Cancer Patients MRI's | Kaggle. https://www.kaggle.com/uzairkhan45/breast-cancer-patients-mris (accessed November 19, 2021).
37. Egala, B. S., Pradhan, A. K., Dey, P., Badarla, V., & Mohanty, S. P. (2023). Fortified chain 2.0: Intelligent block chain for decentralized smart healthcare system. *IEEE Internet of Things Journal*. (Vol. 10, pp. 12308–12321).
38. Aon, S., Sau, A., Dey, P., & Pal, T. (2017). IMOGA/SOM: An intelligent multi-objective genetic algorithm using self organizing map. In *Advances in Computational Intelligence: 14th International Work-Conference on Artificial Neural Networks*, IWANN, Cadiz, Spain, June 14–16, Proceedings, Part I 14 (pp. 40–51). Springer International Publishing.
39. Mukherjee, S., Dey, P., & Pal, T. (2017, July). GFRP cutting parameters optimization using different MOEAs. In *2017 International Conference on Intelligent Computing, Instrumentation and Control Technologies (ICICICT)* (pp. 654–659). IEEE.
40. He, K., Zhang, X., Ren, S., & Sun, J. (2016). Identity mappings in deep residual networks. In *Computer Vision–ECCV 2016: 14th European Conference*, Amsterdam, The Netherlands, October 11–14, Proceedings, Part IV 14 (pp. 630–645). Springer International Publishing.

7 Paddy Leaf Diseases Detection Using Otsu and Yen Thresholding with Deep Convolutional Neural Network

Sk. Hapijul Hossen, Kuntal Mukherjee, Arkaprava Dey, and Sumana Kundu

7.1 INTRODUCTION

Every year we see a huge amount of loss in crop production due to bacterial attacks and diseases. Farmers are not trained enough to detect bacterial diseases. So, the method widely used by government and third-party agencies was an expert to visit the fields and collect samples. After sample analysis, the disease could be detected. But, this method is error-prone and takes a lot of time, so the time available to take appropriate measures is low. Paddy leaf disease prediction, the concept of this research work, centers on replacing human intervention in bacterial disease prediction using deep learning, neural networks, and computer vision concepts.

The proposed methodology works pretty well in classifying a given image. It has three main components. The first component includes reshaping, leaf segmentation, and affected spot segmentation. At first, the given image is reshaped into 128 × 128 × 3 pixels. The first step includes extracting leaves from the background using Yen's thresholding, which works pretty well on segmenting leaves from the background. In the second step, spots will be extracted from the leaf segmented image with the help of Otsu thresholding. The second component contains three sets of convolution, batch normalization, activation, and max pooling layers to extract meaningful information from images to reduce the feature dimension, which saves computational time and space and improves model performance. In the fourth step, the convolutional neural network (CNN) model is used. Here, the CNN model uses filters, precisely known as kernels. These kernels move images to detect useful features. In the fifth step, we predict the image with the help of this model.

 DOI: 10.1201/9781003391456-7

This research work has several contributions to the state of the art. First, most studies feed their images with noisy backgrounds and leaves, some segment the background and affected spots from the image with manual thresholding, while in our approach we use Yen's multilevel thresholding on the saturation channel of the HSV color space of the image to separate the leaf from the background. To segment affected spots from the leaf segmented image, we used Otsu's thresholding technique on the hue channel, which is a global adaptive thresholding method. Further, the processed images were fed to the convolutional network with batch normalization to stabilize the learning process, leading to a reduction in the number of training epochs needed. Last, we detected and classified images using a fully connected deep neural network (FCDNN).

7.2 LITERATURE SURVEY

Many researchers have developed various traditional systems or models for the prediction of rice plant diseases. A few of them are mentioned in the following.

H. B. Prajapati et al. [2] developed a model to predict rice leaf diseases. Based on K-means clustering, the model segmented the disease portion from a leaf image. They used support vector machine on extracted features from color, shape, and texture and achieved 93.33% and 73.33% accuracy on the train and test datasets, respectively. They used a digital camera to take photographs of infected rice plants in a rice field. M. A. Azim et al. [3] developed an XGBoost model on the same dataset and achieved 86.58% accuracy and F1-score of 0.87. There are 120 images of infected rice collected from the UCI Machine Learning Repository. K. Jagan Mohan and M. Balasubramanian [4] developed a model based on a HOG (histogram of oriented gradient) and an SVM approach to detect weed and crop recognition. Their proposed model achieved 97.73% accuracy. R. Sahith et al. [5] developed decision tree–based machine learning algorithms to classify rice plant diseases. According to their work, random forest achieved a 76.19% accuracy rate in its ensemble learning approach. They also used 120 images of infected rice from the UCI Machine Learning Repository: 40 images are bacterial leaf blight, 40 are brown spot, and 40 are leaf smut. R. Deng et al. [6] used a dataset containing 33,026 images. They found three submodels that gave the best performance: DenseNet-121, SE-ResNet-50, and ResNeSt-50, and integrated them into the ensemble model. M. Agarwal et al. used a CNN-based approach to detect tomato leaf diseases [7]. In their model, they used three convolution layers and three max pooling layers followed by two fully connected layers. The accuracy of the proposed model was 91.2%. J. Barbedo et al. [8] developed a deep learning model where no crop had accuracies below 75%. They considered ten diseases. J. Chen et al. [9] implemented the VGGNet pretrained on ImageNet. Inception modules were selected for their approach. The average accuracy of their proposed model was 92.00% for rice plant images. J. Barbedo et al. [10] developed a CNN model in which they considered 12 plant species and 56 diseases. The accuracy varied from 60% to 100% depending on the crop. T. Tawde et al. [11] worked on rice leaf disease prediction using machine learning and deep learning algorithms such as SVM, CNN, and KNN (K-nearest neighbor). Their proposed model predicts diseases like rice blight, rice blast, brown spots, leaf smut, tungro, and sheath blight. T. Islam et al. [12] came up with a model that takes into account the RGB value of the affected portions and then it is simply passed to a naive Bayes model. This method detected three rice diseases: rice brown spot, rice bacterial blight, and rice blast. B. V. Nikith et al. [13] came up with smart farming, which utilizes sensors and machine learning to tackle disease-related losses in agriculture. They compared SVM, KNN, and CNN models for detecting eight leaf diseases. The CNN model achieved 96% accuracy, surpassing KNN (64%) and SVM (76%). S. Omar et al. [14] developed leaf disease detection using CNN. Here, the CNN increased the accuracy of the results. Early detection of disease reduced crop loss and automated systems accelerated convergence and enhanced classification accuracy. H. Jianqing et al. [15] proposed a method based on image processing for detecting banana leaf diseases. It effectively segments disease regions, achieving recognition rates for gray leaf spot (91.7%) and sigatoka leaf spot (90%). S. Datta and N. Gupta [16] observed tea leaf diseases cause significant crop losses. So, they developed a deep CNN model that achieves 96.56% accuracy in classifying tea leaf diseases. S. S. Harakannanavar et al. [17] focused on using machine learning and image processing to detect leaf diseases in tomato plants. Various techniques like resizing, histogram equalization, clustering, and feature extraction were employed. The proposed models – SVM, KNN, and CNN – achieve accuracies of 88%, 97%, and 99.6%, respectively. A. Dash and P. Sethy [18] proposed an image processing method to detect maize leaf diseases like gray-leaf spot, rust, and blight. The proposed method successfully identified infected leaves based on image segmentation and white pixel count. V. V. Srinidhi et al. [19] developed a model using two deep convolutional neural networks (EfficientNet and DenseNet) to automatically detect and classify apple plant diseases with 99.8% and 99.75% accuracy, respectively. Narmadha et al. [20] developed computer vision and deep learning techniques to enable the detection of rice plant diseases. A DenseNet169-MLP model achieved 97.68% accuracy in classifying three diseases: bacterial leaf blight, brown spot, and leaf smut.

7.3 METHODOLOGY

Our methodology aims to develop an efficient system for detecting and predicting paddy plant diseases based on image recognition. This process comprises three main components (Figures 7.1 and 7.2), the first of which assists in preprocessing images before feeding them into the model, including resizing, leaf segmentation, and spot segmentation to remove similar redundant features to utilize the power of convolution. A second component assists in extracting features from preprocessed images through convolution, batch normalization, ReLU activation, and max pooling. A fully connected deep neural network (Figure 7.14) is the third component, which consists of a dense layer, LeakyReLU activation, dropout, and Softmax to classify images.

We have used standard data available at the UCI Machine Learning Repository [1]. The standard database consists of 120 images and 40 samples from each class

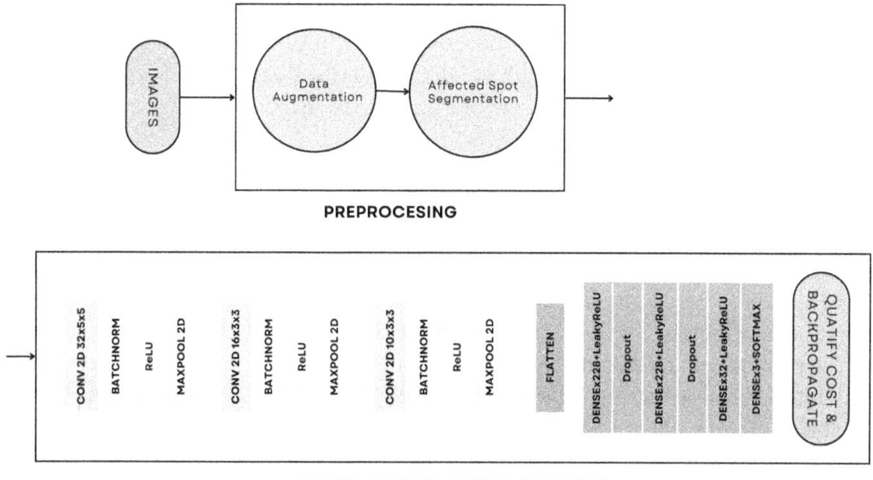

FIGURE 7.1 Architecture of training identification.

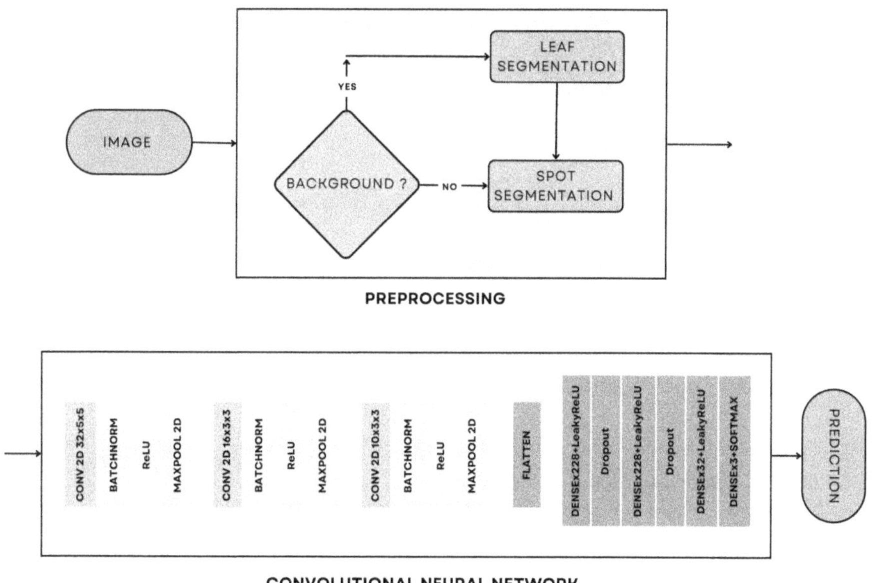

FIGURE 7.2 Prediction Architecture.

(bacterial leaf blight, brown spot, and leaf smut). Since the dataset contains few images, we filled the dataset with images obtained by image augmentation. After augmenting the images, the strength of our dataset was 949 images. The new data set is divided into train sets and test sets, 82% and 18%, respectively.

7.3.1 Database of Paddy Leaf Diseases Images

This database was created separately to classify infected leaves according to different diseases and is available in the UCI Machine Learning Repository. There are three groups of diseases: bacterial leaf blight, brown spot, and leaf smut with 40 photos each (Figure 7.3). All images are in JPG format. It is common for the leaves of the plant to be affected by bacterial leaf blight. Bacteria cause elongated, yellow to white lesions at the tip of the leaves. Infection can cause several inches-long, elongated lesions. Plant leaves frequently suffer from brown spot disease, which is characterized by round to oval shapes and a reddish brown to dark brown appearance. Plant leaves commonly suffer from leaf smut, which causes small, nonuniform spots to appear all over them.

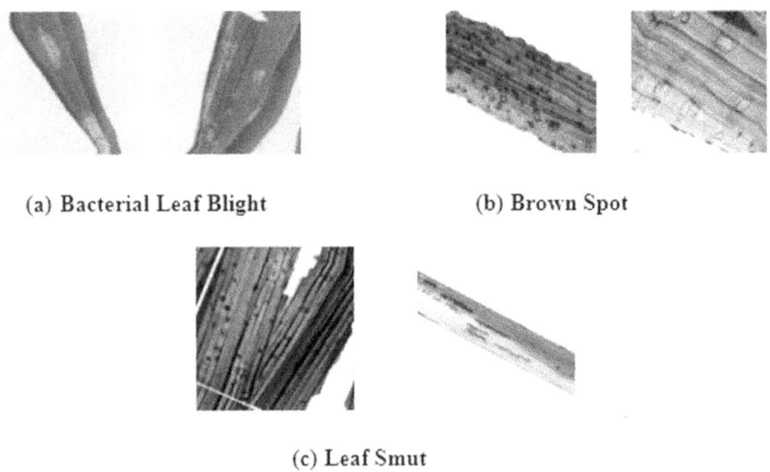

FIGURE 7.3 Samples of a few leaf diseases.

7.3.2 Image Augmentation

First, the image is resized to 128 × 128 × 3 pixels to lessen the number of pixels processed. The standard dataset contains 120 images, 40 for each of the three diseases. More than this is needed to train a model, especially deep learning models. To populate the existing dataset, we augmented images by applying different image transformation techniques such as random contrast, random rotations, random zooming, random crop, and vertical and horizontal flips. By doing so, models are able to learn patterns based on a greater number of examples (Figure 7.4).

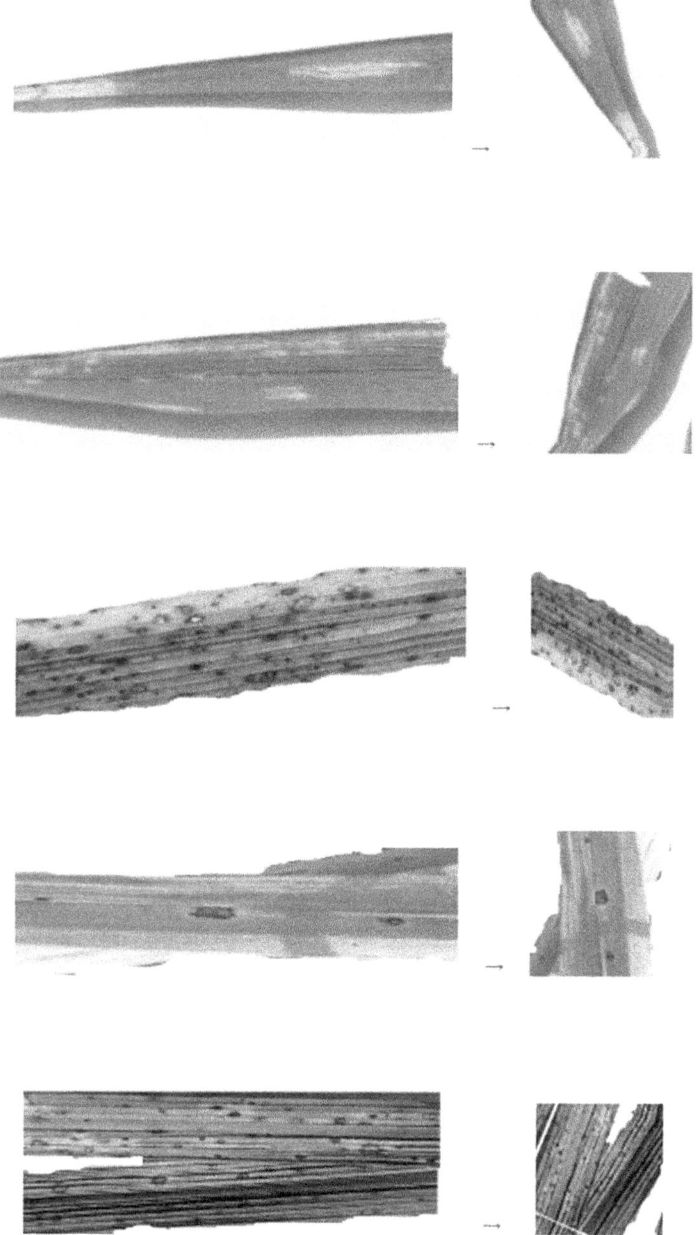

FIGURE 7.4 Samples of some original images to augmented images.

Following is the pseudocode of "Image Augmentation":

Pseudo Code: Image Augmentation

```
1   for class_folder in diseases_folders:
2           for file in class_folder:
3                   image = read(file)

                    # Applies Random Flip - vertical/horizontal
                    new = RandomFlip(image)
                    save(new)

                    # Applies Random Rotation with random angle
                    new = RandomRotate(image, random_rotation_angle))
                    save(new)

                    # Applies Random Zoom with random zoom factor
                    new = RandomZoom(image, random_zoom_factor))
                    save(new)

                    # Applies Random Contrast with random contrast factor
                    new = RandomContrast(image, random_contrast_factor)
                    save(new)

                    # Applies Random Brightness with brightness delta
                    new = RandomBrightness(image, random_brightnesss_delta))
                    save(new)

                    new = RandomSaturation(image, random_saturation_delta)
                    save(new)
4   return
```

7.3.3 Leaf Segmentation

An image with the shape of 128 × 128 × 3 pixels is input into this layer and a segmented leaf image is created. The binarized background mask is created using Yen's thresholding technique after converting the RGB image into HSV (hue saturation value channels). To turn off the background pixels in the original image, we apply a binarized thresholded background mask (Figure 7.5). To adapt thresholding to local characteristics only, the histogram distribution is used. In terms of Yen's definition, the threshold is determined by maximizing the image's entropy, which is ideal for images with variable lighting conditions. Foreground and background areas are separated using a threshold that has the most information. This allows it to handle images with varying lighting conditions and contrasts. It adapts to changes in image intensity levels and is robust to noise and uneven illumination. Image noise or uneven lighting can be solved more effectively with it. As far as our use case is concerned,

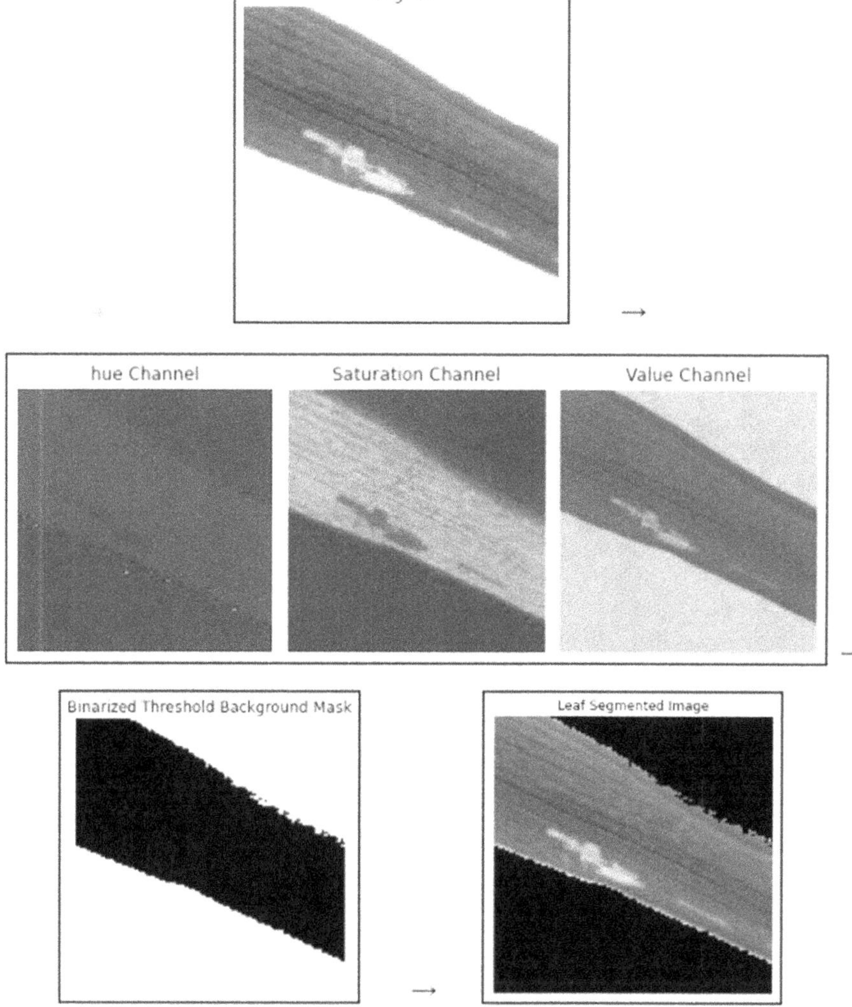

FIGURE 7.5 A sample of the leaf segmentation process.

Yen's thresholding is a reliable solution. It balances simplicity and effectiveness with lightning speed. Yen's thresholding is O(N), where N is the image's pixels. In comparison to other thresholding techniques with higher time complexities, such as O(NlogN) and $O(N^2)$. With its linear time complexity, Yen's thresholding can process large images quickly, making it a great choice for real-time applications. The leaf segmentation process is shown in Figure 7.6.

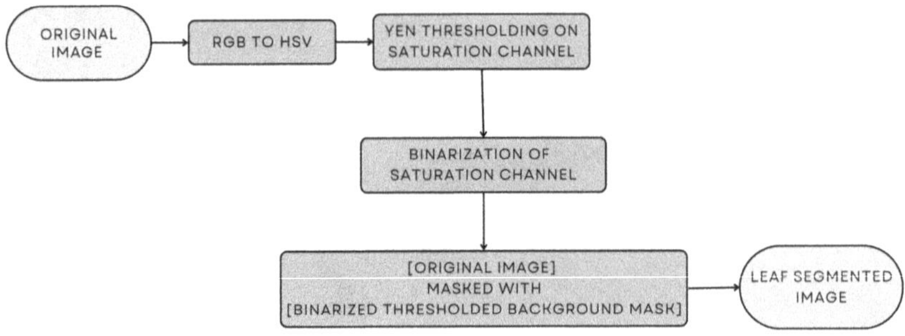

FIGURE 7.6 Block diagram of the leaf segmentation process.

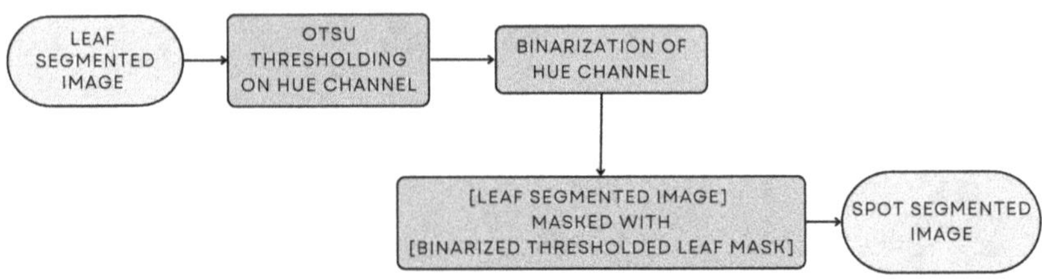

FIGURE 7.7 Block diagram of the affected spot segmentation.

7.3.4 Affected Spot Segmentation

A thresholding and binarization procedure will be used in this layer to separate spots from leaves (Figure 7.8) using Otsu thresholding. After thresholding and binarization of the hue channel, a binarized thresholded leaf mask will be produced. The next step will be to use a binarized thresholded leaf mask with the leaf segmented image to omit all pixels except the ones affected by the disease and to create a segmented image of the spot (Equations 7.1, 7.2, and 7.3). First, Otsu thresholding automatically determines the optimal threshold value without manual input. Second, it is robust to uneven lighting and noise as it considers pixel intensities. Furthermore, it

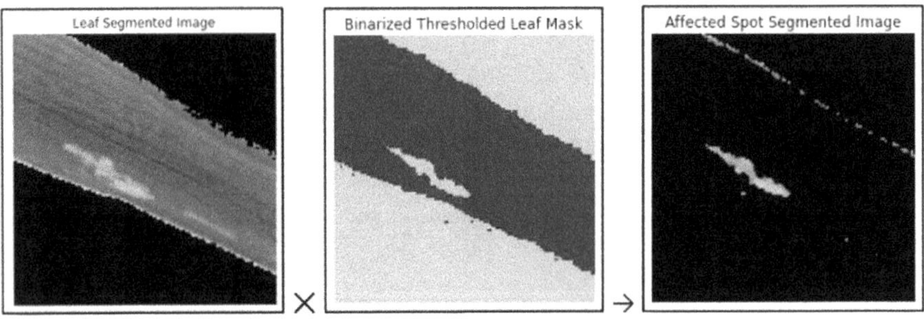

FIGURE 7.8 A sample of the affected spot segmentation process.

adapts to local characteristics to produce reliable segmentation results. This is ideal for bimodal images where the histogram exhibits two distinct peaks. A threshold can be calculated within a single pass of an image histogram, making it suitable for large-scale applications. O(N) time is needed to build the histogram, O(L) time is required to compute the first threshold, O(1) time is required for each subsequent threshold, and L candidate thresholds are needed, totaling O(N + L). The affected spot segmentation process diagram is shown in Figure 7.7.

$$between - class\ variance\ threshold\ as\ t,$$
$$\sigma(t)^2 = \sigma_{bg}^2(t)\omega_{bg}(t) + \omega_{fg}(t)\sigma^2{}_{fg}(t) \tag{7.1}$$
$$each\ class\ at\ threshold\ t\ and\ \sigma^2\ represents\ the\ variance\ of\ color\ values$$

$$each\ class\ at\ threshold\ t\ and\ \sigma^2\ represents\ the\ variance\ of\ color\ values$$

$$\omega_{bg}(t) = \frac{P_{bg}(t)}{P_{all}} \tag{7.2}$$

$$\omega_{fg}(t) = \frac{P_{fg}}{P_{all}} \tag{7.3}$$

$$P_{all} = total\ count\ of\ pixels\ in\ an\ image$$

$$P_{bg}(t) = count\ of\ background\ pixels\ at\ threshold\ t$$

$$P_{fg}(t) = count\ of\ foreground\ pixels\ at\ threshold\ t$$

7.3.5 Convolution Neural Network

7.3.5.1 Convolution 2D

The proposed method of detecting what features are present in an image is based on three convolution layers with 32, 16, and 10 filters. All three convolution layers have the same padding and stride (1,1) (Equations 7.4 and 7.5; Figure 7.9).

$$P_{start} = P_{end} = \left\lceil \frac{S\left\lceil \frac{I}{S} \right\rceil - I + F - S}{2} \right\rceil \tag{7.4}$$

where I is input, F is filter, and S is stride.

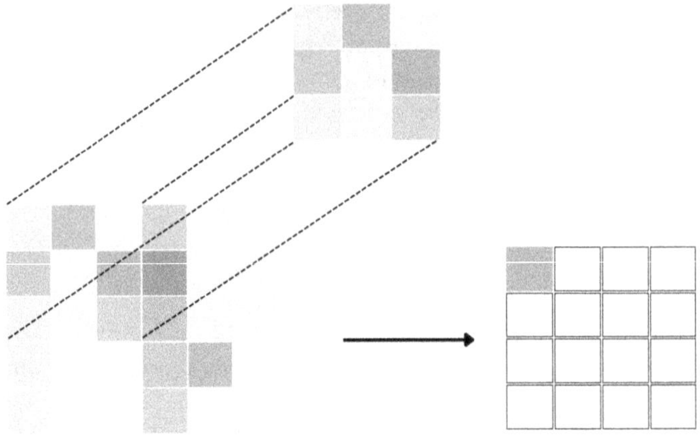

FIGURE 7.9 Convolution 2D.

$$\text{Output O} = \left[\frac{I - F + p_{\text{start}+} \, p_{end}}{S}\right] + 1 \tag{7.5}$$

7.3.5.2 Batch Normalization

To accelerate the training process of CNNs, batch normalization is used after each convolution layer before applying ReLU activation (Equations 7.6–7.10).

$$Minibatch\ B = \Sigma_{\text{i}=1}^{m}\ x_i \tag{7.6}$$

$$Mean\ \mu_{B=} \frac{1}{m} \Sigma_{\text{i}=1}^{m}\ x_i \tag{7.7}$$

$$Variance\ \sigma^2 = \frac{1}{m} \sum_{i=1}^{m} \left(x_i - \mu_B\right) \tag{7.8}$$

$$Normalize\ \hat{x}_i = \frac{x_i - \mu_B}{\sqrt{\sigma^2 + \varepsilon}} \tag{7.9}$$

$$Scale + shift\ z_i = \gamma\ \hat{x}_i + \beta \tag{7.10}$$

3.5.3 ReLU Activation

We used batch normalization followed by ReLU activation to create nonlinearity in the network (Equation 7.11 and Figure 7.10).

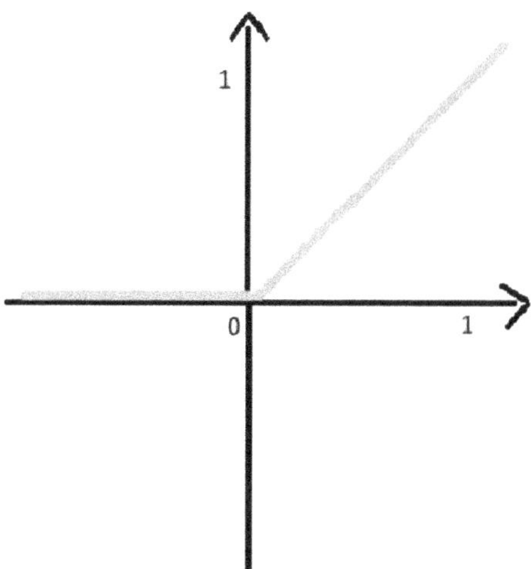

FIGURE 7.10 ReLU.

$$Relu\ g(z) = \max(0,(z)) \tag{7.11}$$

7.3.5.4 Max Pooling

We used max pooling followed by the ReLU activation layer to minimize the computational cost by reducing the number of parameters learned in order to overcome overfitting issues (Figure 7.11).

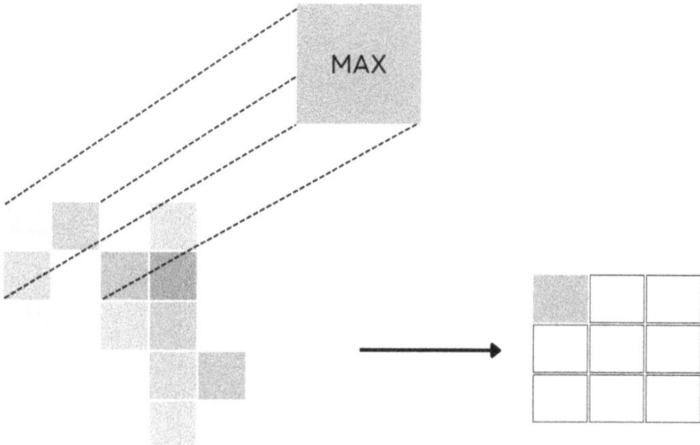

FIGURE 7.11 Max pooling.

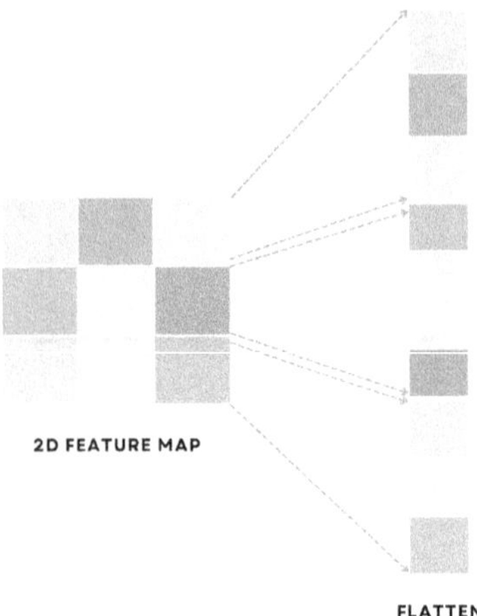

FIGURE 7.12 Flatten.

7.3.5.5 Flatten Layer

The flatten layer (Figure 7.12) takes a convoluted 2D features map and flattens it into 1D features, before feeding it to a fully connected deep neural network for classification. It makes features easy to interpret and less prone to overfitting as compared to normal fully connected layers.

7.3.5.6 Fully Connected Deep Neural Network

7.3.5.6.1 Dense Layer

In the proposed method, we have three dense layers that have 228, 128, and 32 neurons each activated by LeakyReLU (Equation 7.12), and the last dense layer has three neurons activated by Softmax (Equation 7.13) to activate one of the neurons.

7.3.5.6.2 LeakyReLU Activation

In the proposed method, each dense layer neuron's output will pass through LeakyReLU (Equation 7.12) activation. The reason we used LeakyReLU was that we wanted to increase the number of epochs to improve performance, and LeakyReLU worked better than other activation methods (Figure 7.13).

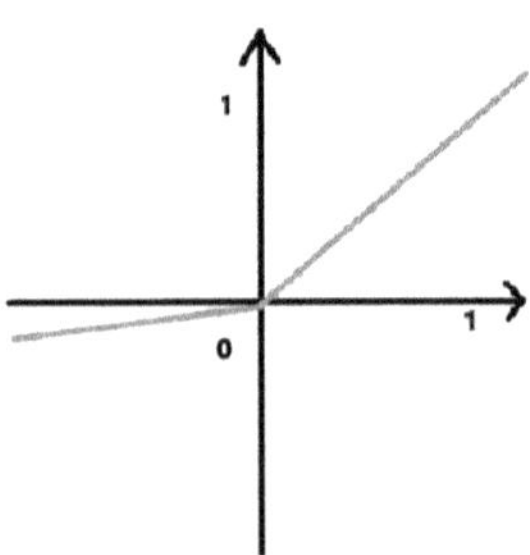

FIGURE 7.13 LeakyReLU.

$$LeakyRelu\ g(z) = \max(\varepsilon z, z) \tag{7.12}$$

7.3.5.6.3 Dropout

In order to regularize a neural network, we used the dropout layer. The proposed methodology applies dropout after the first two dense layers to make the network performance better on the test dataset.

7.3.5.6.4 Softmax

The final layer of the proposed network is a dense network of three neurons with Softmax activation. This layer is the output layer, which will give probability values for each of the three classes. A neuron out of three with the highest probability will be activated as the output (Equation 7.13).

$$p = [p_0, p_2, \ldots . p_n]\ where \qquad p_i = \frac{e^x i}{\Sigma_{j=1}^{n} e^x j} \tag{7.13}$$

The fully connected deep neural network is shown in Figure 7.14.

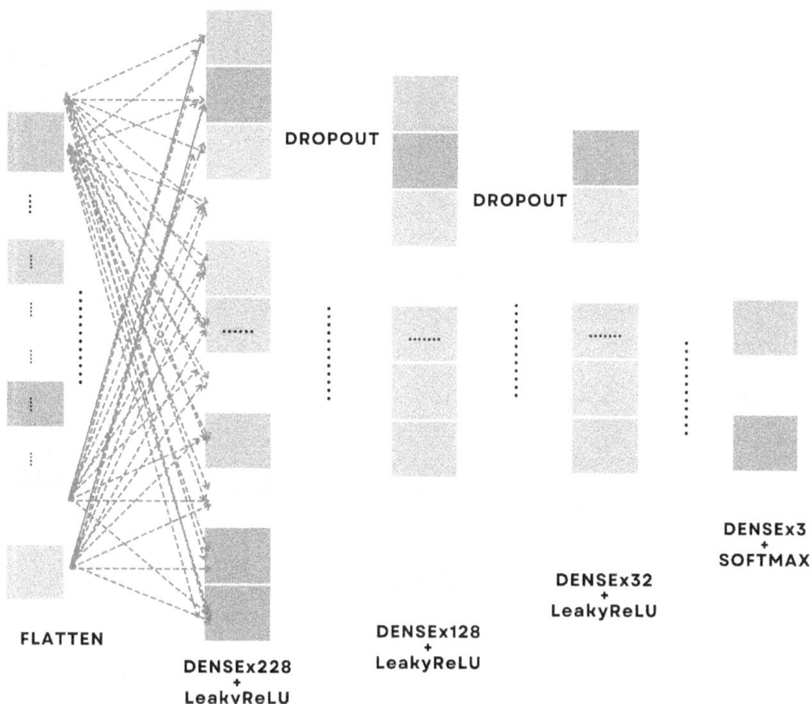

FIGURE 7.14 Fully connected deep neural network.

7.4 RESULTS AND ANALYSIS

The working model achieved 98% train accuracy and 91% test accuracy. A score of 0.99 on the train set and a score of 0.92 on the test set correspond to the F1-scores.

Metrics included for result analysis are categorical cross-entropy loss, accuracy, precision, recall, and F1-score. Table 7.1 shows statistics on loss and accuracy over the last ten epochs.

TABLE 7.1
Last Ten Epochs Stats

	Mean	Std	Min	50%	Max
Loss	0.094195	0.033585	0.038901	0.100562	0.149872
Accuracy	0.980754	0.007300	0.964889	0.982445	0.989597
val_loss	0.417216	0.016687	0.391864	0.418794	0.444246
val_accuracy	0.910556	0.006651	0.900000	0.911111	0.922222

7.4.1 Categorical Cross-Entropy

When there are more than two categories, categorical cross-entropy loss is used (Equation 7.14 and Figure 7.15).

$$Categorical\ Cross\ Entropy\ Loss = -\frac{1}{N}\sum_{i=1}^{N}\sum_{c=1}^{M} y_{ic} \times \log\left(p_{ic}\right) \tag{7.14}$$

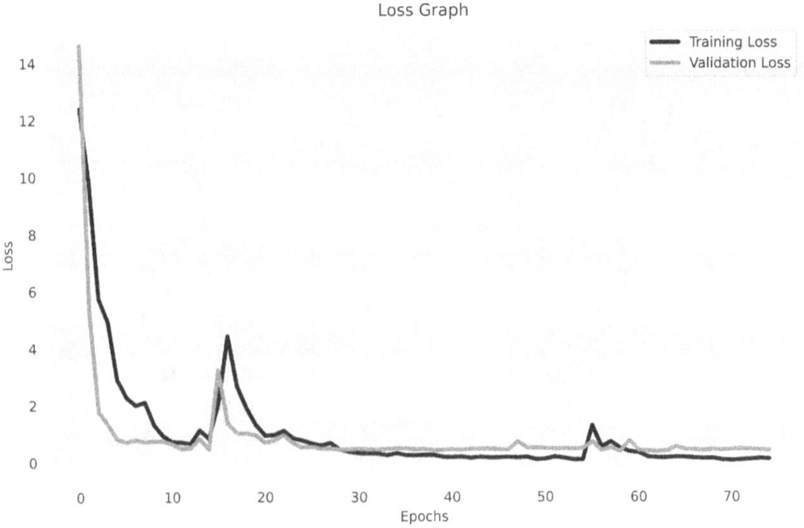

FIGURE 7.15 Loss graph.

where N is the sample count, M is the class count, y is the actual, and p is the probability.

7.4.2 Accuracy

Accuracy is a metric that describes the model performance over all classes. It becomes useful when all classes are equally important. We successfully achieved 98% train accuracy and 91% test accuracy with our methodology (Equation 7.15 and Figure 7.16).

$$Accuracy = \frac{True_{BLB} + True_{LS} + True_{LS}}{True_{BLB} + False_{BLB} + True_{BS} + False_{BS} + True_{LS} + False_{LS}} \quad (7.15)$$

where *BLB* is bacterial leaf blight, *BS* is brown spot, and *LF* is leaf smut.

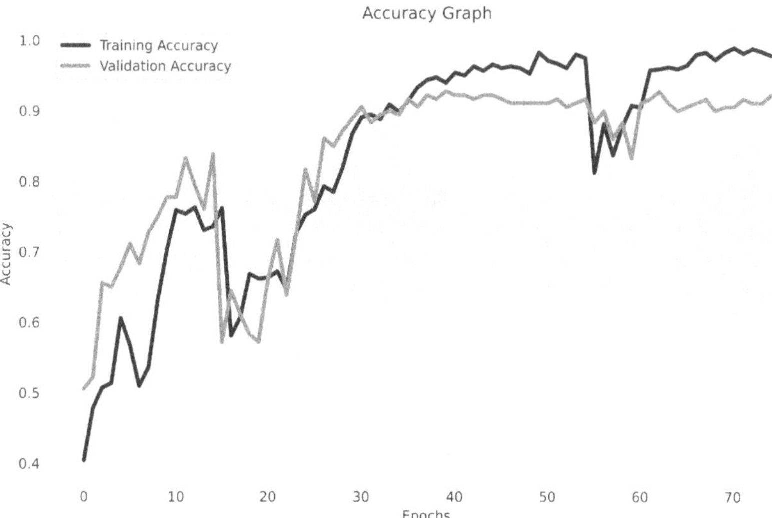

FIGURE 7.16 Accuracy graph.

7.4.3 Precision

An estimate of precision is obtained as a ratio between a class's correct prediction and total number of times predicted as the class. The precision metric determines how accurate a model is in classifying a group, category, or class (Equation 7.16).

$$Precision = \frac{True_{PredictedCategory}}{True_{PredictedCategory} + False_{PredictedCategory}} \quad (7.16)$$

7.4.4 Recall

An estimate of recall is obtained as a ratio between the correct predictions of the class and total actual count for that class. The recall metric only cares about how a particular class is correctly classified and doesn't care about how accurately other classes are classified (Equation 7.17).

$$Recall = \frac{True_{category}}{True_{category} + False_{others}} \tag{7.17}$$

7.4.5 F1-Score

An estimate of F1-score uses precision and recall as its core blocks. The main aim of the F1-score is to consolidate precision and recall into a single generalized metric. F1-scores give a single value to evaluate the model's performance, which is the computed harmonic mean of precision and recall (Equation 7.18).

$$F1\,Score = 2 \times \frac{Precision \times Recall}{Precision + Recall} \tag{7.18}$$

Hence, it is evident from the preceding figures and tables that our model has good accuracy and robustness. Our model is trained on 769 images (bacterial leaf blight = 254, brown spot = 254, leaf smut = 254) and tested on 180 images (60 images for each class). Our model achieved an average F1-score of 0.99, precision 0.99, and recall 0.99 on the train set and an average F1-score of 0.92, precision 0.92, and recall 0.92 on the test set. Because we have trained our model on more samples through image augmentation, it is more robust when it comes to detecting and classifying images. As part of our methodology, we also used Yen's thresholding technique for leaf segmentation and Otsu's thresholding technique for spot segmentation by removing unnecessary features from images during preprocessing. Therefore, these noises won't deceive the model (Table 7.2 and Table 7.3).

TABLE 7.2
Performance on Train Set

	Precision	Recall	F1-Score
BLB	1.000000	1.000000	1.000000
BS	0.992337	0.992337	0.992337
LS	0.992126	0.992126	0.992126
Macro avg	0.994821	0.994821	0.994821
Weighted avg	0.994798	0.994798	0.994798

TABLE 7.3
Performance on Test Set

	Precision	Recall	F1-Score
BLB	0.916667	0.948276	0.932202
BS	0.916667	0.948276	0.932203
LS	0.933333	0.87500	0.903226
Macro avg	0922222	0.923851	0.922544
Weighted avg	0.922593	0.922222	0.921900

7.4.6 Comparative Analysis

Based on Table 7.4 and Figures 7.17, 7.18, and 7.19, we can see that our approach has a performance edge over those proposed by K. J. Mohan and M. Balasubramanian, M. A. Azim, and K. Ahmed. Our method is robust because it is trained on more images obtained from image augmentation, and it is free of noise because only important parts of the image are provided by segmentation. Convolution and FCDNNs are used to detect and classify images.

TABLE 7.4
Comparative Analysis on Accuracy

	Proposed Method	Reference [4]	Reference [3]	Reference [2]	Reference [5]
Accuracy	98.075	97.730	86.580	93.333	76.190
F1-score	0.995	0.933	0.870	NA	0.760
Precision	0.9947	0.9333	NA	NA	0.7823
Recall	0.9947	0.9333	NA	NA	0.7723

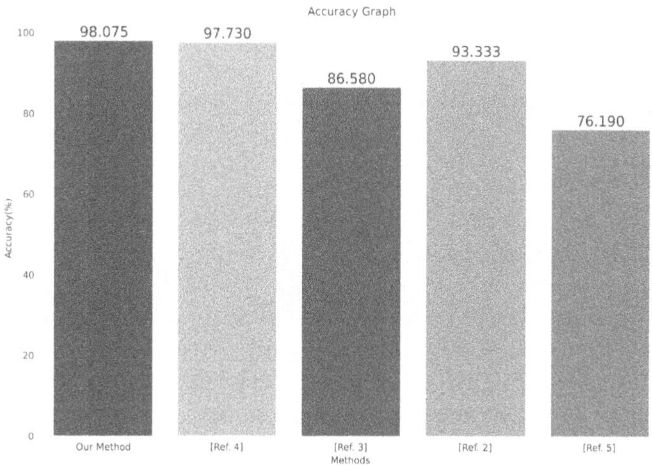

FIGURE 7.17 Comparative Analysis on Accuracy.

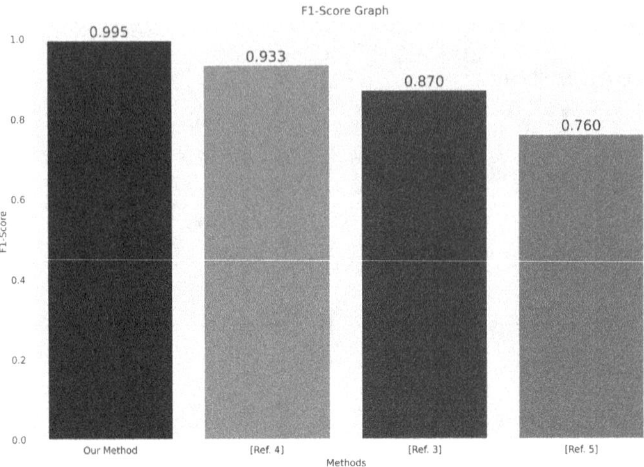

FIGURE 7.18 Comparative analysis on F1-score.

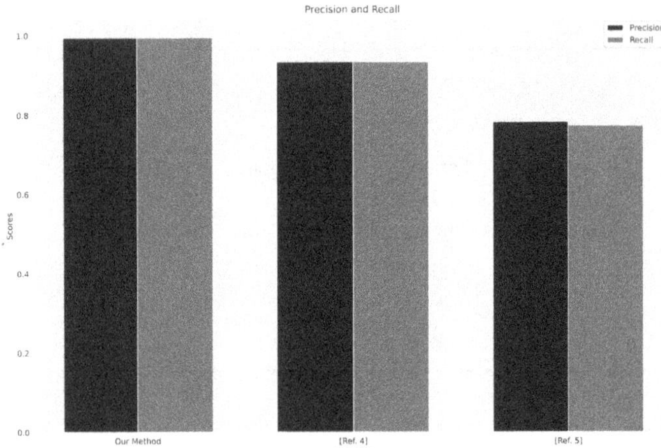

FIGURE 7.19 Comparative Analysis on Precision and Recall.

7.5 CONCLUSION

This work aimed to develop a model to detect paddy leaf diseases. Models were built in three major components (Figure 7.1). From preprocessing to denoising, the first component focuses on reducing unnecessary noise from the images. Further, four parts within the second component extract features from segmented images, including convolution, batch normalization, activation, and max pooling. The third component includes an FCDNN that focuses on classification. The proposed method is well suited for large-scale and real-time applications.

As a further development, our vision is to build an API service that can be used by different web and mobile applications, where a person can click or upload images from their respective devices, and then the deployed model will predict the disease from the images accordingly.

REFERENCES

1. Prajapati, H. B., Shah, J. P., Dabhi, V. K., "Rice Leaf Diseases Data Set", Distributed by UCI Machine Learning Repository (2019). https://archive.ics.uci.edu/ml/datasets/Rice+Leaf+Diseases.
2. Prajapati, H. B., Shah, J. P., Dabhi, V. K., "Detection and Classification of Rice Plant Diseases", *Intelligent Decision Technologies* (2017) 11(3), 357–373.
3. Azim, M. A., Islam, M. K., Rahman, M. M., Jaha, F., " An Effective Feature Extraction Method for Rice Leaf Disease Classification", *Telkomnika: Telecommunication, Computing, Electronics and Control* (2021) 19(2), 463–470.
4. Mohan, K. J., Balasubramanian, M., "Recognition of Paddy Plant Diseases Based on Histogram Oriented Gradient Features", *International Journal of Advanced Research in Computer and Communication Engineering* (2016) 5(3), 1071–1074.
5. Sahith, R., Reddy, P. V. P., Nimmala, S., "Decision Tree-Based Machine Learning Algorithms to Classify Rice Plant Diseases", *International Journal of Innovative Technology and Exploring Engineering* (2019) 9(1), 5365–5368.
6. Deng, R., Tao, M., Xing, H., Yang, X., Liu, C., Liao, K., Qi, L., "Automatic Diagnosis of Rice Diseases Using Deep Learning", *Technical Advances in Plant Science, Frontiers in Plant Science* (2021). https://doi.org/10.3389/fpls.2021.701038.
7. Agarwal, M., Singh, A., Arjaria, S., Sinha, A., Gupta, S., "ToLeD: Tomato Leaf Disease Detection Using Convolutional Neural Network", *Procedia Computer Science* (2020) 167, 293–301.
8. Barbedo, J. G. A., "Plant Disease Identification from Individual Lesions and Spots Using Deep Learning", *Biosystems Engineering* (2019) 180, 96–107.
9. Chen, J., Chen, J., Zhang, D., Sun, Y., Nanehkaran, Y. A., "Using Deep Transfer Learning for Image-Based Plant Disease Identification", *Computers and Electronics in Agriculture* (2020) 173, 105393.
10. Barbedo, J. G. A., "Impact of Dataset Size and Variety on the Effectiveness of Deep Learning and Transfer Learning for Plant Disease Classification", *Computers and Electronics in Agriculture* (2018) 153, 46–53.
11. Tawde, T., Deshmukh, K., Verekar, L., Reddy, A., Aswale, S., Shetgaonkar, P., "Rice Plant Disease Detection and Classification Techniques: A Survey", *International Journal of Engineering Research and Technology* (2021) 10(7), 560–567.
12. Islam, T., Sah, M., Baral, S., Roychoudhury, R., "A Faster Technique on Rice Disease Detection Using Image Processing of Affected Area in Agro-Field", *Proceedings of the International Conference on Inventive Communication and Computational Technologies* (2018), 62–66.
13. Nikith, B. V., Keerthan, N. K. S., Praneeth, M. S., Amrita, T., "Leaf Disease Detection and Classification", *International Conference on Machine Learning and Data Engineering. Procedia Computer Science* (2023) 218, 291–300.
14. Omar, S., Jain, R., Bali, V., "Leaf Disease Detection Using Convolutional Neural Network", *2022 International Conference on Machine Learning, Big Data, Cloud and Parallel Computing (COM-IT-CON)* (2022, 26–27 May).

15. Jianqing, H., Qi, Y., Debing, L., Jiarong, Z., "Research on Banana Leaf Disease Detection Based on the Image Processing Technology", *2022 IEEE 5th International Conference on Computer and Communication Engineering Technology* (2022), 53–56.
16. Datta, S., Gupta, N., "A Novel Approach for the Detection of Tea Leaf Disease Using Deep Neural Network", *International Conference on Machine Learning and Data Engineering* (2023) 218, 2273–2286.
17. Harakannanavar, S. S., Rudagi, J. M., Puranikmath, V. I., Siddiqua, A., Pramodhini, R., "Plant Leaf Disease Detection Using Computer Vision and Machine Learning Algorithms", *Global Transitions Proceedings* (2022) 3(1), 305–310.
18. Dash, A., Sethy, P. K., "Detection of Defected Maize Leaf Using Image Processing Techniques", *2022 International Conference on Inventive Computation Technologies (ICICT)*, 271–275.
19. Srinidhi, V. V., Sahay, A., Deeba, K., "Plant Pathology Disease Detection in Apple Leaves Using Deep Convolutional Neural Networks Apple Leaves Disease Detection Using EfficientNet and DenseNet", *2021 5th International Conference on Computing Methodologies and Communication (ICCMC)* (2021), 1119–1127.
20. Narmadha, R. P., Sengottaiyan, N., Kavitha, R. J., "Deep Transfer Learning Based Rice Plant Disease Detection Model", *Intelligent Automation and Soft Computing* (2022) 31(2), 1257–1271.

8 Applications of IoT-Enabled Systems in Healthcare Industry

T. Venkat Narayana Rao and S. Tabassum Sultana

8.1 INTRODUCTION

A term with many applications, technologies, standards, and initiatives is the Internet of Things (IoT). It primarily consists of an internet-connected network of objects. This includes IoT-enabled physical objects and IoT-enabled devices. The foundation and core of IoT are things and data. IoT assets and devices have electronic parts and software for data collection, organization, and sharing. It was Kevin Ashton who coined the phrase "Internet of Things". He considered radio frequency identification (RFID) in the late 1990s, a technology that enables tiny radio frequency tags to be integrated into diverse objects, comprised of information and being readable from a distance [1]. It permits, for instance, tracing the shipment of goods, enhancing the stock management system, and preventing thefts. It's a tiny sticker or special label in a plastic unit. In the commercial sector, these RFID tags are now frequently used. Ashton predicted that every single thing in the IoT would have a digital complement serving as its practical illustration.

Nowadays, a wider range of industries are using RFID technology. This technology is widely used to automate industrial processes, particularly in the complex manufacturing of automobiles and appliances (e.g., washing machines and refrigerators). Certain libraries, like the Vatican Library, which has more than 2 million reproductions of books in its collection, have adopted RFID to expedite book and catalog searches, automate book deliveries, and aid in preventing theft. Many public libraries around the world are utilizing this technology. Many nations now include RFID tags in passports. E-passports with a chip that contains the same data as the printed version are known as biometric passports. This technology is increasingly captivating the medical domain. Patients who require ongoing supervision are frequently followed wherever they go in conventional hospitals. The idea of a wireless sensor network was recently developed, and it can trace and manage objects by linking the tracking machine to the display of heart rate devices. To support the current IoT concept, these devices communicate and integrate with smartphones, cloud platforms, social networks, and predominant technology like big data analytics.

DOI: 10.1201/9781003391456-8

In the early 2000s, the number of hardware devices linked to the internet increased rapidly, and IoT has been actively developing. Concerns about user privacy are raised by the IoT's massive use of big data. The protection of users' rights is the main objective of the General Data Protection Regulation (GDPR). The challenges of implementing GDPR requirements in IoT were examined by Alexia Kounoudes and coauthors. To investigate the issue of user privacy more thoroughly, the authors undertook a methodical literary analysis[2].

The management strategy and proper endorsements of artificial intelligence (AI) trustworthiness designed by the European Commission as well as the Group of 20 (G20), the Organization for Economic Cooperation and Development's (OECD) Principles on Artificial Intelligence, and general human rights should be taken into deliberation while working with IoT. Particularly, the following interrelated principles should be obeyed: human-centric values and justice; justifiable development and fortune; reliability, protection, and security; and transparency, precision, and accountability[3, 4].

IoT requires a dedicated environment that includes various "smart" devices armed with network access, sensors, provision for supervising the network, data transfer, devices, and applications. This ensures that work is done continuously and, consequently, of a high standard. This system won't function if any one of these parts is missing. The industries dealing with mobile and internet service providers, federal governments, and even normal users must work closely together to fully realize the prospective of IoT capabilities[4, 5].

To examine the IoT's foundation in the healthcare system, this chapter focuses on how IoT technologies can be applied to the rapidly developing field of personalized health. It covers cutting-edge and complex IoT-derived methods as well as well-known health examples. The ethical, technical, and financial barriers to creating a better medical structure that can identify and diagnose ailments early are also a major focus of this study. Such cutting-edge health systems could be used effectively by healthcare providers to provide precise information about the correct number of patients at the appropriate time. This would induce quickly and effectively manageable medical situations. In this study, we intend to cover the function and a few uses of IoT technologies in the field of healthcare. We then present carefully chosen medical cases that highlight IoT-enabled healthcare systems, and then a discussion of the potential complications associated with using IoTin the field of healthcare[18, 21].

8.2 IOT-ENABLED HEALTHCARE

One of the most beneficial uses for IoT is in the healthcare industry. Internet-based medical services are made possible by IoT. The distance between the patient and the physician can be radically cut down due to portable IoT-based health supervising devices, as shown in Figure 8.1. IoT empowers us to approach every patient separately, assess their health, and apply a specific course of treatment. Doctors are able to monitor their patients' health remotely and respond in real time with the help of portable sensors, as shown in Figure 8.1A. Real-time metrics, on the other hand,

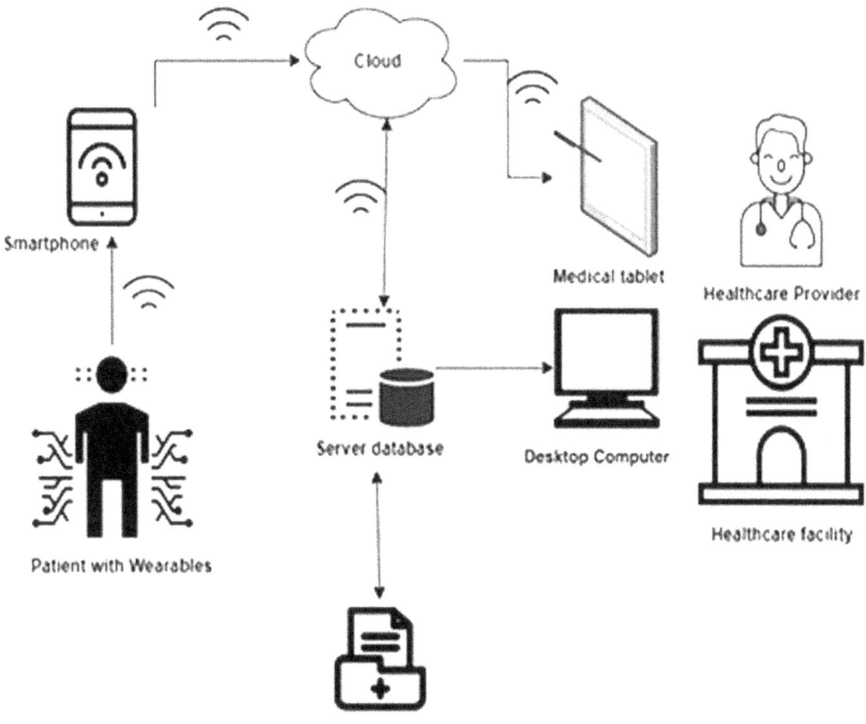

FIGURE 8.1A Healthcare and IoT.

necessitate a stable internet connection. Even though IoT in healthcare is rapidly developing, some medical industries are still not fully utilizing it. The creation of suitable internet applications for conventional medicine still faces some challenges. IoT will likely result in attracting more applications in the upcoming years as there is an enormous increase in medical research. The need to gather a lot of data, analyze it, and interpret it is something that modern medical professionals must deal with to make enlightened and individualized decisions. It all requires a lot of time and work for real-time decisions. This process can be stepped up and made easier by new IoT technologies[17]. A budding extent of digitized medicinal data is realized in association with the pervasive initiation of automated health cataloging. It takes a long time to fully view and evaluate all of this data. Additionally, it is necessary to train medical staff in AI-based technology, which is closely related to the IoT. Doctors might enhance treatment methods for patients through synchronized deliberations of digital technologies such as AI and IoT. These technologies make it possible to process a lot more data, store it, and analyze it to track a specific disease or process development in great detail. The management of healthcare will improve as a result of skillfully fusing logical, personal know-how with the potential of novel

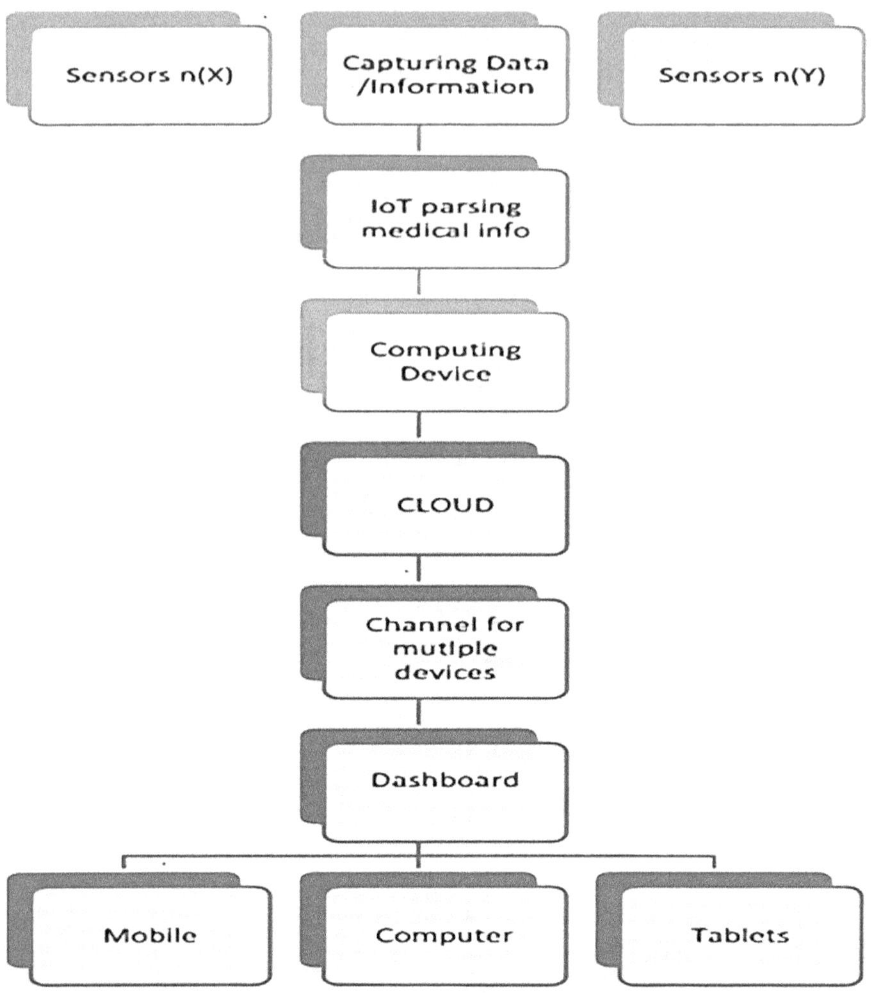

FIGURE 8.1B Phases of Healthcare and IoT.

approaches to diagnosis, gathering, and investigation. The IoT in healthcare concept is introduced in Figure 8.1B.In the end, the IoT presents network-assisted expertise, linking wearable and convenient devices that can be activated, detected, collaborative, and associated with other comparable media across the internet. Data production, use, and distribution are being fundamentally altered by the IoT. In contrast to IoT technologies, which routinely gather and process ecological data that influences a person's health, regular patients often use these systems to review their dietary ingestion, resting poster, vital signs, workouts, and other bodily conditions. This interoperability has eventually sparked a new wave of innovative medical alternative production[5, 6].

8.3 APPLICATIONS OF IOT IN HEALTHCARE

IoT applications in healthcare can significantly advance clinical care and research administration of patients. It also has numerous related applications when taken in a broader sense in the industrial and insurance sectors. In each of these situations, three key principles form the foundation of IoT contributions. The collection of data, the first guiding principle, is supported by networked equipment like cameras, sensors, monitors, detectors, and equalizers. Data conversion is the second principle. The analog inputs of sensors and other related devices must be prepared for further processing, and should be converted into digital form. In the third guideline, data storage, is normally accomplished by a cloud-based system. Data processing using advanced analytics modalities gives users the knowledge they require to make decisions. The majority of healthcare practices already follow the aforementioned principles, i.e., handwritten patient records to databases that are shared among several laboratories. The continuous flow of data is what makes them distinctive in the IoT context. The results of IoT-based decisions may be immediate. Wearable technology dominates IoT infrastructure for patients. Depending on the patient's history and the parameters that need to be monitored, this may include pulse/heart rate, oxygen saturation, blood pressure, and blood sugar level monitors. In the event of an urgent condition, these devices can guarantee individualized care or decline over time. If they are physically connected, they can also serve as reminders. IoT offers a direct connection to medical professionals in real-time to patients, coworkers, and visitors to their lab or clinic. A doctor could be informed if an arrhythmia affecting a patient or if they are being threatened by hypoglycemia. The patient can receive immediate assistance and medical advice. Device monitoring can also be useful to inform if patients are not following their medical care. The frequency with which pillboxes are opened each day can be tracked. There is evidence that IoT device datasets can help doctors identify the most effective management technique and course of treatment for their patients. There is an impact that is significant to personalized healthcare. On a larger scale, this is a big data approach. Treatment outcome studies could use this data as a starting point. Hospitals and research facilities on a larger scale serve as incubators for IoT applications[1, 7, 8].

This occurs as a result of the substantial load and variety of data required because of their accountability to be processed and the portion of the money they get. In addition to keeping an eye on inpatients and outpatients, IoT can be used in hospitals, labs, and the previously mentioned areas of health to protect tools like oxygen, nebulizers, defibrillators, and wheelchairs pumps. Additionally, research facilities can keep an eye on how experiments are progressing the deployment of tools and the ongoing accessibility of resources in a laborious way. Sensor and communication technologies are eventually used with greater trust. In several instances, multidimensional information technology solutions help researchers and clinicians to utilize the expanding IoT techniques to create novel structures and healthcare alternatives. The importance of IoT-related health research, which involves superior and effective preventive care, is profoundly lower cost. In many scholarly and commercial fields, especially in medicine, the Internet of Things is gaining ground as a cutting-edge

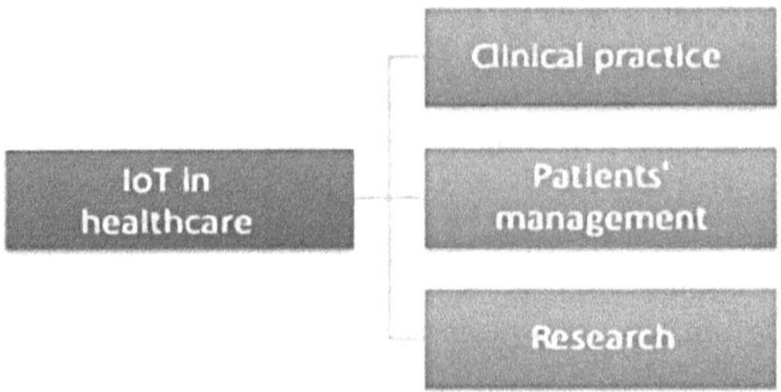

FIGURE 8.2 IOT key applications.

research topic. The acceptance of wearable technology, including smartphones, in general, are transforming healthcare from a conventional hub-centered system to one of more personalized healthcare programs. Individualized medical services have recently been made available to patients using e-health[9].

The era of big data has seen significant advancement thanks to IoT, which supports several current technical software to improve services in the present day. Medical systems are employing IoT data analytics as an input source to learn more about the identification of early diseases and choose crucial situations to improve life value. IoT devices can instantly gather and share data with other cloud platforms, enabling the gathering, processing, storage, and analysis of enormous amounts of data. IoT devices would be useful for remote environmental monitoring or computerizing local business processes. IoT applications in the healthcare sector show promise to improve patient access to care, cut costs, and, most important, improve quality of life. As well as improving their work, the healthcare industry and insurance programs can, through means of IoT applications, store data, assess products, and assess patients. IoT could be used to support quicker compensation services. The crucial are as utilizing IoT in the medical field are depicted in Figure 8.2. Such applications, however, may run into significant obstacles with legal challenges brought on by the interference and the data protection policy.

8.4 CASES OF EMPLOYING IOT IN HEALTHCARE

Symptom monitoring is now possible, thanks to mobile applications and wearable technology medical education, physical fitness, cooperative illness management, and coherence care. Analytics software programs could greatly improve data interpretation and reduce the amount of time needed to put the data back together.

The electronic evolution of medicine would be facilitated by research into big data business practices and choosing a time due to the growing global elderly population. It would be crucial to improve comprehension and inferring of health data; reduce chronic diseases, and diseases caused by diet; and improve mental abilities, mental health, and lifestyles. We will give a brief overview of the most well-known IoT healthcare applications; it would be impossible to list all of them. This is apparent from looking at the scientific literature and some commercial resources.

Wearables for cancer care systems have already undergone clinical trials. In 2018, a randomized medical trial was revealed at the American Annual Meeting and Society of Clinical Oncology. The research focus was on neck and head injury victims. A Bluetooth-empowered weight scale and blood pressure monitor were used to keep an eye on patients with a cancer cuff and a symptom-tracking app that sent both regular and needed messages to medical professionals. The study included about 400 patients, and the patients who utilized the IoT-based system reported having less severe symptoms compared with the control group, which underwent a weekly physical examination[4, 6].

Diabetes is a classical disease for evaluating treatment adherence and self-monitoring in a variety of settings, including oral pharmacotherapy, insulin injections, and blood among other things that need monitoring of glucose levels and blood pressure. Numerous current devices can be used to monitor glucose continuously. Even so, the majority of the time requires constant observation and prompt action[9, 10].

Increasing evidence suggests that type 1 diabetes mellitus (T1D) patients may be more. Patients may avoid complications with prompt or even constant monitoring. A smart insulin pen is a useful tool for gauging the treatment compliance of people with diabetes[19, 20].

Analogous devices could be employed for pillboxes as with insulin injections. Apps for smartphones can connect to wearables, and doctors can regularly evaluate them. Physicians might be informed if these modalities were included in an IoT context for patients who are delaying treatment and take appropriate action. Systems for administering insulin (automatically) have been long awaited in T1D care. The introduction of such facility has been hampered by possible regulatory and management flawed equipment used in clinical practice. Patients and doctors have engaged in a number of advocacy efforts. Networks have already been observed while accounting for potential IoT contributions important to overcoming such challenges. Despite the need for numerous steps, a closed-loop automation and IoT security can be crucial, and diabetic ketoacidosis is a risk for T1D patients. Asthma is a chronic illness treated with exaggerations, as opposed to diabetes that provides a favorable environment for IoT-enabled healthcare. The heavy liability is represented for hundreds of millions of individuals worldwide[11, 22].

IoT wearable devices that perform early detection are greatly aided by warnings of the presence of common allergens, and future exacerbation and its management. IoT-based inhalers are shown in the same frame could deliver trustworthy data about adherence to the patient's doctors and the patient's capacity to use the device safely. Both mental health disorders and asthma have chronic components. IoT can improve patient support in addition to the monitoring options already mentioned. IoT can offer helpful chatbots when combined with AI modalities for a wide range of objectives, including regular cognitive function and the detection of suicidal thoughts, and treatment for patients with dementia or slight cognitive impairment. We have highlighted a few instances of IoT deployments in this section such as cancer treatment, patient-oriented self-assessment practices, and medication. The asthma exacerbations are managed, along with delivery and adherence tracking support services for mental health conditions that are deteriorating, as depicted in Figure 8.3. Such methods

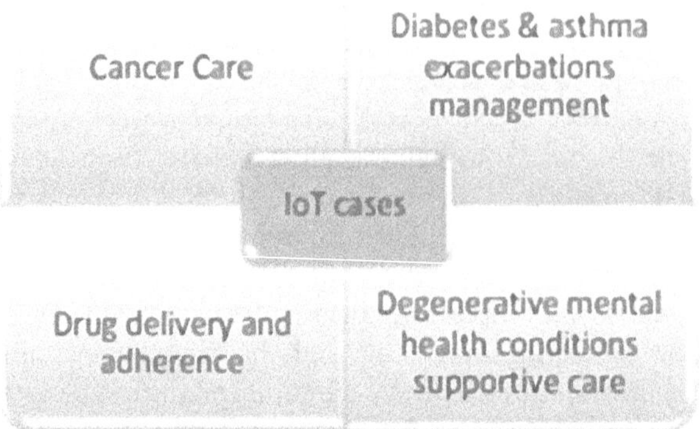

FIGURE 8.3 Select cases of IoT implementations in healthcare industry.

demonstrate how IoT has the potential to transform patient care and clinical practice, and if developed further and hopefully applied, management and research[12, 11].

8.5 CHALLENGES OF IOT IN HEALTHCARE

A revolution in healthcare is anticipated thanks to IoT. But there is no revolution without conflict. In actuality, it is a conflict between moral and technical standards that sculpts how innovation is applied. The issues of IoT in healthcare can be subdivided into three categories: ethical, technical, and financial[23, 24].

8.5.1 Technical Challenges

Since IoT is still not a common practice in daily life, there are technical considerations. Fifth-generation wireless technology (5G) and then the Internet of Things are used in the majority of nations. There are no services offered. Patients are included, but so is the vast majority of healthcare. IoT is not well understood by researchers and practitioners. What can IoT accomplish in daily life aside from healthcare? It is said that 5G could be regarded as IoT's first technical hurdle for the healthcare industry. The installation of numerous antennas required for 5G implementation is expensive, time-consuming, and thought to pose a threat to health. However, more research needs to be done because there is not enough evidence to support this claim to prove that the widespread use of 5G technology is safe, addressing international issues, consequences of 5G, influencing decision-makers, and altering with the assistance provided. The public view can take as much time as safety studies, if not more. The potential advantages of IoT use in healthcare can be a strong argument against the deployment of 5G. There are many different wearables in the healthcare industry as well as data gathering tools that are difficult to change into an integrated pattern of gathering data for technical, operational, and financial reasons. Manufacturers still follow the current standards and communication protocols have not been agreed upon. Different wearables that target the disease can be used by diverse patients with the dissimilar ailments. Patients with ailments such as diabetes might employ various glucose and sign-observing systems in addition to a dissimilar insulin pump with a closed-loop system. This would work for at least 3 different patient's data, despite the fact that these data will ultimately be managed and will take additional time, which may be problematic for conditions that are already acute. When multiplied by a huge number, management has also been a problem[12, 13, 25, 27].

8.5.2 Financial Challenges

In terms of the IoT's financial aspects, we intend to go into more detail. The International Data Corporation (IDC) estimates that Europe's existing budget for remote health monitoring is €10.41 with a previous budget of €12.4 billion that initially started with 1% billion only. It may look good to have such a budget concerning the implementation of IoT in healthcare. But there are complexities. Many potential investors have already been put off by IoT implementation. Third-party service providers may be involved to warrant the financial instability of IoT capabilities and the connectivity network that supports them. According to empirical findings, both public and private healthcare providers would be reluctant to be without data and experience from other healthcare systems/countries, and funding would not be provided for the creation of an IoT healthcare network[26, 28].

In 2014, the size of the healthcare marketplace was projected to be $60 billion. It is anticipated by the year 2021 to have a total worth of $136 billion. Notably, the healthcare IoT compound annual growth rate (CAGR) is anticipated to stretch or even surpass 120.5%during the forecasted period. This upward shift depends on the ability of the healthcare system and the outsourced suppliers to establish and uphold a sufficient level of consideration and collaboration. IoT has the possibility to lower healthcare costs if it is adopted. Costs associated with healthcare are typically broken down into direct and indirect costs. The latter comprise of healthcare costs and healthcare recipients' expenses, such as lost wages from missing work, the use of family members or other entities, as well as unpaid treatment costs. Since IoT healthcare services are not yet available everywhere, a cost-effective model of healthcare development based on IoT has been highlighted by economists that includes proactive asset management, inventory control, rigorous quality assurance, improved product packaging, and supply[14, 15]. In order for the Internet of Things to be financially successful, chain management has been acknowledged. However, as of now, these ideas seem more industrial than healthcare-related. They will need to work closely together to adapt to clinical practice between healthcare managers, clinicians, and economists until there is a deep understanding[29, 30].

8.5.3 Ethical Challenges

Data management and care are the roots of the IoT ethical debate in the healthcare paradigm. The three main contentious issues in the supervision of delicate health-related data are informative confidentiality, autonomy, and data sharing. In healthcare standards, the segregation and null interaction of doctor–patient interaction, the decontextualization of healthiness and well-being, and the danger of receiving unqualified medical staff are raising red flags in ethical guidelines. Policymaking in this area may be impacted by ethical repercussions. Universal law should be adhered to by any relative legislation including national and regional standards and the Universal Declaration of Human Rights. In the European Union, this is termed the General Data Protection Regulation (GDPR). In addition, it anticipates that ethical barriers to policy making could come from governmental policy makers in the domain of IoT implementation for medical field. This includes the guidelines stipulated by GDPR.

IoT research in the field of healthcare can be significantly influenced by the European Union. It is crucial to examine some actual scenarios in the IoT healthcare context and recognize the ethical responsibility[17, 18]. People will have sensors following them to and from work, become ingrained in daily life, and might even be overlooked by their users. All moments in the lives of medical sensor users, including typical variations in heart rate during a fight or a joyful occasion, will be recorded. Private conversations may also be "overheard" by sensors that detect and analyze the sound made by the consumer or staff members. Even if the users give their consent, out of concern for their welfare, the privacy of their relatives, friends, and coworkers may be violated by monitoring. Researchers have already developed remedies that promise a selective memory of IoT-linked sensors. Daily family disputes or silenced discussions of controversial actions occult hypertension or arrhythmia symptoms of the user. If the sensors are unable to determine what is important, a clinician or data scientist should. In order to make a choice, there must be a privacy violation relying on data chosen by sensors and only collected by them at the same time. It carries a heavy ethical burden to make potentially risky decisions. Assume a case if a monitoring system that is powered by IoT enabled set up to rise the anticoagulation dosage, it could be argued that studying causes extensive gastrointestinal bleeding[16, 31, 32].

By using sensors, the required evidence-based recommendations will be enabled. The patients need not do anything but just might have to respond to the queries posed by the monitoring system effortlessly.

IoT healthcare services should not ignore the importance of cybersecurity. Cloud-mediated services are necessary for data processing and storage despite all the moral issues surrounding outsourcing healthcare services. When it comes to who will have access to this data, hacking is still a significant risk. Insurance firms and human resources divisions are responsible for the potential for unfair treatment. Employees might violate biometric and medical history information. In similar circumstances, any other organization or person may assert financial or other claims to prevent interpreting sensible data.

8.6 PROPOSED METHODOLOGIES AND TECHNOLOGICAL PROCEDURES FOR IOT-ENABLED HEALTHCARE

Numerous studies concerning an electronic health system's development have a primary focus on delivering healthcare service through distant patient monitoring:

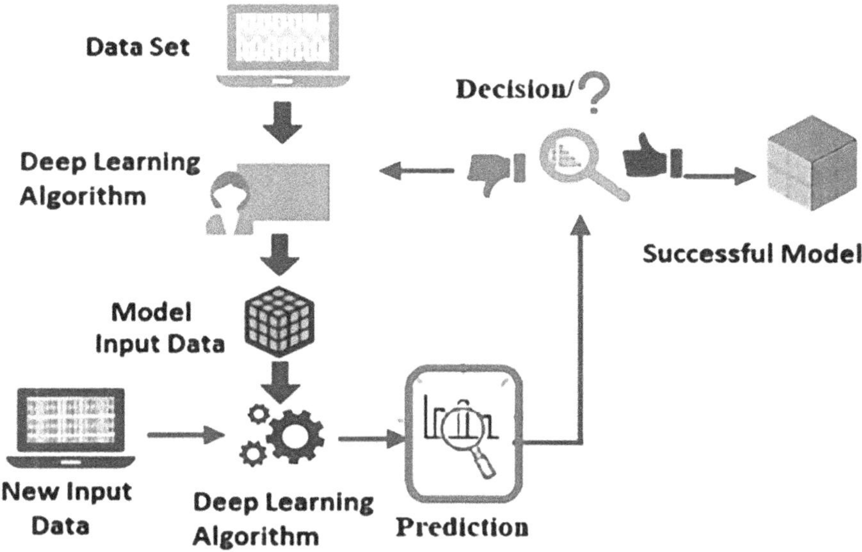

FIGURE 8.4 Learning algorithm–based step for assessment support.

- Wearable devices for patient monitoring
- Utilization of Message Queuing Telemetry Transport (MQTT)with IoT
- Integration of MQTT Protocol applied to IoT servers
- Implementation of decision enabling and support server

MQTT serves as an OASIS messaging protocol for the Internet of Things. Engineered as an exceedingly lightweight subscribe/publish messaging transport process, it efficiently connects distant devices with minimal code tracking and conserves internet bandwidth. Refer to Figure 8.4 for an illustration of the learning algorithm–based step for assessment support in the server.

The decision support service employs a categorization procedure, an AI or ML (machine learning) tool, to aid physicians in making informed choices. By analyzing data emanating from medical sensors transmitted via the Internet of Things, the server deciphers the patient's condition, thereby facilitating communication of the patient's status to medical professionals, hospitals, clinics, and healthcare centers.

8.7 USEFUL TOOLS AND FEATURES OF MACHINE LEARNING IN HEALTHCARE

8.7.1 Clinical Support Systems for Decision-Making

Clinical decision support systems (CDSS)aid in analyzing huge volumes of data to classify diseases, to decide and determine the next treatment stages, and to remedy patient care proficiently. The CDSS is an authoritative tool that helps doctors do their jobs resourcefully and swiftly, and it decreases the probability of acquiring the incorrect analysis or prescribing unproductive treatment.

The utility of ML in the healthcare industry has been evident for a while, it but has recently become extra extensive. The motive is the wide recognition of the electronic health record system and the digitalized state of numerous datasets and medical images[33].

8.7.2 Smarter Recordkeeping Process

Ensuring that patients' details are updated frequently is a challenging process, though it is important for active decision-making and improved patient supervision. One such tool used by machine learning as input is the optical character recognition (OCR) method for faster data entry and recording and later data can be analyzed to improve decision-making and treatment[34].

8.7.3 Machine Learning in Medical Imaging

Medical images have been dealt with as analog entities. This has restricted the usage of technology for abnormality recognition, segmenting into groups, and complete ailment examination. The digitalization procedure has led to more prospects with data investigation, which includes aid from machine learning algorithms. The ML tools are cable of viewing and analyzing the images with more accuracy with regard to 3D radiological images.

8.7.4 Personalized Medicine

The medical field is a complex and resource-demanding area in which every case has its specific priorities. So, complex judgments must be built on effective treatments, dealing with drugs to be taken, and reducing possible side effects. IBM's Watson Oncology system utilizes a patient's previous record to yield a number of multiple effective treatment alternatives[35, 36].

8.7.5 Behavior Changes

Avoidance of disease is a vital entity in healthcare, examination, and treatment. This includes modifying individual behavior to dispose of harmful habits and initiate a healthy and vigorous way of life.ML-enabled applications monitor a patient's everyday actions and list their insentient practices and repetitive instincts so as to enable them to forgo such behavior.

8.7.6 Predictive Approach to Treatment

Identifying rare and challenging diseases at early stages can considerably better the chances of life-saving treatment. ML in healthcare can be employed to effectively foresee certain dreaded diseases in high-risk patients. This might include recognition of possible liver diseases, diabetes, kidney diseases, and cancer.

8.7.7 Collection of Data

Data collection is a crucial task that physicians have to perform accurately while gathering a patient's history. Employing ML in healthcare, healthcare experts can ask pertinent questions of a patient based on numerous parameters. This will aid in collecting appropriate data and estimating the most prospective conditions for treatment.

8.7.8Care for Senior and Low-Mobility Groups

Machine learning would assist low-mobility humans, i.e., the elderly and patients who are immovable, with smart reminders and well-developed plans to help predictand evade potential physical harms by recognizing hindrances and defining the optimum course, and obtaining comfort as early as possible.

8.7.9 Robotic Surgery Process

Surgical actions need great accuracy, flexibility in varying situations, and a stable method for a long period. Qualified doctors have all these traits. However, one of the opportunities envisaged for ML in healthcare is to make use of robots to fulfill these actions. It is very well evident that robotic surgeries area vital aid and simplify surgical tasks for surgeons.

8.7.10 Drug Discovery and Production

Upon acquiring the data of vigorous elements in drugs and the extent they tend to affect the human body, ML algorithms could design a lively component that would work to study similar diseases. Such a method could be implemented to generate personal treatment for patients with rare diseases or certain distinct traits. In the future, this machine learning approach could be used with nanotechnology for improved medication provision[38].

8.7.11 Clinical Research

Clinical investigation and trials are expensive and long procedures. There is a purpose for this: new medical measures and drugs should be established to be harmless before being used extensively. However, there are times when treatment needs to be released rapidly, like the vaccines for COVID-19. Interestingly, there is an approach to make the process shorter with the aid of ML systems. It can be implemented to find out the precise model for the trial, collect extra points, examine the persistent information from the trial contributors, and diminish data-related inaccuracies[37].

8.7.12 Communicable Disease Eruption Estimation

The COVID-19 epidemic has shown how unprepared we were for a communicable disease spread of this magnitude. Specialists in the area have cautioned governments about the likelihood of such a situation for ages.

In current times, we have recognized that ML tools can aid in identifying signs of an epidemic ahead of time. The algorithm inspects the satellite data, societal media reports, and news sources to envision whether the infection is threatening to spread out of control[41].

8.8 STATE-OF-THE-ART TECHNOLOGIES INTEGRATED WITH IOTIN HEALTHCARE INDUSTRY

In the contemporary world, global startups are investing in revolutionary technology to optimize operations. Medical facilities must harness cutting-edge software to expedite healthcare delivery and navigate increasing competition. Presented next are notable technological advancements aiding physicians in streamlining their day-to-day operations:

i. **Artificial intelligence**: AI holds transformative potential for the healthcare sector. It empowers healthcare providers with improved decision-making capabilities, reducing the likelihood of errors. This advanced technology has led to more precise and efficient interventions, ranging from cancer diagnosis using radiology tools to the identification of infectious diseases. As technology continues to evolve, its impact on healthcare spans treatments, diagnostics, and care processes.

ii. **Telehealth**: The pandemic prompted a shift to online patient care, and telemedicine has since become a favored option for appointments. Beyond the pandemic, the flexibility and convenience of telehealth are set to make it a lasting choice. Patients in remote areas or those who travel for work can easily engage with physicians via technology, ensuring healthcare access without compromising well-being.

iii. **Hospital information system**: An efficient and cost-effective system is the backbone of healthcare. Hospital information systems offer a multitude of advantages, including revenue generation, improved decision-making, enhanced data security, technical advancement, error reduction, data monitoring, heightened patient care efficiency, and improved hospital reputation.

iv. **Blockchain**: Blockchain presents a user-centric approach to gathering, verifying, and sharing information securely. It safeguards patient data, allowing alterations only through registered user actions. This protection ensures data anonymity when necessary.

v. **Health chatbots**: Chatbots have become integral to hospitals, facilitating automated conversations to assist patients. They reduce administrative costs and offer information and support without direct interaction with healthcare providers. Their versatility spans diagnosis, customer service, patient organization, emergency aid, and medication management.

vi. **Cloud technology**: Cloud technology's role surpasses data storage, enabling hospitals to automate data sharing through applications. It ensures compliance with healthcare industry regulations while providing access to artificial intelligence capabilities, enhancing systems.
vii. **Advanced diagnostic technology**: Timely and precise diagnoses are pivotal to effective treatment. Technological innovations like blockchain, AI, ML, and IoT have revolutionized diagnostic capabilities. Laboratory automation streamlines test reporting, even during challenging scenarios like a pandemic.
viii. **Mobile health and Internet of Medical Things (IoMT)**: Mobile health tools empower healthcare providers with access to patient information, facilitating efficient data utilization for optimal care decisions. Mobile health integration enables tasks such as updating charts, ordering tests, and managing prescriptions.
ix. **Centralized monitoring of hospital**: Centralized monitoring of patients combats alarm fatigue by providing an additional set of eyes on patients. High-definition cameras and sensors enable remote tracking of vital signs, generating alerts when necessary and enhancing caregiver communication.
x. **Interoperability**: Seamless patient data exchange is essential for protecting identities. Interoperability secures data transfer, reducing clinicians' information search time and enhancing patient care while lowering overall costs.

8.9 DISCUSSION OF ADAPTABILITY AND FUTURE OF IOT

IoT aids in ensuring decision-making and execution rely on gathering and preprocessing of a vast volume of data. Additionally, the technology can help manage such a massive volume of dynamic information. People have created AI technology in response to change. One of the primary benefits of IoT is the process of widespread application of the technological revolution. One of the biggest innovations of this century will be IoT based humanity service. IoT is becoming increasingly popular as a result of the previous two years' explosive growth centuries. A projection of IoT in healthcare is depicted in Figure 8.5. It is well known that important decisions call for careful consideration of all factors, many different topics, and things that are unrelated to the subject in great detail. Basically, the choice should be as close to real time as possible due to particular physiological and cognitive factors. Due to such restrictions, people are not always able to react quickly and make wise choices. IoT and AI are important technologies through which the medical industry can gain a lot post implementation[21, 39].

IoT is a technology that is increasingly used in the modern healthcare sector. IoT has a direct impact on people's lives and demonstrates the significance of the medical field within contemporary society. One of the most promising systems is the medical industry in important areas where big numbers are consumed in information flow. It is not possible to use it or transform it into a particular end product, interactive

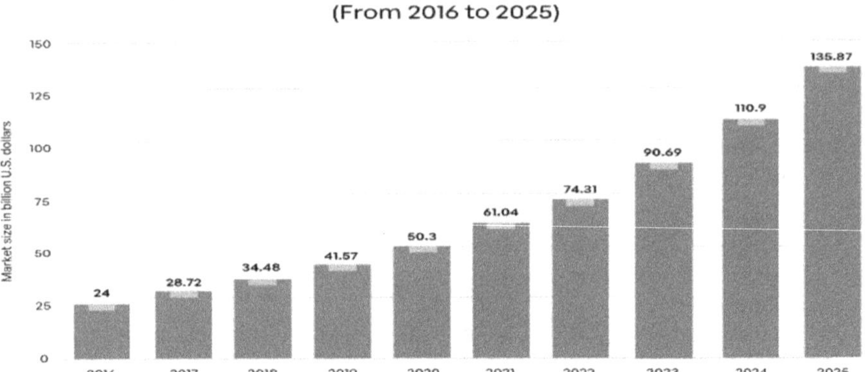

FIGURE 8.5 Future perspective of IoT in healthcare.

content, and cutting-edge technologies. Scientific research indicates that the majority of the leaders in the health sector think that the Internet of Things will bring about a revolution in the upcoming years. The three areas primarily involved in this are the prevention of chronic disease flare-ups, remote patient health monitoring, and data gathering. The IoT's fastest-growing sector is the health sector. Scientists predict that over the next ten years, there will be a tenfold increase in the number of connected medical devices. According to several analytics, there will be 92 million wearable medical sensors available worldwide in the next two years. Systems are designed to facilitate and optimize but not replace doctors and nurses. Using internet-based technologies, doctors can provide remote care for patients, especially crucial when the epidemiological system is deteriorating. IoT makes it possible to assess the health of each patient and to determine a customized course of action[17, 40].

As a result of the computerization of data collection in medicinal establishments and the optimization of the medical workforce, IoT can also make medical care easier by monitoring the patient's condition and providing more precise disease diagnosis and the progression of the illness in real time. IoT can also advance how well diseases can be predicted and prevented. It is conceivable that the number of medical errors is a sensible and rational application of AI and IoT. Significant reductions in practice are required in order to save more patients. There have been numerous discussions recently regarding the development and prevalent use of AI in many areas of human activity. There are some risks and obstacles in the development of IoT technology. Lack of is one of the primary systemic obstacles to knowledge of IoT's benefits. As a result, something is missing or imperfect in the company's development plan. Political risks and barriers are also an important combination of technological, legal, educational, and economic factors[42]. The protection of personal information, technology compatibility, and normalization with standards is very vital. These obstacles require more research to determine countermeasures, since they are the origin of a variety of threats when using IoT.

8.10 CONCLUSION

The chapter focuses on recent technologies that are quickly becoming useful in the area of healthcare devices to regularly monitor health biometrics or handle health-related data. These devices include healthcare using internet-based expertise and widely available smartphones. Health management apps are being used by both patients and providers combining the Internet of Things. In a field like healthcare, big data techniques are essential. The chapter reviews how IoT in the healthcare sector is transforming the development of efficient healthcare provision and building a platform for providing digital support at each step of communication between various healthcare segments. It further adds value in enabling quick adaptation of contemporary medicine to meet the demands of patients and adherence to time. As a result, it is possible to make medical decisions effectively. But AI has also been widely used in numerous areas of human movement.

This chapter has offered fresh perspectives on the functions and uses of IoT technologies in healthcare. Also described were some medical options that stress an IoT-driven healthcare system and the upcoming difficulties relating to it in the medical field. More studies should be initiated on AI and IoT or any other topic connected to the various elements of their creation and application, and as a means of providing healthcare in the future, use is encouraged.

The development of IoT technology faces certain barriers and risks. Systemic barriers include inadequate comprehension of IoT's value and an imperfect or lack of development strategy. Overcoming these challenges necessitates further investigation and the formulation of strategies. This chapter introduces innovative insights into IoT's role and applications in healthcare, with showcased medical cases highlighting IoT-driven healthcare systems and associated prospective challenges. Encouragement is given for more research in the realm of AI, IoT, and their multifaceted development, implementation, and utilization, as a pathway toward future healthcare enhancements.

REFERENCES

1. Li, S., Xu, L.D., Zhao, S. The internet of things: A survey (2015). https://doi.org/10.1007/s10796-014-9492-7
2. Kounoudes, A.D., Kapitsaki, G.M. A mapping of IoT user-centric privacy preserving approaches to the GDPR. IoT. 11, 100179 (2020). https://doi.org/10.1016/j.iot.2020.100179
3. Sadoughi, F., Behmanesh, A., Sayfouri, N. Internet of things in medicine: A systematic mapping study. *J. Biomed. Inform.* 103, 103383 (2020). https://doi.org/10.1016/j.jbi.2020.103383
4. Paranjape, K., Schinkel, M., Nanayakkara, P. Short keynote paper: Mainstreaming personalized healthcare-transforming healthcare through new era of artificial intelligence. *IEEE J. Biomed. Health Inform.* 1 (2020).https://doi.org/10.1109/JBHI.2020.2970807
5. Ergen, O., Belcastro, K.D. Ai driven advanced internet of things (Iotx2): The future seems irreversibly connected in medicine. *Anatol. J. Cardiol.* 22(Supplement 2), 15–17 (2019).

6. Gopal, G., Suter-Crazzolara, C., Toldo, L., Eberhardt, W. Digital transformation in health-care—Architectures of present and future information technologies. *Clin. Chem. Lab. Med.* 57, 328–335 (2019). https://doi.org/10.1515/cclm-2018-0658
7. Mittelstadt, B. Ethics of the health-related internet of things: A narrative review. *Ethics Inf. Technol.* 19, 157–175 (2017).https://doi.org/10.1007/s10676-017-9426-4
8. Psiha, M.M., Vlamos, P. IoT applications with 5G connectivity in medical tourism sector management: Third-party service scenarios. *Adv. Exp. Med. Biol.* 989, 141–154 (2017). https://doi.org/10.1007/978-3-319-57348-9_12
9. Latif, S., Qadir, J., Farooq, S., Imran, M.A. How 5G wireless (and concomitant technologies) will revolutionize healthcare. *Future Internet* 9, 93 (2017). https://doi.org/10.3390/fi9040093
10. O'Brolcháin, F., de Colle, S., Gordijn, B. The ethics of smart stadia: A stakeholder analysis of the Croke Park project. *Sci. Eng. Ethics* 25, 737–769 (2019). https://doi.org/10.1007/s11948-018-0033-5
11. Gope, P., Hwang, T.BSN-Care: A secure IoT-based modern healthcare system using body sensor network. *IEEE Sens. J.*16, 1 (2016)
12. Li, D. 5G and intelligence medicine—How the next generation of wireless technology will reconstruct healthcare? *Precis.Clin.Med.* 2, 205–208 (2019). https://doi.org/10.1093/pcmedi/ pbz020
13. Chai, P.R., Zhang, H., Jambaulikar, G.D., Boyer, E.W., Shrestha, L., Kitmitto, L., Wickner, P.G., Salmasian, H., Landman, A.B.An Internet of Things buttons to measure and respond to restroom cleanliness in a hospital setting: Descriptive study. *J. Med. Internet Res.*21 (2019). https://doi.org/10.2196/13588
14. Stefano, G.B., Kream, R.M.The micro-hospital: 5G telemedicine-based care. *Med. Sci. Monit. Basic Res.*24, 103–104 (2018). https://doi.org/10.12659/MSMBR.911436
15. Joyia, G.J., Liaqat, R.M., Farooq, A., Rehman, S.Internet of medical things (IOMT): Applications, benefits and future challenges in healthcare domain. *JCM* (2017). https://doi.org/10. 12720/jcm.12.4.240-247.
16. Sharma, L., Garg, P.K.*Artificial Intelligence: Technologies, Applications, and Challenges*. CRC Press, 2021.
17. Mohammadi, F.G., Shenavarmasouleh, F., Arabnia, H.R.Internet of Things (IoT) in healthcare: Applications, challenges and solutions. *2021 International Conference on Computational Science and Computational Intelligence (CSCI)*, IEEE Xplore, June 2022.
18. Mohd, J., Khan, I.H. Internet of Things (IoT) enabled healthcare helps to take the challenges of COVID-19 pandemic. *J. Oral Biol. Craniofac. Res.*11(2, April–June), 209–214 (2021).
19. Bhatia, H., Panda, S.N., Nagpal, D.Internet of Things and its applications in healthcare-a survey. *2020 8th International Conference on Reliability, Infocom Technologies and Optimization (Trends and Future Directions) (ICRITO)*. IEEE, 04–05 June 2020.
20. Phani Praveen, S., Hasan Ali, M., Musa Jaber, M., Buddhi, D., Prakash, C., Rani, D.R., Thirugnanam, T.IoT-enabled healthcare data analysis in virtual hospital systems using industry 4.0 smart manufacturing. *Intern. J. Pattern Recognit. Artif. Intell.*37(02), 2356002 (2023).
21. Tkachenko, N. Machine learning in healthcare: 12 real-world use cases to know, October 6, 2021.
22. Greengard, S.*The Internet of Things*. The MIT Press, Cambridge, MA, 2015.
23. Kounoudes, A.D., Kapitsaki, G.M.A mapping of IoT user-centric privacy preserving approaches to the GDPR. *Internet Things*11, 100179 (2020).
24. Fullerton, K.Coordinated plan on artificial intelligence (COM(2018) 795 final) (2018).

25. Paranjape, K., Schinkel, M., Nanayakkara, P.Short keynote paper: Mainstreaming personalized healthcare-transforming healthcare through new era of artificial intelligence. *IEEE J. Biomed. Health Inform.*1, 1203–1216 (2020).
26. Ergon, O., Belcastro, K.D.Ai driven advanced internet of things (Iotx2): The future seems irreversibly connected in medicine. *Anatol. J. Cardiol.*22(Supplement 2), 15–17 (2019).
27. Gopal, G., Suter-Crazzolara, C., Toldo, L., Eberhardt, W.Digital transformation in health-care—Architectures of present and future information technologies. *Clin. Chem. Lab. Med.*57, 328–335 (2019).
28. Mittelstadt, B.Ethics of the health-related internet of things: A narrative review. *Ethics Inf. Technol.*19, 157–175 (2017).
29. Latif, S., Qadir, J., Farooq, S., Imran, M.A.How 5G wireless (and concomitanttechnologies) will revolutionize healthcare?*Future Internet*9, 93 (2017).
30. Gape, P., Hwang, T.BSN-Care: A secure IoT-based modern healthcare system using body sensor network. *IEEE Sens. J.* 16, 1 (2016) 22, 65–76 (2018). https://doi.org/10.1089/omi.2017.0194
31. Li, D.5G and intelligence medicine—How the next generation of wireless technology will reconstruct healthcare?*Precis. Clin. Med.*2, 205–208 (2019).
32. Russell, C.L.5 G wireless telecommunications expansion: Public health and environmental implications. *Environ. Res.*165, 484–495 (2018).
33. Chai, P.R., Zhang, H., Jambaulikar, G.D., Boyer, E.W., Shrestha, L., Kitmitto, L., Wickner, P.G., Salmasian, H., Landman, A.B.An Internet of Things buttons to measure and respond to restroom cleanliness in a hospital setting: Descriptive study. *J. Med. Internet Res.*21 (2019).
34. Stefano, G.B., Kream, R.M.The micro-hospital: 5G telemedicine-based care. *Med. Sci. Monit. Basic Res.*24, 103–104 (2018).
35. Joyia, G.J., Liaqat, R.M., Farooq, A., Rehman, S.Internet of medical things (IOMT): Applications, benefits and future challenges in healthcare domain. *JCM* (2017).
36. Gruson, D.Ethics and artificial intelligence in healthcare, towards positive regulation. *Soins Rev. Ref. Infirm.* 64, 54–57 (2019).
37. Nikus, K., Lähteenmäki, J., Lehto, P., Eskola, M.The role of continuous monitoring in a 24/7 telecardiology consultation service–a feasibility study. *J. Electrocardiol.*42, 473–480 (2009).
38. Baker, S.E., Xiang, W., Atkinson, I.M.Internet of things for smart healthcare: Technologies, challenges, and opportunities. *IEEE Access* (2017) January 2021, DOI:10.1007/978-981-15-9897-5_1.
39. Tyagi, S., Agarwal, A., Maheshwari, P.A conceptual framework for IoT-based healthcare system using cloud computing. In *2016 6th International Conference—Cloud System and Big Data Engineering, Confluence* (2016). DOI:10.1109/CONFLUENCE.2016.7508172
40. Sharma, M., Singh, G., Singh, R.An advanced conceptual diagnostic healthcare framework for diabetes and cardiovascular disorders. *ICST Trans. Scalable Inf. Syst.*5, 154828 (2018).
41. Zhang, P., Schmidt, D.C., White, J., Mulvaney, S.Towards precision behavioral medicine with IoT: Iterative design and optimization of a self-management tool for type 1 diabetes. In *2018 IEEE International Conference on Healthcare Informatics (ICHI)* (2018), DOI:10.1109/ICHI.2018.00015.
42. Parmentier, F.Healthcare data and artificial intelligence: A geostrategic vision. *SoinsRev.Ref. Infirm.* 64, 53–55 (2019).

9 Enhancing Health and Environmental Monitoring

Open-Source IoT-Enabled SCADA System with Node-RED, InfluxDB, Grafana, and Raspberry Pi

Rajib Das

9.1 INTRODUCTION

Air pollution has profound effects on both physical and mental health, with long-term exposure increasing the risk of cardiovascular and respiratory diseases. This critical environmental issue not only impacts human health but also disrupts the natural ecosystem. According to the World Health Organization (2016), approximately 4.2 million premature deaths worldwide are attributed to air pollution. Therefore, understanding human behavior becomes crucial in identifying high-risk areas and times of air pollution exposure [1].

In the present era, the healthcare industry is experiencing a paradigm shift, thanks to the emergence of the Internet of Things (IoT), which enables real-time monitoring of patient health and environmental parameters. IoT-based healthcare and environmental monitoring systems offer promising prospects for improving patient outcomes, reducing healthcare costs, and enhancing access to healthcare services. To overcome the challenges in existing systems related to cost, complexity, and power consumption that hinder their implementation in remote monitoring [2, 6], real-time data analysis, and generating alerts, an open-source SCADA-based IoT-enabled health and environmental monitoring system with Node-RED, InfluxDB, Grafana, ESP32, and Raspberry Pi has been proposed.

This system aims to monitor essential health parameters, including body temperature, blood oxygen saturation (SpO_2) levels, temperature, humidity, air pressure, dew point, gas resistance, and air quality within healthcare environments. Leveraging

DOI: 10.1201/9781003391456-9

supervisory control and data acquisition (SCADA), the system enables real-time data exchange between field devices and a central control/monitoring center [3].

Open-source SCADA systems provide a flexible and cost-effective alternative to proprietary solutions, offering benefits in terms of scalability and adaptability [4]. The responsibilities of a SCADA system encompass data gathering, display, supervisory control, networked data communication, alarm processing, historical data archiving, data trending and reporting, and remote monitoring [5].

This work explores the development and implementation of the proposed open-source SCADA-based IoT-enabled health and environmental monitoring system. It discusses the challenges of existing healthcare monitoring systems, highlights the advantages of an open-source solution, and presents an overview of SCADA system functionalities and architecture.

By delving into this topic, readers will gain insights into the potential benefits and practical applications of open-source SCADA systems in IoT-enabled healthcare and environmental monitoring. This knowledge will contribute to the advancement of efficient, cost-effective, and accessible monitoring solutions, ultimately leading to improved healthcare outcomes and environmental sustainability.

9.2 LITERATURE REVIEW

In recent years, there has been a significant increase in the use of IoT in healthcare. Several researchers have proposed various IoT-based healthcare monitoring systems. For example, Rahmani et al. [14] proposed the use of smart e-health gateways at the edge of healthcare IoT systems to improve data processing and reduce latency. The study utilized fog computing, a form of edge computing, to enable real-time data processing and analysis at the edge of the network, which can improve the efficiency and reliability of healthcare IoT systems.

Hariz Hasshim et al. [15] proposed an IoT-based health monitoring system designed to monitor the vital signs of elderly patients, including heart rate, body temperature, and blood pressure, and send alerts to caregivers in case of any abnormalities. The study showed that the system was reliable and could provide continuous monitoring without being intrusive.

Islam et al. [16] developed a smart healthcare monitoring system that included sensors for monitoring heart rate, blood pressure, body temperature, blood oxygen level, CO, and CO_2. The condition of the patient is conveyed via a portal to medical staff, where they can process and analyze the current situation of the patient.

Polu's [17] system was designed to monitor patients' vital signs, medication adherence, and lifestyle factors, and provide real-time feedback to patients and caregivers. The study showed that the system was effective in improving patient outcomes and reducing healthcare costs.

Selvaraj et al. [18] conducted a systematic review of challenges and opportunities in IoT healthcare systems. The study emphasized the need for secure and private data storage and transmission, as well as the need to ensure the interoperability of different devices and systems.

Abdulmalek et al. [19] conducted a review of IoT-based healthcare monitoring systems and identified several key features that such systems should possess, including real-time monitoring, remote access, data analytics, and data security. The review explores the latest trends in healthcare monitoring systems by implementing the role of the IoT.

Qian et al. [20] developed a real-time wearable fall detection system that was designed to detect falls and provide immediate assistance to patients. The system utilized wearable sensors and machine learning algorithms to detect falls and determine the severity of the fall. The study showed that the system was effective in detecting falls and could provide timely assistance to patients.

Another example is the work done by Tsao et al. [7], who proposed an IoT-based smart system that included various wearable devices that monitor the wearer's vital signs such as body temperature, head temperature, heart rate, blood pressure, and blood oxygen saturation. The system also included a user interface that displays the collected data and provides real-time alerts and notifications.

There is no local storage or edge device for sensor data for data analytics and professional visualizations that has been found in the previous literature. Moreover, there is also no concept of SCADA that introduces automation and alert features in healthcare smart systems. This work overcomes these limitations in an efficient way.

9.3 OBJECTIVES

Designing and implementing an open-source IoT-enabled SCADA-based health and environmental monitoring system for smart healthcare systems using Node-RED, InfluxDB, Grafana, and Raspberry Pi is the main goal of this work. The proposed system is designed to measure various health parameters such as body temperature and SpO_2, and environmental parameters such as temperature, humidity, air pressure, dew point, gas resistance, and air quality. The proposed monitoring system is built using a Raspberry Pi 4 IoT server, ESP32, MQTT, Node-RED, InfluxDB, and Grafana. The Raspberry Pi 4 IoT server acts as a central hub for the monitoring system, providing connectivity to the sensors, data storage, and data visualization tools. The ESP32 serves as a low-power microcontroller that collects data from the sensors and transmits it to the Raspberry Pi 4 using the MQTT protocol. Node-RED is used for data processing and analysis, while InfluxDB is used for data storage and retrieval. Grafana is used for data visualization, enabling users to easily view and analyze the collected data. The system will also generate alerts or send notifications based on sensor data threshold values and allow smart control of healthcare appliances using a four-channel relay module.

Technical reasons for choosing the development infrastructure include implementing an open-source smart edge device (local IoT physical server) for healthcare systems. In the cloud, data are easily stored, processed, and connected but with some considerations like latency, connectivity costs, privacy, and security concerns. Node-RED was chosen for gathering sensor data using the Mosquitto broker and handling supervisory monitoring, remote control of healthcare smart appliances, and generating alerts based on sensor data. Moreover, Grafana was chosen to enhance the data analytics and professional monitoring capabilities of sensor data.

9.4 DEVELOPMENT METHODOLOGY

The development process for the suggested system is covered in this section. The proposed system is designed to be a low-power, portable, open-source SCADA-based IoT-enabled health and environmental monitoring system for healthcare systems. The system uses the Raspberry Pi 4 IoT server, ESP32, MQTT, Node-RED, InfluxDB, and Grafana.

The proposed system comprises several subsystems that work together to achieve its goals. These subsystems include the hardware subsystem, software subsystem, and network subsystem.

The hardware subsystem is composed of a Raspberry Pi 4 IoT server, ESP32, and several sensors. The Raspberry Pi 4 is used as the main controller and server for the system. It is connected to the internet through Wi-Fi or Ethernet. The ESP32 is used as the sensor node and communicates with the Raspberry Pi 4 through MQTT. The sensors used in the system include the DS18B20 for body temperature measurement; MAX30102 for SpO_2 measurement; BME680 for temperature, humidity, air pressure, dew point, and gas resistance measurement; and MQ135 for air quality monitoring.

Node-RED, InfluxDB, and Grafana make up the software subsystem. Node-RED is a flow-based programming tool that is used to develop the data acquisition and control system. It is set up on the Raspberry Pi 4 and is used to acquire data from the sensors, process the data, and control the healthcare appliances. InfluxDB is a time series database that is used to store the data collected from the sensors. Grafana is a data visualization tool that is used to display the data collected from the sensors in real time.

The network subsystem is used to connect the different components of the system. The ESP32 communicates with the Raspberry Pi 4 through MQTT. The Raspberry Pi 4 communicates with the internet through Wi-Fi or Ethernet.

The proposed system will be built using the Raspberry Pi 4 IoT server, ESP32, MQTT, Node-RED, InfluxDB, and Grafana. The system will use the DS18B20 sensor to measure body temperature; MAX30102 particle sensor to measure SpO_2; BME680 sensor to measure temperature, humidity, air pressure, gas resistance, and dew point; and MQ-135 gas sensor to measure air quality. The data collected from the sensors will be transmitted to the IoT server using the MQTT protocol. Node-RED will be used to create the dashboard and set up the alert system. The data will be stored in the InfluxDB database, and Grafana will be used for data visualization. For portability, the system will be powered by a lithium-ion battery and a 5V power supply. Email notification features will also be included in the system.

9.5 SYSTEM OPERATION

The proposed system operates as follows:

1. The sensors measure health and environmental parameters, such as body temperature, SpO_2, temperature, humidity, air pressure, dew point, gas resistance, and air quality.
2. The ESP32 microcontroller sends the sensor data to the Raspberry Pi 4 IoT server using the MQTT protocol.
3. Node-RED receives the sensor data and stores it in the InfluxDB time series database.
4. Node-RED compares the sensor data with the threshold values configured by the user through the GUI. If the sensor data exceeds the threshold values, Node-RED generates an alert or notification through email.
5. Grafana creates interactive dashboards to visualize the sensor data in real time.

9.6 SYSTEM ARCHITECTURE AND DESIGN

The proposed system architecture consists of three major components, namely, hardware, software, and a physical IoT server. Figure 9.1 shows the overall system architecture.

9.6.1 Hardware Architecture

The hardware architecture consists of an IoT physical server module (Raspberry Pi 4), client modules using (ESP32 DOIT KIT v1), and a laptop or tablet or smartphone along with different sensors and actuators such as MAX30102, DS18B20, BME680, MQ-135, buzzer, bulb, four-channel 5V relay module, DC fan, jumper wires, and AC and DC power source for valuable operation. Brief descriptions of the prototype hardware are discussed herewith.

The hardware architecture of the proposed system comprises various sensors, actuators, the physical server module Raspberry Pi 4, client modules ESP32 (ESP32 DOIT KIT v1), and a laptop or tablet or smartphone. The sensors used in this system include a temperature sensor (DS18B20); a particle sensor (MAX30102); a gas sensor (MQ-135); a BME680 sensor for measuring humidity, temperature, air pressure, and gas resistance; and a relay module for controlling appliances or generating alerts, or sending the necessary signals to actuators (AC bulb, DC fan, buzzer). All these sensors and actuators are connected to the ESP32 modules. The Raspberry Pi 4 serves as the main processing unit for the system. It runs on the Raspbian operating system and provides the necessary computing power for the system. The ESP32 module is used for wireless communication with the sensors and actuators and for sending or receiving data to or from the local physical IoT server using the MQTT protocol. Brief descriptions of the prototype hardware are as follows.

9.6.1.1 Raspberry Pi 4

The Raspberry Pi, a credit card-sized computer, does not have a separate CPU, RAM, or GPU. Instead, they are all squeezed into one component called a system-on-chip, or SoC, unit. It is open hardware with the exception of its primary chip,

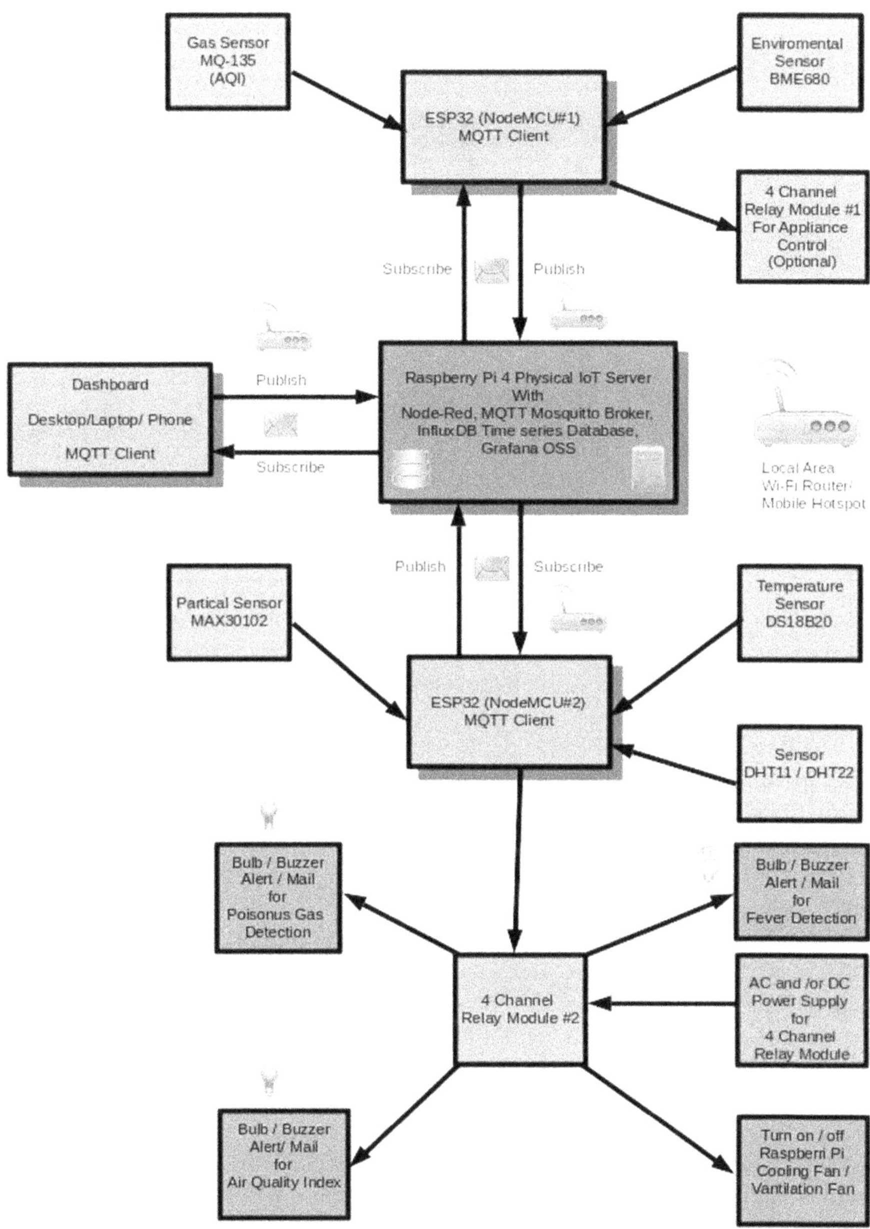

FIGURE 9.1 Building block representation of the proposed IoT-enabled SCADA system.

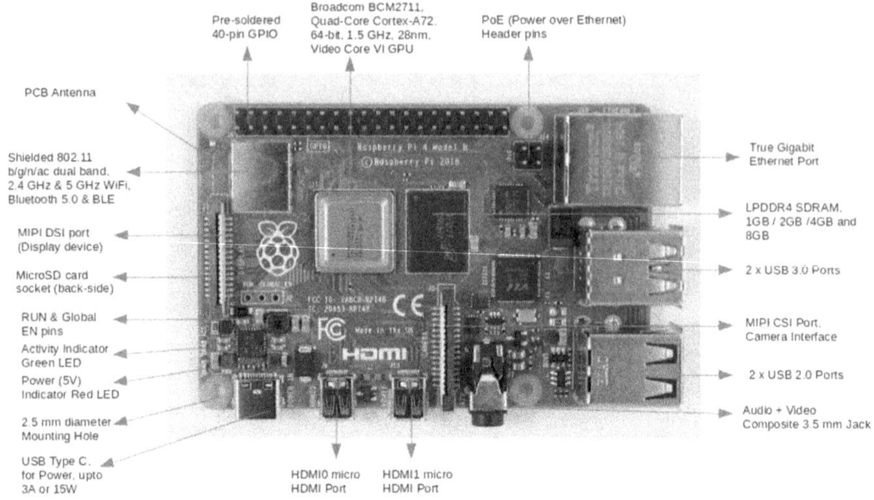

FIGURE 9.2 Raspberry Pi 4 Model B single-board computer.

the Broadcom SoC, which runs the main components of the board's CPU, graphics, memory, and USB controllers. It is slower than a modern laptop or desktop but is still a complete Linux computer and can provide all the expected abilities that implies but at a low-power level.

The Raspberry Pi 4 (RPi4) Model B, as shown in Figure 9.2, includes a system-on-chip (SoC Broadcom BCM2711) single-board microcomputer (SBC), central processing unit (CPU core 1.5GHz 64/32 bit quad-core ARM Cortex-A72). The RPi4 computer board's SoC, which uses Broadcom VideoCore VI as its graphics processor, has 40 GPIO pins, two HDMI ports for connecting to LCDs, a display connector (DSI), camera connector (CSI), four USB ports, a 5V power supply port, SD card slot on the back side of the board for storing data and installing the operating system (Windows 10 IoT Core, RISC OS, FreeBSD and additional distributions of Linux such as Raspbian Bullseye), audio video jack, and Ethernet port [8]. It is a cheap yet incredibly strong and efficient tool for IoT applications that simultaneously interface with several devices.

Overall, the Raspberry Pi 4 provides a powerful and versatile platform for developing IoT applications in healthcare systems. Its combination of processing power, RAM, connectivity options, and input/output options makes it well-suited to collecting and processing health data, managing patient information, and controlling medical devices.

9.6.1.2 ESP32 DOIT Development Kit

The 30-pin ESP32 DOIT Development Kit V1 is a powerful development board designed for IoT applications. It is widely used in various industries, including healthcare. In this context, the ESP32 development kit is used to build IoT-based healthcare systems that can remotely monitor patients' health conditions and provide timely assistance.

The ESP32 DOIT Development Kit V1 comes with the following features that make it suitable for IoT healthcare systems [9]:

1. Dual-core Tensilica LX6 processor
2. Integrated 520 KB SRAM and 4 MB flash memory
3. Wi-Fi and Bluetooth connectivity
4. 30 programmable GPIO pins
5. Hardware accelerated encryption (AES, SHA2, ECC, RSA)
6. Low power consumption
7. Integrated Li-ion battery management system
8. USB OTG interface
9. On-board JTAG programming/debugging interface

The ESP32 DOIT Development Kit V1 is a powerful development board that can be used in various IoT applications, including healthcare. Its Wi-Fi and Bluetooth connectivity, low power consumption, and integrated battery management system make it suitable for remote monitoring of patients' health conditions. With its powerful processor and ample memory, the ESP32 development kit can handle complex data processing tasks and can be programmed to perform specific functions required in healthcare systems.

9.6.1.3 Four-Channel 5V Relay Module (Active Low)

The four-channel relay module is a versatile and reliable component of a smart healthcare and environmental monitoring system. Its high switching capacity, compact size, and compatibility with the GPIO protocol make it an ideal choice for controlling multiple devices and appliances in healthcare and environmental monitoring applications.

A microcontroller like the ESP32 can control any of the four independent relay channels that make up the relay module. Each channel of the relay module has a maximum switching voltage of 250V AC or 30V DC and a maximum switching current of 10 A. It is designed to operate on a 5V DC input voltage, which is standard in most microcontroller-based systems. The relay module is compact and has dimensions of 75 mm × 50 mm × 18 mm, making it easy to integrate into existing systems. It is an essential component of a smart appliance control system, allowing healthcare IoT professionals to control the operation of medical devices and appliances remotely. It also plays a vital role in alert generation by enabling the system to switch on and off warning indicators, such as sirens or flashing lights, in case of an emergency.

In this work, a four-channel relay module board was used to interface the ESP32 with electrical appliances/bulbs/buzzer/fan. Input IN1, IN2, IN3, IN4 of the relay module are active low signal lines. The relay can be operated by a separate power supply, i.e., JD-VCC [8].

Features:

- Module can be controlled directly by Microcontroller ESP32 (or Raspberry Pi, Arduino, 8051, AVR, PIC, DSP, ARM, ARM, MSP430, TTL logic)
- Easy to install and fix
- Optically isolated relays to protect the microcontroller from damage if the equipment being controlled fails
- 5V four-channel relay interface board and each one needs a 15–20 mA driver current
- Four screw holes, hole diameter 3.1 mm
- Relay status indicator light, release status LED is off
- Relay maximum output: DC 30V/10A, AC 250V/10A

9.6.1.4 MAX30102 Particle Sensor

The MAX30102 particle sensor is a highly integrated pulse oximeter and heart rate sensor module designed for healthcare applications. It can measure SpO_2 and heart rate (HR) with high accuracy and reliability, making it suitable for use in medical devices such as fitness trackers, medical monitors, and wearables [8].

Features:

- High accuracy and reliability for SpO_2 and HR measurements
- Low power consumption and compact size
- Integrated ambient light rejection technology for improved accuracy in outdoor environments
- Easy to use with I^2C interface
- Built-in LED driver for pulse oximetry and heart rate applications
- Supports multiple LED colors (red and infrared) for different applications
- Flexible programming options for customization and optimization
- Advanced signal processing algorithms for noise reduction and motion artifact detection
- Real-time data streaming and remote monitoring capabilities through Wi-Fi and Bluetooth connectivity

The MAX30102 particle sensor, when combined with the ESP32 microcontroller, provides a powerful and flexible solution for healthcare applications. The advanced signal processing algorithms enable accurate and reliable SpO_2 and HR measurements, even in challenging environments. Real-time data streaming and remote monitoring capabilities through Wi-Fi and Bluetooth connectivity make it possible to develop sophisticated and connected medical devices. Overall, the MAX30102 particle sensor with ESP32 microcontroller is an ideal solution for healthcare applications that require reliable and accurate SpO_2 and HR monitoring.

9.6.1.5 DS18B20 Temperature Sensor

The DS18B20 digital temperature sensor is a versatile and cost-effective solution for temperature measurement in healthcare monitoring applications with ESP32. Its one-wire interface allows multiple sensors to be connected to a single wire, making it easy to set up and use. The sensor has a wide temperature range of –55°C to

+125°C with a temperature resolution of 0.0625°C and an accuracy of ±0.5°C (from –10°C to +85°C). The DS18B20 sensor operates on a power supply of 3.0V to 5.5V DC and has a current consumption of 1 mA (max) [8].

One of the main advantages of the DS18B20 sensor is its high accuracy, making it suitable for monitoring critical temperature conditions in healthcare applications. Additionally, the sensor is waterproof, making it ideal for use in environments where moisture is a concern. The DS18B20 is also easy to use and has a long lifespan.

The DS18B20 sensor can be connected to an ESP32 microcontroller for wireless data transmission. This allows for real-time temperature monitoring and alerts, enabling healthcare providers to take appropriate actions when necessary.

In summary, the DS18B20 digital temperature sensor is an advanced, cost-effective solution for healthcare monitoring with ESP32. Its high accuracy, waterproofing, and wireless connectivity make it an ideal choice for temperature monitoring in healthcare applications.

9.6.1.6 BME680 Environmental Sensor

The BME680 environmental sensor is a state-of-the-art sensor designed to detect various environmental conditions. It operates on a low voltage of 1.8V to 3.6V and consumes only 0.15 mA in standard operation mode. The sensor can operate over a wide temperature range of –40°C to 85°C, making it suitable for use in extreme environments [8].

The BME680 sensor uses MEMS (microelectromechanical system) technology that enables it to detect VOCs with high accuracy. The sensor has an integrated heater that can increase the temperature inside the sensor, which accelerates the desorption of VOCs from the surface of the sensing material. The sensor then measures the resistance change of the sensing material, which is proportional to the concentration of VOCs in the environment. It has a built-in I^2C (Inter-Integrated Circuit) interface, which makes it easy to interface with microcontrollers and other digital devices. The sensor also has a flexible configuration that allows users to customize the measurement parameters, such as the sampling rate and filter settings, to meet their specific application requirements.

In summary, the BME680 environmental sensor is a highly advanced sensor that can detect temperature, humidity, pressure, and volatile organic compounds (VOCs) with high accuracy and precision. It is a versatile sensor that can be used in various applications, including healthcare monitoring systems, due to its compact design, low power consumption, and flexible configuration.

9.6.1.7 MQ-135 Sensor

The MQ-135 sensor is designed to detect a wide range of gases, including benzene, alcohol, smoke, and other harmful gases. It has a high sensitivity to toxic gases and is commonly used to detect harmful gases in industrial settings, homes, and vehicles, and can detect even low levels of pollutants in the air [8].

It is used to monitor and measure the air quality of a given environment. The Air Quality Index (AQI) is a metric that indicates the level of pollution in the air and is used to determine the health risks associated with exposure to pollutants. It operates on the premise that gases and sensing materials interact chemically. When the gas comes in contact with the sensing material, it causes a change in resistance, which is then measured and converted into a readable signal. The sensor is widely used in IoT healthcare systems because of its low cost, high accuracy, and ease of integration with other IoT devices. It can be easily connected to the cloud, allowing healthcare providers to monitor air quality in real time, and take necessary actions to ensure patient safety.

9.6.1.8 Local 4G LTE Wi-Fi or Wireless Dongle

To retrieve the sensor data, we must send data to the Raspberry Pi using the MQTT protocol over an 802.11n Wi-Fi dongle or hotspot. This cutting-edge device makes use of MIMO technology to speed up WLAN operations and improve the consistency and range of broadcasts. A 4G LTE Wi-Fi dongle can be used to create a 150 Mbps Wi-Fi hotspot. Figure 9.3 shows a symbolic portable Wi-Fi hotspot.

9.6.2 Software Architecture

The software architecture of the proposed system consists of several software components, such as an integrated development environment (IDE), MQTT protocol,

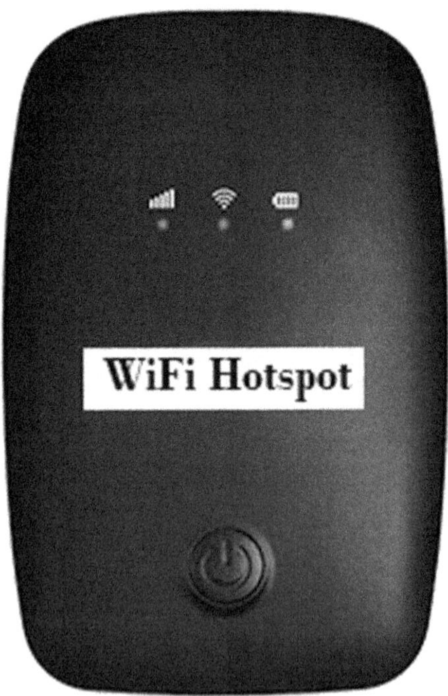

FIGURE 9.3 A symbolic portable Wi-Fi hotspot device.

Node-RED, InfluxDB, and Grafana OSS. Node-RED is used as the main programming environment for the system. It provides a user-friendly graphical interface for designing the IoT system. For storing the data produced by the sensors, InfluxDB is used as the database. It is a high-performance distributed time series database that is optimized for handling high write and query loads. Grafana is used as the visualization tool for the system. It provides a rich set of features for creating custom dashboards and visualizations.

9.6.2.1 Integrated Development Environment (IDE)

Arduino IDE is an open-source powerful tool for programming microcontrollers. It can be used to program the ESP32 microcontroller, which is commonly used in IoT applications for health and environmental monitoring systems, using the ESP32 board package. The IDE provides an easy-to-use platform for uploading code, monitoring serial output, and debugging programs. The IDE also provides a library of prebuilt functions that can be used to interface with sensors and devices. It is compatible with MAC OS, Windows, and Linux-based operating systems. The Arduino and ESP32 board can be uploaded and compiled using IDEs that have distinctive capabilities including finding and replacing text, copying and pasting, highlighting syntax, brace matching, and automatic formatting and indenting. It can significantly simplify the development of IoT applications, making it an essential tool for researchers and developers in this field.

9.6.2.2 Message Queuing Telemetry Transport (MQTT)

To efficiently manage the massive amounts of data generated by IoT devices, the Message Queuing Telemetry Transport (MQTT) protocol has emerged as a popular protocol for data transmission. The MQTT protocol is a lightweight, simple, and scalable protocol that enables IoT devices to exchange data in a reliable and efficient manner. It uses a publish–subscribe model to transmit data, where a publisher sends data to a broker, and subscribers receive data from the broker. This model minimizes the bandwidth required for data transmission and enables devices with limited processing power to participate in the network.

In healthcare and environmental monitoring applications, the MQTT protocol plays a crucial role in collecting and transmitting data from a wide range of sensors and devices. It enables real-time monitoring of vital signs and environmental factors such as air quality, temperature, and humidity, and provides timely alerts and notifications in case of emergencies.

Moreover, the MQTT protocol provides end-to-end security and ensures the confidentiality, integrity, and availability of data transmitted across the network. It supports authentication and authorization mechanisms, data encryption, and data compression, ensuring secure and efficient data transmission. It enables efficient health and environmental monitoring, provides real-time data analysis, and ensures secure and reliable data transmission. The use of the MQTT protocol in IoT applications can lead to improved healthcare outcomes, better environmental management, and a sustainable future.

One of the key features of MQTT is its quality of service (QoS) levels, which ensure that messages are delivered in a reliable and efficient manner. These QoS levels are QoS 0, QoS 1, and QoS 2.

The MQTT protocol makes supervisory control and data acquisition possible in this study.

QoS Level	Delivery	Description
QoS 0	At most once	● The message is delivered at most once. ● It does not guarantee delivery and may result in message loss. ● Suitable for applications that can tolerate occasional message loss.
QoS 1	At least once	● The message is delivered at least once. ● If the subscriber does not acknowledge the message, the publisher will send the message again until it receives an acknowledgment. ● Provides reliable message delivery but may result in duplicate messages. ● Suitable for applications that require reliable data transmission.
QoS 2	Exactly once	● The message is delivered exactly once. ● It uses a four-step handshake process to ensure that the message is delivered without duplicates or loss. ● Provides the most reliable message delivery but may result in higher latency and bandwidth usage. ● Suitable for applications that require real-time and reliable data transmission.

The selection of QoS level depends on the specific requirements of the application and the importance of the message being transmitted. By selecting the appropriate QoS level, IoT applications can ensure reliable and efficient data transmission, leading to improved healthcare outcomes, better environmental management, and a sustainable future.

The MQTT architecture and MQTT protocol are shown in Figure 9.4 and are relevant to this work [8]. It is a good option for this design because it enables straightforward communication between the clients (the ESP32 microcontroller, computers, and/or mobile devices with Node-RED client) and the server (the Raspberry Pi MQTT broker). Any type of data can be published or subscribed to by clients. The data is then made available to all clients who have subscribed to that topic by the broker. The local server (Raspberry Pi4) is running the Eclipse Mosquitto software as a broker. In this work, the ESP32 microcontroller publishes sensor data along with specific topics to the MQTT broker (Mosquitto broker), and desktop computers, smartphones, and other devices subscribe to the topics in order to view the published data on the server. The MQTT protocol makes the supervisory control possible in this work.

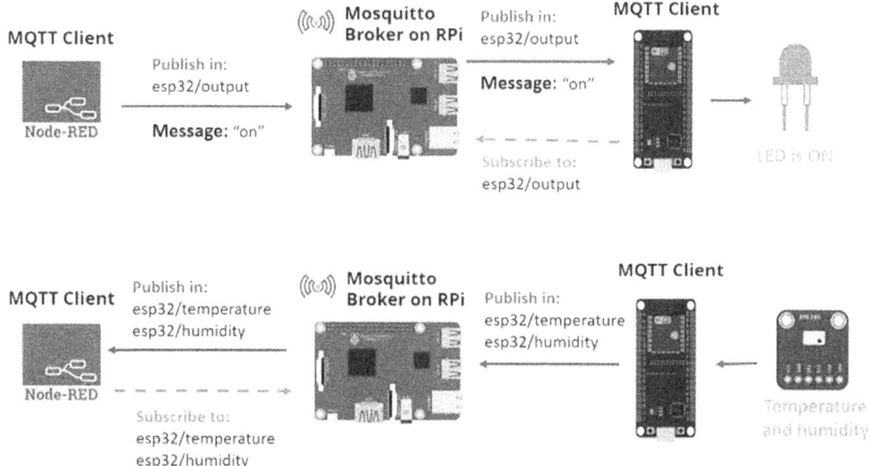

FIGURE 9.4 MQTT Architecture and MQTT Protocol with Mosquitto Broker on RPi and MQTT Client [8].

9.6.2.3 Node-RED

Node-RED is an open-source platform that provides a visual programming interface, making it an excellent choice for developing IoT-based healthcare systems. Its visual interface simplifies the process of integrating various devices and sensors, making it more user-friendly and functional. Additionally, it offers scalability, supporting a range of protocols, and real-time data processing and analysis, enabling healthcare professionals to monitor and analyze patient data continuously. Node-RED's support for machine learning algorithms and data visualization tools simplifies the interpretation of complex data, enabling healthcare professionals to make informed decisions. Furthermore, Node-RED integrates seamlessly with third-party tools, simplifying the storage and management of patient data. Overall, Node-RED offers significant advantages for healthcare professionals and developers looking to create efficient and effective healthcare systems [10–11]. These features are listed in the following table.

Feature	Summary
Visual programming	Node-RED provides a web-based visual programming interface that enables users to drag and drop prebuilt nodes, allowing for easy development of complex flows. This makes it ideal for building IoT-based healthcare systems, as it can help users quickly connect and integrate different devices and sensors.
Scalability	Node-RED is highly scalable and can be deployed across multiple devices and platforms, making it ideal for large-scale IoT-based healthcare systems. It also supports a wide range of protocols, including MQTT, HTTP, and TCP, making it compatible with various IoT devices and platforms.

Real-time data processing	Node-RED enables real-time data processing and analysis, making it ideal for healthcare systems that require continuous monitoring and analysis of patient data. It also supports machine learning algorithms, enabling users to build predictive models and algorithms to detect anomalies and identify trends in patient data.
Data visualization	Node-RED supports various data visualization tools, such as graphs and charts, that enable users to visualize and analyze data in real time. This makes it easier for healthcare professionals to monitor and analyze patient data and make informed decisions.
Integration with third-party tools	Node-RED integrates seamlessly with various third-party tools, such as cloud services and databases, making it easier for users to store and manage patient data. This also enables users to integrate Node-RED with other healthcare systems, such as electronic health record (EHR) systems.

9.6.2.4 InfluxDB

InfluxDB is a powerful and versatile time series database that is well-suited for IoT applications. Its features, including time series data storage, high write and query performance, a SQL-like query language, support for retention policies, built-in visualization, and integrations with other tools, make it an ideal choice for storing and analyzing IoT data. With its open-source license and active community, InfluxDB is a cost-effective and reliable solution for researchers and practitioners in the IoT space. Some of the key features of InfluxDB that make it well-suited for IoT include [12]:

1. **Time series data storage**: It is specifically designed for storing and querying time series data. This means that it is optimized for handling large volumes of data that are generated at regular intervals, such as sensor readings.
2. **High write and query performance**: It is designed to handle high write and query loads, making it ideal for IoT applications that generate a lot of data. It uses a columnar storage format and a distributed architecture to achieve high performance.
3. **SQL-like query language**: It uses a SQL-like query language called InfluxQL, which makes it easy to query and analyze time series data.
4. **Support for retention policies**: It allows you to define retention policies that specify how long data should be stored and when it should be automatically deleted. This is useful for managing the storage requirements of IoT applications that generate a lot of data.
5. **Built-in support for visualization**: It comes with a built-in visualization tool called Chronograph, which allows creation of custom dashboards for monitoring and analyzing IoT data.
6. **Integrations with other tools**: It has integrations with a wide range of other tools and platforms, including Grafana, Prometheus, and AWS IoT Core. This makes it easy to build end-to-end IoT solutions using InfluxDB as the data store.

9.6.2.5 Grafana Dashboard

Grafana Dashboard is an advanced tool that provides various features essential in IoT healthcare applications. Its ability to monitor and visualize data in real time, customization, alerting, data analytics, integration, multiuser support, security, and scalability make it a popular choice among healthcare professionals. It is a widely used tool in IoT healthcare applications due to its ability to visualize large amounts of data in real time. The key features of Grafana Dashboard in IoT healthcare applications are [13]:

1. **Data visualization**: Grafana Dashboard provides a powerful visualization tool that can display complex data from multiple sources. It supports different types of charts, graphs, and tables that enable the user to quickly identify trends, patterns, and anomalies in the data.
2. **Real-time monitoring**: It allows users to monitor data in real time. This feature is essential in IoT healthcare applications where continuous monitoring of patients' vital signs, such as heart rate, blood pressure, and temperature, is critical for timely intervention.
3. **Customization**: It allows users to customize the dashboard according to their needs. Users can choose from a wide range of plugins and themes that can be integrated into the dashboard to enhance its functionality and appearance.
4. **Alerting**: It provides a powerful alerting system that enables users to receive notifications when specific conditions are met. This feature is critical in IoT healthcare applications where prompt action is necessary to avoid adverse outcomes.
5. **Data analytics**: It provides data analytics tools that enable users to perform advanced data analysis on the data. The dashboard supports different types of queries, such as SQL, and can also integrate with machine learning tools to provide predictive analytics.
6. **Integration**: It can integrate with various data sources, including databases, APIs, and IoT devices. This feature enables users to collect and monitor data from different sources, providing a comprehensive view of the system being monitored.
7. **Multiuser support**: It supports multiple users, enabling teams to collaborate on the same dashboard. This feature is beneficial in IoT healthcare applications where multiple healthcare professionals need to monitor and analyze data simultaneously.
8. **Security**: It provides robust security features, including user authentication and authorization, data encryption, and access control. This feature makes sure that the monitored data is secure and that only authorized personnel can access it.
9. **Scalability**: It is highly scalable and can handle large amounts of data. This feature is crucial in IoT healthcare applications, where data is generated continuously, and the system needs to accommodate the growing volume of data.

9.6.3 Physical IoT Server Architecture

The IoT server architecture of the proposed system includes an MQTT broker (Mosquitto), Node-RED, InfluxDB, and Grafana OSS that are installed on a Raspberry Pi 4 to set up a local physical server. The MQTT broker is used for message queuing and delivery between the sensors and the local server. The local server is used for data storage, analysis, and visualization. It is hosted on a Raspberry Pi 4 platform. The data generated by the system is transmitted to the local IoT server using the MQTT protocol.

9.7 EXPERIMENTAL SETUP

The proposed system was designed as shown in Figure 9.1. The figure shows the realized embedded open-source IoT-enabled SCADA-based health and environmental monitoring prototype system with its components for reading and monitoring different health and environmental parameters. Each component of a system, like the Raspberry Pi and ESP32, is powered by a power source. The ESP32, the device's brain, controls the sensor and actuator blocks that are used for measurements, observations, and controlling the devices.

The Raspberry Pi 4 with its OS Bullseye was used to build a physical IoT server for the proposed system, along with Node-RED, Mosquitto Broker, InfluxDB, and Grafana. There are three MQTT clients in the system. Data acquisition of the AQI from the MQ-135 gas sensor and several environmental parameters, including temperature, humidity, air pressure, dewpoint, and gas resistance from the BME680 sensor, are both done using a single MQTT client (NodeMCU#1). This client published different measured values as an individual topic using the MQTT protocol. Another MQTT client (NodeMCU#2) is used for measuring SpO_2 and body temperature using the MAX30102 particle sensor and DS18B20 temperature sensor, respectively. This client can also be used to measure the ambient temperature and humidity if required, but it was optional in this work. Different alerts for poisonous gas detection, fever detection, and air quality status are generated with the turn on/off exhausted fan or bulb or buzzer using a four-channel relay module through ESP32. This client published and subscribed to different topics and acted accordingly to turn on the buzzer/fan/bulb based on the sensor's threshold data to generate the respective alert. On the other hand, another MQTT client (dashboard of laptop/tablet/smart mobile phone) is used to subscribe to different topics to visualize that on the dashboard and publish supervisory control signals to control the on/off of the healthcare appliances over the internet with the help of MQTT which is built on the TCP protocol, and Wi-Fi technology, which establishes internet connectivity among the ESP32 clients, Raspberry Pi–IoT server and Node-RED, InfluxDB, or Grafana Dashboard client. In this way, the SCADA system was built with the enabling technology of IoT.

9.8 RESULTS AND DISCUSSION

The different health and environmental parameters were measured using the proposed SCADA-based IoT-enabled healthcare prototype system for 48 hours (6–7 March

2023). Measurements were performed in the Control System and Instrumentation Lab of the Electronics and Communication Engineering Department at Cooch Behar Government Engineering College in Cooch Behar, West Bengal, India. Figures 9.5a–k show different aspects of the prototype system.

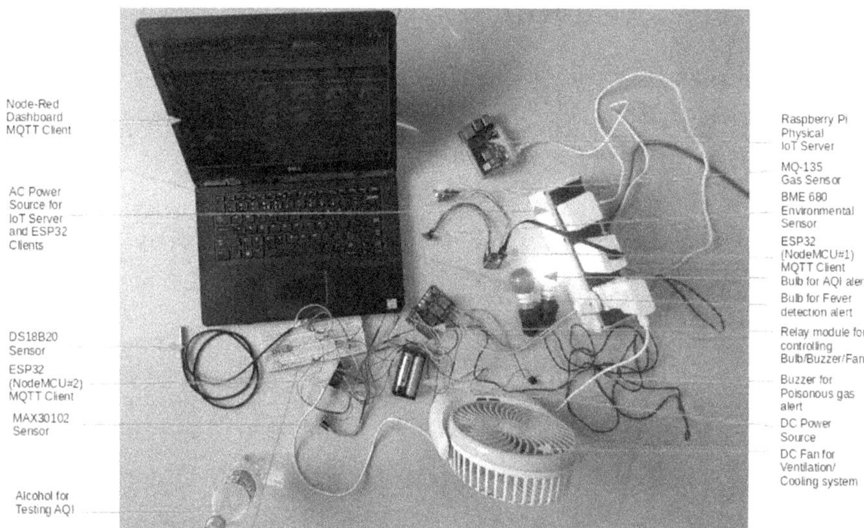

FIGURE 9.5A Experimental setup of IoT-enabled SCADA prototype system.

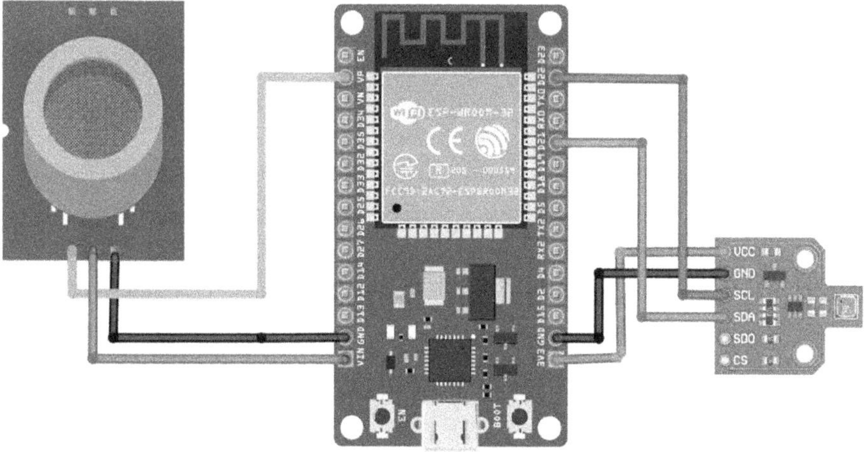

FIGURE 9.5B Wire diagram of the prototype system for the ESP32 (NodeMCU#1) MQTT client.

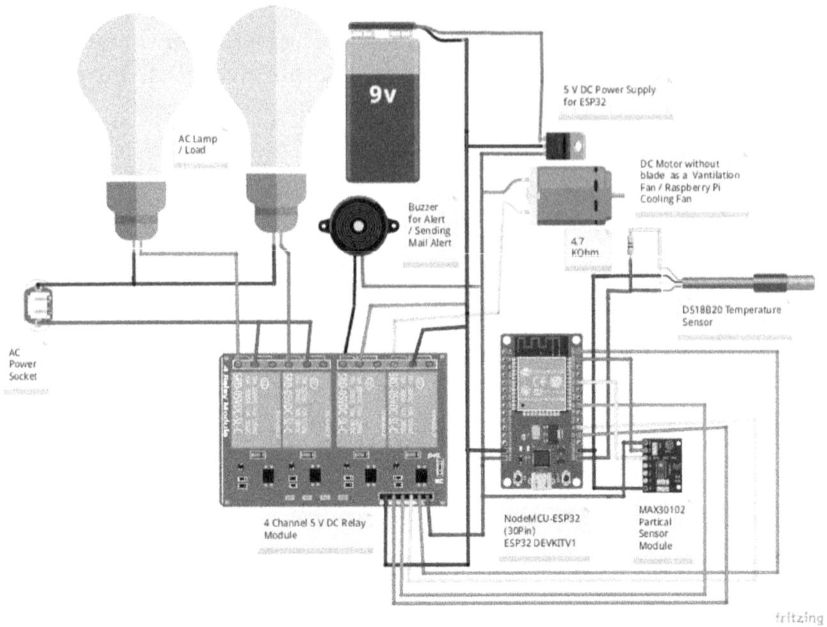

FIGURE 9.5C Wire diagram of the prototype system for the ESP32 (NodeMCU#2) MQTT client.

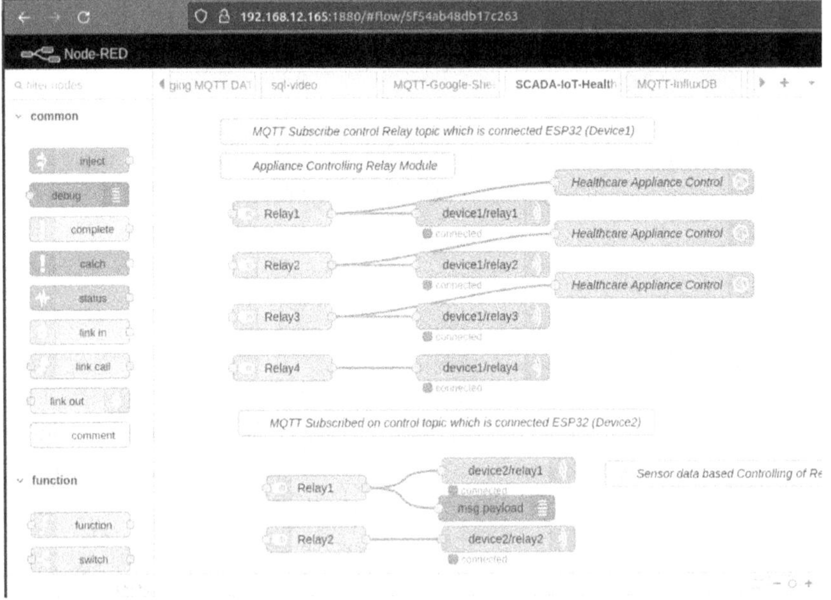

FIGURE 9.5D Node-RED flow for healthcare appliance control and related information stored in InfluxDB.

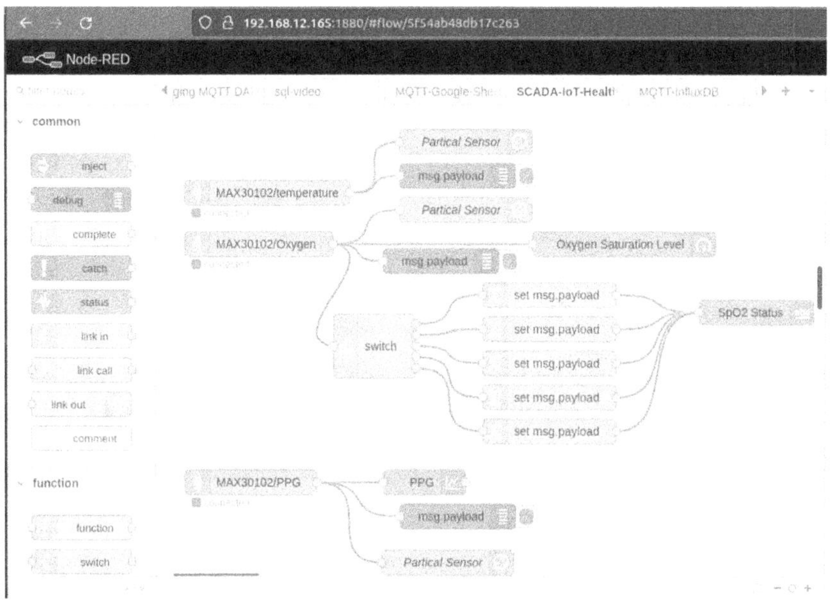

FIGURE 9.5E Node-RED flow for body temperature and SpO_2 measurement value, SpO_2 status generation for alert, and their related information stored in InfluxDB.

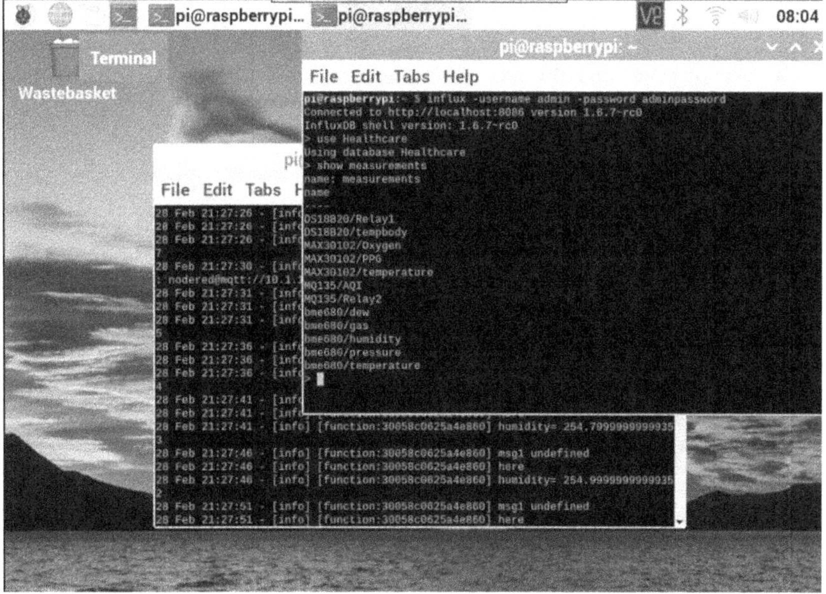

FIGURE 9.5F The Raspberry Pi IoT server that runs an MQTT broker (Mosquitto) and database (InfluxDB).

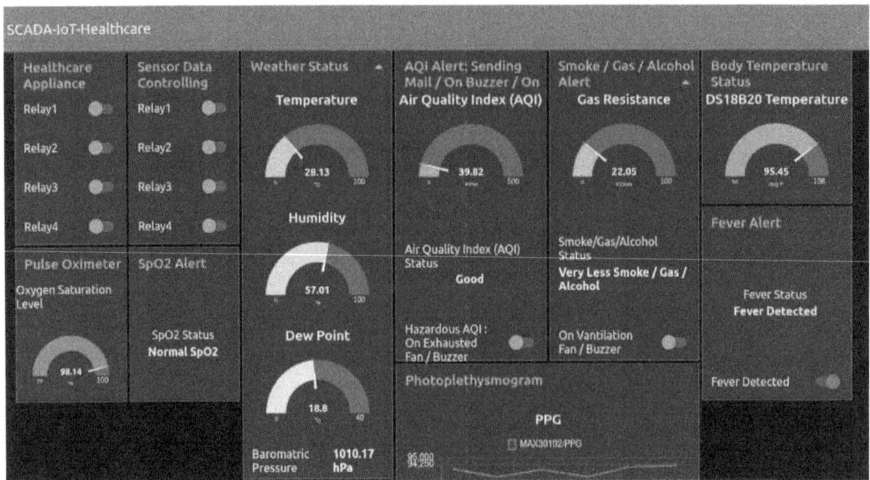

FIGURE 9.5G Node-RED dashboard where SpO_2 level status is normal, and the weather status is as shown. The AQI is 39.82 PPM and the related AQI status is good. Gas resistance is 22.05, which indicates very little smoke/gas/alcohol and no need to turn on the ventilation fan or buzzer. Body temperature is at 95.45 with a fever status of "fever detected" and the related mail alert is on. The fever detection alert is set at 95°C for this prototype system.

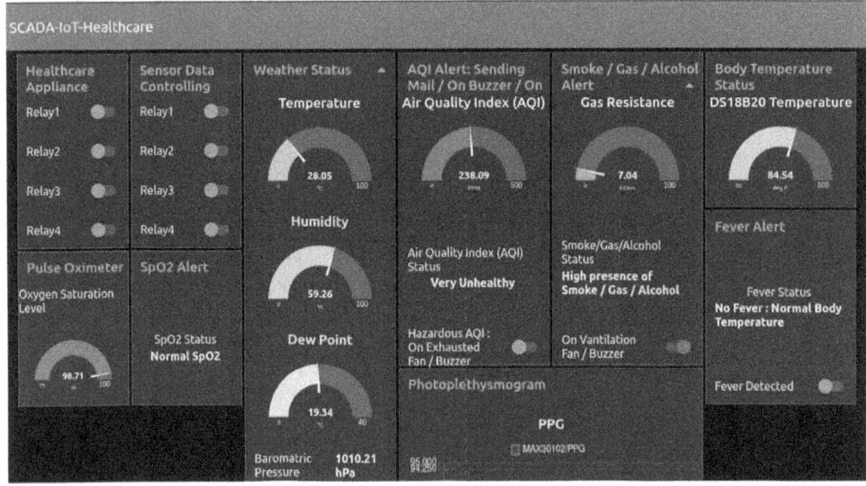

FIGURE 9.5H Node-RED dashboard where SpO_2 level status is normal, and weather status is as shown. The AQI is 238.09 PPM and the related AQI status is very unhealthy. The gas resistance is 7.04, which indicates a high presence of smoke/gas/alcohol and the need to turn on the ventilation fan or buzzer. The body temperature is 84.54 with fever status as "no fever: normal body temperature"; the related mail alert is off. The gas resistance threshold value is set below 10 KOhm for this prototype system.

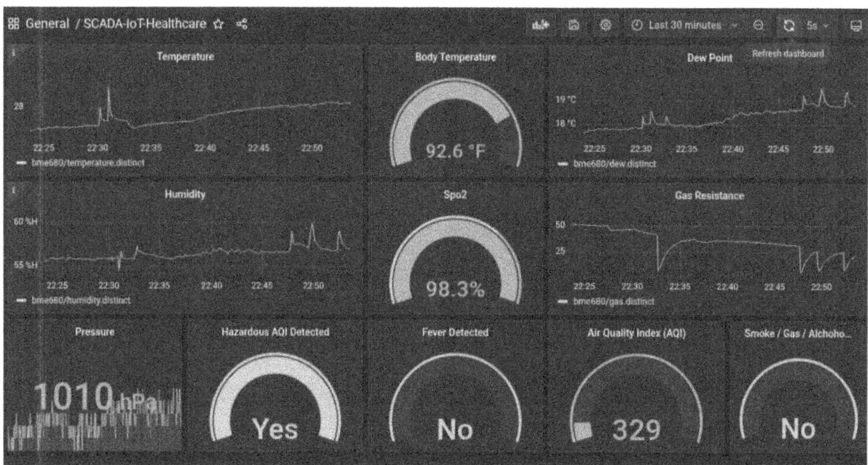

FIGURE 9.5I The Grafana dashboard of the proposed system with measurements of different health and environmental parameters. Here, the AQI is 329 PPM due to the alcohol present close to the MQ-135 gas sensor, which is tested using an alcohol sample bottle as shown in Figure 9.5a. The AQI status for hazardous is set at 300 PPM.

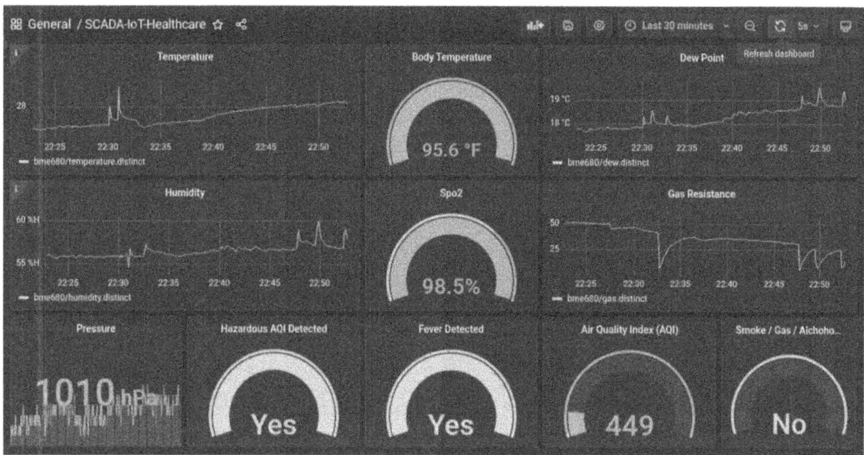

FIGURE 9.5J The Grafana dashboard of the proposed system with measurements of different health and environmental parameters. Here, the AQI is 449 PPM due to the alcohol present close to the MQ-135 gas sensor, which is tested using an alcohol sample bottle as shown in Figure 9.5a. The AQI status for hazardous is set at 300 PPM, and a fever is detected as informed in Figure 9.5g.

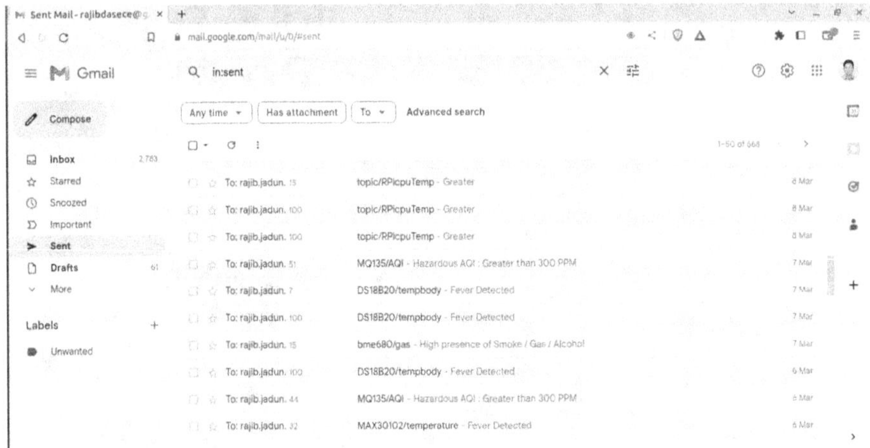

FIGURE 9.5K The email notification for different scenarios of the alert generation.

9.9 CONCLUSION AND FUTURE WORK

In this work, an open-source IoT-enabled SCADA-based health and environmental monitoring system was been successfully implemented with RPi4, ESP32, MQTT, Node-RED, InfluxDB, and Grafana. This framework can be transferred to other SACDA-based IoT applications. In this study, all sensor data taken from the different sensors was raw data. In future work, sensors will be calibrated for more accurate and practical implementation. Other environmental parameters, such as PM2.5, PM10, SO2, and noise level, could also be monitored using the specific sensors. This work can be extended to long rang (LoRa)-based SCADA-enabled sustainable smart environmental monitoring system applications in the future.

DECLARATIONS

The author affirms that the publication of this work does not present any conflicts of interest.

REFERENCES

1. Alvear-Puertas, V. E., et al. (2022). "Smart and Portable Air-Quality Monitoring IoT Low-Cost Devices in Ibarra City, Ecuador." *Sensors*, 22(18), 7015. https://doi.org/10.3390/s22187015
2. Malche, T., Maheshwary, P. and Kumar, R. (2019). "Environmental Monitoring System for Smart City Based on Secure Internet of Things (IoT) Architecture." *Wireless Personal Communications*, 107, 2143–2172. https://doi.org/10.1007/s11277-019-06376-0
3. Mohammad, N. and Shahjahan, M. (2019). "Design and Development of IoT based Supervisory Control and Data Acquisition System." *2019 5th International Conference on Advances in Electrical Engineering (ICAEE)*, Dhaka, Bangladesh, pp. 306–311. https://doi.org/10.1109/ICAEE48663.2019.8975695

4. Uddin, S. U., Jabbar, M. Baig, A. and Iqbal, M. T. (2022). "Design and Implementation of an Open-Source SCADA System for a Community Solar-Powered Reverse Osmosis System." *Sensors*, 22(24), 9631. https://doi.org/10.3390/s22249631
5. Aghenta, L. O. and Iqbal, M. T. (2019). "Design and Implementation of a Low-Cost, Open Source IoT-Based SCADA System Using ESP32 with OLED, ThingsBoard and MQTT Protocol." *AIMS Electronics and Electrical Engineering*, 4(1), 57–86. https://doi.org/10.3934/ElectrEng.2020.1.57
6. Kent, L. Y. and Kamsin, I. F. B. (2021). "Implementation of IoT in Patient Health Monitoring and Healthcare for Hospitals." *Proceedings of the 3rd International Conference on Integrated Intelligent Computing Communication and Security (ICIIC 2021), Atlantis Highlights in Computer Sciences*, Volume 4. https://doi.org/10.2991/ahis.k.210913.059
7. Tsao, Y.-C., et al. (2022). "An IoT- Based Smart System with an MQTT Broker for Individual Patient Vital sign Monitoring in Potential Emergency or Prehospital Application." *Hindawi, Emergency Medical International*, 2022, Article ID 7245650. 13 Pages. https://doi.org/10.1155/2022/7245650
8. https://randomnerdtutorials.com
9. https://www.mischianti.org/2021/02/17/doit-esp32-dev-kit-v1-high-resolution-pinout-and-specs/
10. Node-RED Official Website. https://nodered.org/
11. Olsson, J. and Asante, J. (2016). "Using Node-Red to Connect Patient, Staff and Medical Equipment." https://liu.diva-portal.org/smash/get/diva2:949264/FULLTEXT01.pdf
12. https://docs.influxdata.com/influxdb/v2.7/get-started/
13. https://grafana.com/docs/grafana/latest/introduction/
14. Rahmani, A. M., et al. (2018). "Exploiting Smart e-Health Gateways at the Edge of Healthcare Internet-of-Things: A Fog Computing Approach." *Future Generation Computer Systems*, 78(Part 2), 641–658. https://doi.org/10.1016/j.future.2017.02.014
15. Hariz Hasshim, M., et al. (2019). "IoT Based Health Monitoring System for Elderly Patient." *Journal of Electronic Voltage and Application*, 1(2) (2020), 27–36 https://doi.org/10.30880/jeva.2020.01.02.004
16. Islam, M. M., Rahaman, A. and Islam, M. R. (2020). "Development of Smart Healthcare Monitoring System in IoT Environment." *SN Computer Science*, 1(3), 185. https://doi.org/10.1007/s42979-020-00195-y
17. Polu, S. K. (2022). "Design of Remote Patient Monitoring System for Chronic Diseases." *IJARCCE*, 11(3). https://doi.org/10.17148/IJARCCE.2022.11308
18. Selvaraj, S., et al. (2020). "Challenges and Opportunities in IoT Healthcare Systems: A Systematic Review." *SN Applied Sciences*, 2, 139. https://doi.org/10.1007/s42452-019-1925-y
19. Abdulmalek, S., Nasir, A., Jabbar, W. A., Almuhaya, M. A. M., Bairagi, A. K., Khan, M. A. and Kee, S. H. (2022). "IoT-Based Healthcare-Monitoring System Towards Improving Quality of Life: A Review." *Healthcare (Basel, Switzerland)*, 10(10), 1993. https://doi.org/10.3390/healthcare10101993
20. Qian, Z., et al. (2022). "Development of a Real-Time Wearable Fall Detection System in the Context of Internet of Things." *IEEE Internet of Things Journal*, 9(21), 21999–22007. https://doi.org/10.1109/JIOT.2022.3181701

10 Transfer Learning for Healthcare

Anindita Saha and Moumita Roy

10.1 OVERVIEW OF IOT-BASED HEALTHCARE APPLICATION

The rapid advancement of information technology (IT) and communication techniques in the last decade has triggered the advent of the novel concept of the Internet of Things (IoT). It plays a key role in enabling automation in various fields including smart healthcare systems. Nowadays, the branch of IoT focused on medical science is popularly known as the Healthcare Internet of Things (HIoT) [1]. HIoT promotes a network of interactive and interconnected medical devices, sensors, and healthcare resources such as doctors, hospitals, and rehabilitation centers along with patients for the continuous real-time data transfer. The end-to-end network of a typical HIoT system comprises three primary operational layers: data collection layer, data storage layer, and data processing layer. The data collection layer focuses on the collection of health data through various body sensor nodes attached to the human body. Further, the data storage layer mainly deals with the storage of big data accumulated from various sensors and transmitted through the internet. Finally, the data processing layer analyzes the data stored in servers through the application of computing algorithms in order to take the necessary actions.

The notion of HIoT has revolutionized the existing medical infrastructure to a great extent. It brings about a pragmatic change by transforming traditional healthcare systems into Healthcare 4.0, which is dependent on data and focuses on the welfare of the patients [2]. The incorporation of cutting-edge technologies such as IoT [3] and body area networks operated by state-of-the-art emerging branches of artificial intelligence such as machine learning (ML) or deep learning (DL) have enabled real-time analysis of health data that was not possible for doctors a few years ago. If remote patient monitoring becomes feasible, healthcare services could be made available to more people at a minimal cost. Further, communication between patients and doctors can become more reliable and easier through various applications of HIoT. Diverse areas of healthcare services, including diagnosis, prognosis, and spread control, developing assistive systems, and continuous monitoring of health parameters particularly for chronic diseases can benefit from the application of HIoT [1, 4].

 DOI: 10.1201/9781003391456-10

10.2 SURVEY OF ML-BASED AND DL-BASED TECHNIQUES BASED ON HEALTHCARE APPLICATIONS

Research says the key concerns for all applications of healthcare IoT are data gathering and processing [1]. Due to the vast multitude and complex nature of the large amount of data involved in healthcare, analysis using ML or DL algorithms has proven to be of vital importance in recent years. These algorithms extract worthy information from the acquired data and draw useful inferences. Since ML or DL models can give the desired levels of accuracy when trained in the appropriate environment, several contemporary research efforts explore a new dimension of applications of ML or DL algorithms to HIoT systems and estimate their suitability for these systems. Some of the relevant research is presented in Table 10.1. For instance, Chen et al. [5] streamlined machine learning algorithms for effective prediction of chronic disease outbreaks in disease-frequent communities. The authors proposed a novel convolutional neural network (CNN)-based multimodal disease risk prediction algorithm that utilizes structured and unstructured data from the hospital. A study was conducted by Ginantra et al. [6] where the authors predicted and diagnosed acute respiratory infections in a person following the symptoms caused by using the machine learning approach. Further, Hadi et al. [7] presented a multidisciplinary approach by interconnecting big data analytics and radio resource optimization, along with electronic healthcare in a multitier 5G network. Here, a patient-centric heterogeneous network was proposed where three ML algorithms – naïve Bayes (NB), logistic regression (LR), and decision tree (DT) – are employed to function as an ensemble classifier system to examine the medical records of patients with a history of stroke. However, while these ML techniques typically require less training data for the model compared to DL algorithms, the quality of the data is more significant in order to achieve the desired accuracy. In addition, developing such an ML system necessitates domain expertise and human engineering to design feature extractors that can transform raw data into suitable representations from which a learning algorithm can detect patterns.

Besides, the ML techniques, the state-of-the-art literature review also establishes the contribution and efficiency of deep learning techniques for medical diagnostics over the years. For instance, Liu et al. [8] aimed to make a comparative analysis between the diagnostic accuracy of deep learning algorithms and healthcare professionals in classifying diseases using medical imaging. Further, a B5G framework was presented by Rahman et al. [9] that supports COVID-19 diagnosis, considering the low-latency, high-bandwidth features of the 5G network at the edge. Here, the authors proposed a distributed DL-based model, which enables every COVID-19 edge to make use of a DL framework that is specific to its domain, apart from deploying a three-phase reconciliation with the globally accepted DL framework. A DL-based healthcare framework was developed by Sharma et al. [2] for IoT-based assistance of Alzheimer patients. Here, a scheme based on recurrent neural network (RNN) for prediction of Alzheimer disease that works in three phases was presented. First, sensor-based motion data was utilized for predicting Alzheimer disease in patients using RNN. Then an ensemble approach for abnormality tracking for

TABLE 10.1
Relevant ML and DL Approaches for IoT Healthcare Applications

Year	Reference	Description	Technique Used	Algorithm
2016	[11]	Classification of Alzheimer disease using fMRI data	DL	CNN was used to classify Alzheimer brain from normal healthy brain.
2018	[12]	Classification using for brain tumors	DL	A deep neural network classifier was used.
2019	[13]	A DL-based approach to pneumonia classification in healthcare	DL	A CNN model was developed to extract features from x-ray images of the chest to diagnose the existence of pneumonia and perform prediction through classification.
2020	[9]	5G-based framework for COVID detection	DL	A distributed DL paradigm was proposed that enables every edge to make use of a domain-specific DL framework along with deployment of a three-phase reconciliation in sync with a globally accepted DL framework.
2020	[2]	Healthcare framework for IoT-based assistance of Alzheimer patients	DL	A recurrent neural network–based Alzheimer prediction scheme was proposed and an ensemble approach for abnormality tracking was introduced comprising of an emotion detection system that relies on CNN as well as a natural language processing (NLP)-based scheme based on timestamp window.
2020	[6]	Acute respiratory infection prediction	ML	Prediction and diagnosis of the presence or absence of acute respiratory infection using KNN, SVM, naïve Bayes, along with neural network.
2020	[7]	Prediction of the likelihood of an imminent stroke	ML	Usage of naïve Bayesian (NB) classifier, logistic regression (LR), and decision tree (DT) that operate as an ensemble system to examine the medical records of patients who have suffered from stroke and readings from body-attached IoT sensors.
2021	[1]	Applications of ML algorithms in HIoT	ML	Reviews and compiles the various state-of-the-art ML applications that are being integrated with HIoT, as well as analyzes the systems that utilize the combination of artificial intelligence and IoT for an accurate and predictive healthcare system, especially with structured and unstructured data from hospital.

Alzheimer patients was designed, which consisted of two parts: a CNN-based emotion detection scheme and a timestamp window-based natural language processing (NLP) scheme. Third, an IoT-based assistance mechanism for Alzheimer patients was presented. These DL techniques are a form of representation learning. Unlike ML, here the system is provided with raw data and develops its own representations required for pattern recognition that consists of multiple layers of representations. Because such deep learning systems can undertake multiple data types as input, this is typically suitable for healthcare applications with heterogeneous health data [10].

10.3 ROLE OF TRANSFER LEARNING IN HEALTHCARE

Artificial intelligence has garnered worldwide attention through a wide range of applications due to the quick advancements in computer and communication techniques over the past few decades. A wide range of applications has been developed using ML [14] and DL [15], demonstrating outstanding performance in a number of fields, including speech recognition, natural language processing, and computer vision. Apart from these, context-aware human activity recognition can also be performed using DL, with the help of metaheuristic techniques for improved performance metrics [16]. The most effective and efficient application of DL is image classification, which aims to identify images and assign them to one of the several potential categories. However, recent research has revealed that the image classification problem can be resolved using TL [17, 18], which can aid in building accurate models that take less time and improve predictive analysis to a substantial extent. The basic concept, architecture, and applications of TL are explained in more detail in the subsequent sections.

10.3.1 Concept of Transfer Learning

Human beings possess a natural capacity to learn, recognize, and categorize objects using their various sense organs from various sources of available data. Machines also need data to learn and develop the ability to identify as well as classify objects with the help of labels with which it was trained during the training phase. This is successfully conducted by building a model with a sufficient amount of training data as input and state-of-the-art learning techniques prevalent in literature, which is the currently popular paradigm for ML. This paradigm of learning is referred to as isolated learning since it disregards any other relevant information and prior knowledge.

Training from scratch necessitates the classifier to be trained on an extensive dataset containing millions of data points to ensure a significant performance metric, such as accuracy. However, this is a cumbersome process as it requires huge computational power apart from being time-consuming in execution. TL [17] partially resolves the limitations of the isolated learning paradigm that is mostly used in deep learning today for improved performance metrics.

In deep neural networks, the transferring or reusing of the learned parameters of a previously trained network on a specific task (called a pretrained network) to another

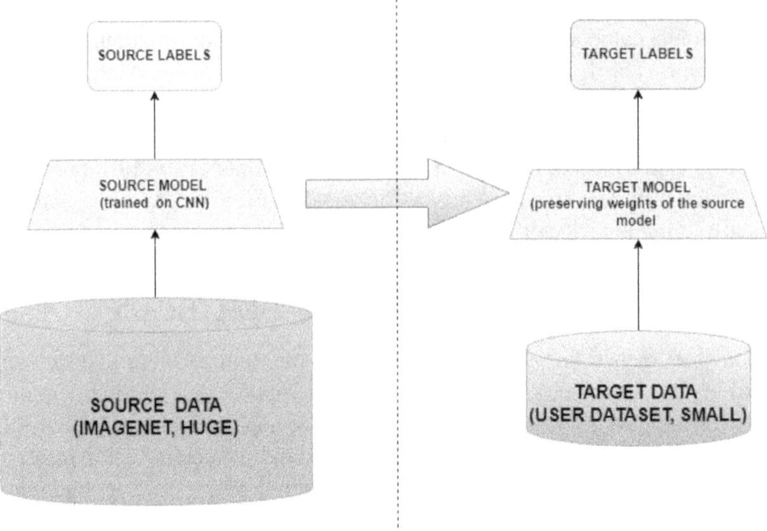

FIGURE 10.1 Basic architecture of transfer learning.

network for a related but different task can be conducted. This successfully eliminates the need for training the new model from scratch and still can deliver optimum results with those learned parameters. This also acts as an optimization for allowing rapid progress during the modeling of the second task and for higher accuracy even with only a small amount of data. Simply put, in TL, a source base network is trained on a base dataset with a source task (problem), and then the learned features are repurposed or transferred to a second target network to be trained on a target dataset with a target task (problem). Thus, the machine exploits the knowledge gained from a previous task *A*, with a lot of available data to improve the generalization of task *B*, which doesn't have much data for training [19]. Figure 10.1 shows the basic concept of TL.

Mathematically, if P_s is considered to be a source problem that was solved by a model M_s trained on dataset D_s, then the learned parameters of this M_s (which is now known as a pretrained model) can be used to solve a target problem using the concept of TL.

10.3.2 Definition of Transfer Learning

TL can be appropriately defined with the proper concept of a domain and a task [20].

Definition 1 (Domain): A *domain D* consists of two parts: *X*, which is a feature space, and a marginal probability distribution ( ) over the feature space, and

D may be represented as *D*= {*X*, ( )}. The feature set *X* may be defined as *x* {*x* |$x_i \in X$, $i = 1, \ldots, n$}. Definition 2 (Task): Given a domain *D* = {*X*, *P*(*X*), a task T, is represented as $T' = Y, f(x)$, where *Y′* is a label space and $f(x)$ is an implicit decision function $f(x)$, which is usually learned from the sample data in the given dataset.

The function, which is also a conditional probability function represented as P($y|x$) and can be mathematically expressed as {xi, yi} where $x \in X$ and $y \in Y$. The function is also known as a prediction function since it can predict the corresponding label $f(x)$ for a new instance of x. In most of the research, single-source domain DS and single-target domain DT are considered. A domain is usually observed by several instances with or without the label information. Conventionally, the source domain data DS is denoted as DS = {($xS1$, $yS1$)…($xsns$, $ysns$)}, where $xSi \in XS$(data instance) and $yS \in YS$ (corresponding class labels). Similarly, target domain data may be specified as DT = {($xT1$, $yT1$)…($xTns$, $yTns$)}, where the input $xT \in XT$ and $yT \in YT$ is the corresponding output.

Definition 3 (Transfer learning): Given a source domain D_s, a corresponding source task T_s, with a target domain D_T and a target task T_T, the primary objective of TL is to improve the performance of the objective function f_T (.) for the target task T_T, by discovering and learning hidden knowledge from D_s and T_T, where $D_s \neq D_T$ or $T_s \neq T_T$ [21].

10.3.3 Transfer Learning versus Traditional Deep Learning

TL was introduced to overcome several shortcomings that were prevalent in traditional machine learning or deep learning approaches [22]. Traditional models allow machines to learn from input data without being programmed explicitly. The models can recognize patterns from the training data to generate predictions with the unseen data and achieve higher performance in general. However, such effective and efficient predictive analysis can be obtained only when they are trained on a huge amount of data. At times, it is challenging to collect such a huge dataset for accurate results. Further, it is imperative to train these traditional models from scratch, which is expensive computationally. Moreover, there are isolated training approaches suitable for traditional algorithms, where every model is specifically trained for a certain target task with no dependency on past knowledge. A huge amount of time is required to train traditional models with such huge datasets from scratch, which also is a major concern in real scenarios. TL can overcome the limitations set by these traditional approaches. Here information is extracted through a pretrained neural network, preferably CNN, from given and related data and transferred to solve a new but related task with a new dataset. These pretrained models are already well trained on large datasets, which are partially retrained with a smaller dataset for solving the new problem and also render higher accuracy. This also allows them to be computationally faster, as the features learned from the pretrained models are reused and eliminate the need to train the entire model from scratch. This concept is illustrated in Figure 10.2.

Based on the research findings, most of the pretrained TL models rely on CNNs [23], a popular DL model most widely used for image classification. Since CNN can extract critical properties of an input image, it is popular among researchers to build a pretrained model because the availability of data for constructing a pretrained model for the initial training is an essential component in TL. It is imperative

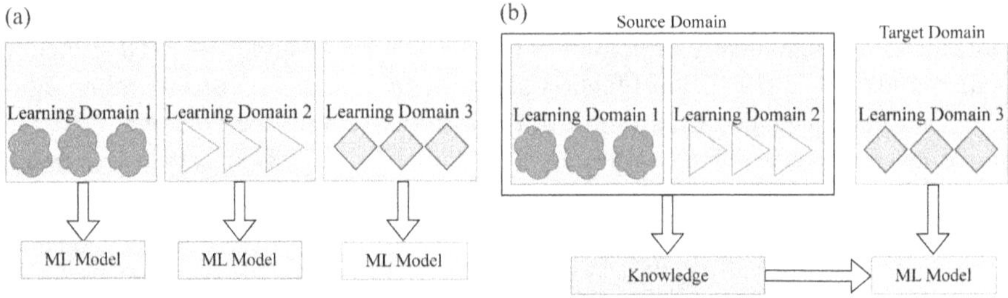

FIGURE 10.2 Traditional models versus transfer learning models.

to possess a basic knowledge of CNN before learning about image classification through TL, which is discussed in detail in the subsequent section.

10.3.4 CNN

Owing to the effectiveness of deep learning algorithms in image classification, target identification, and object recognition, popular and basic DL algorithms like artificial neural networks (ANNs) [24] have successfully been employed in IoT-based smart healthcare to predict and diagnose diseases with outstanding accuracy [25]. Other potential DL models like CNN [26] have performed exceptionally well in the healthcare domain [27–29]. It is the most extensively used neural network class and has been acknowledged as the highest-performing model across all datasets, particularly in the case of analyzing visual images using deep learning.

The core component of CNN [26] is a multilayered neural network that offers solutions, particularly for the analysis, classification, and recognition of images and videos. A sequence of convolutional and pooling layers, some fully connected layers, and a normalizing layer (such as the softmax function) make up the basic framework of a CNN. The convolutional and pooling layers essentially provide the learning of the model, while the fully connected layer offers the classification. The convolutional layer allows the model to learn about the properties of the input which is a 2D image with $a \times b$ pixels. In each layer of convolution, there are 2D metrics of fixed size called kernels, which are unique and can identify some features of the image, by analyzing for a specific pattern. Assuming the filter to be an $m \times n$ matrix, the same $m \times n$ matrix can be selected from the input and an elementwise cross-product may be performed for both matrices. The SOP, or summation of all products, then creates the correlated elements in the newly created matrix known as a feature map. At this point, activation functions such as sigmoid, tanh, or ReLU may be used for the purpose. The feature map is then filled with the output of that specific filter in that specific convolutional layer after swiping the kernel across the image [30]. The mathematical equation of the convolution process is shown next.

For a 2D input image, I, and a 2D kernel filter, K, the calculation of the convoluted image, S, is calculated as follows:

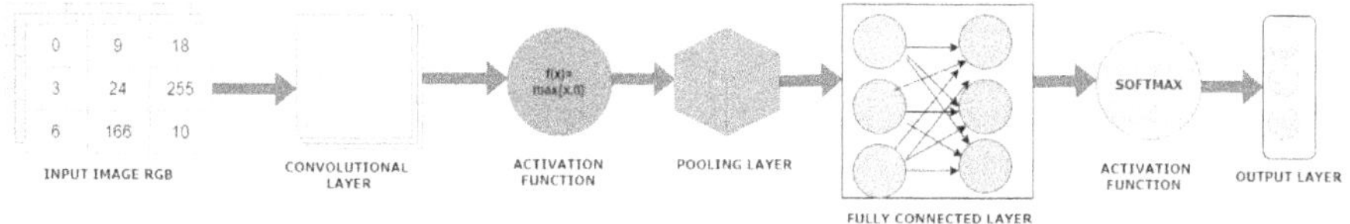

FIGURE 10.3 Basic architecture of CNN.

$$(i, j) = (I * K)(i, j) = \sum\sum I(m, n)K(i - m, j - n) \tag{10.1}$$

where $m \times n$ is the dimension of the kernel K and I and j are the coordinates of the matrix from which the calculation of the convolution is done [31].

Pooling layers are generally applied between convoluted layers, perform subsampling, and diminish the feature map size with the selection of the most essential features, which eventually decreases the computational power needed to process the model. They also aid in effective training of the model, as the invariable as well as dominant features are also eradicated through the procedure. In general, the neurons of the CNN layers are connected only to the partially overlapping and spatially mapped previous layers neurons. This generates a necessity for the fully connected (FC) layer of the CNN architecture, where all neurons from the preceding layers form a dense network with one or more such layers before the final output layer, that performs the actual classification. At this stage, output classes are obtained by calculating the probability distributions of the output using softmax regression. Figure 10.3 gives an idea about the traditional CNN model in brief.

10.3.5 Pretrained Model

As discussed in the previous sections, TL thrives on the concept of pretrained models, which are constructed using powerful CNNs, capable of achieving higher accuracy for predictions with extremely large datasets. However, in real life, it is cumbersome to collect specific datasets for industrial or commercial applications. Hence, most of the data that are available in practical platforms are diminutive. To address this issue, researchers have modeled a few pretrained models using ImageNet [32, 33], which is an organized database of 14,197,122 annotated images, as per the WordNet hierarchy and most commonly used for CNN model training, for object detection and image classification.

Being large enough, ImageNet is capable of creating a generalized CNN model as observed in an annual competition called ImageNet Large Scale Visual Recognition Challenge (ILSVRC), which was conducted from 2010 to 2017 [32]. The competition was based on two tasks, where the first challenge was to detect objects within an image, belonging to 200 classes popularly known as object localization. The second task comprised image classification, each of which was labeled with 1000 categories. This competition witnessed some trailblazing DL models, popularly termed pretrained models, submitted by well-known researchers all across the globe.

TABLE 10.2
Prevalent Pretrained Models: Keras Applications

Model	Size (in MB)	Parameters (in Millions)	Top 5	Accuracy (in %)
Xception	88	22.9	81	94.5
VGG16	528	138.4	16	90.1
VGG19	549	143.7	19	90.0
ResNet50	98	25.6	107	92.1
INCEPTIONV3	92	23.9	189	92.8
INCEPTIONResNetV2	215	55.9	449	95.3
MobileNet	16	4.3	55	89.5
DenseNet201	80	20.2	402	93.6
NASNetLarge	343	88.9	533	96.0
EfficientNetB7	256	66.7	438	97.0

These pretrained models are publicly accessible, along with their parameters such as weights, and later can be used to perform a similar but different task, thus forming the crux of TL. This saves the researcher from training the current model from scratch, saving time and cumbersome efforts required to train huge datasets. Training at times becomes unfeasible during real-life applications due to a scarcity of data as well. Hence, pretrained models are preferable options in comparison. Interestingly, a substantial number of pretrained models are provided by Keras, a deep learning library that can be used for several tasks such as classification, prediction, or even feature extraction from different datasets. A detailed list of a few frequently used pretrained models trained on an ImageNet dataset is in Table 10.2.

10.3.6 Steps to Conduct Transfer Learning with Pretrained Models

To build hierarchical representations of the data, deep learning systems are frequently constructed using a series of convolutional layers and max pooling layers. These layers serve as feature extractors that are coupled to the final layers and carry out particular tasks, such as classification or regression. Typically, the neurons in these top layers are fully linked. As deep learning models learn hierarchical representations, the first layers frequently identify basic representations like edges and corners, while the succeeding layers learn more sophisticated representations like the components of things. In order to conduct TL, the entire model is trained on the ImageNet dataset [32], and the learned weights of the CNN model are trained to learn several patterns in the input image which can be reused at ease to conclude the classes of newly fed images, and thus TL generalizes images outside the ImageNet dataset [32] with the help of pretrained models.

In general, TL can be implemented in two ways depending on a base neural network, which is trained on a large dataset: the first n layers are copied to the first n

layers of the target network, and the remaining layers are initialized and trained according to the target task. There are two ways to implement TL depending on the distribution of the data: the number of parameters in the first n layers of the base network, and the size of the target dataset [34, 35]. In the first approach, all weights of all layers of the convolutional layer in the pretrained model are frozen, signifying that they remain unchanged during the training with the target dataset for the new task.

This approach is commonly known as feature extraction, where only the last layer or fully connected layer is removed and replaced with a customized layer to be trained on a new dataset. During training, only the weights of the newly added fully connected layer are retrained, retaining the weights of the frozen convolutional layers. This solution is typically useful for extremely small datasets (1000 images) with a large number of parameters. Further, this approach is useful for scenarios where the base dataset is similar to the target dataset in output labels. Figure 10.4 gives an idea of the same.

In the second approach, weights of some convolutional layers are frozen instead of all, and the unfrozen convolutional layers along with the newly added, customized fully connected layers are retrained with the target dataset, at a very low learning rate. Commonly known as fine-tuning, this method of TL is often conducted on moderate and large-sized target datasets (10,000–100,000 images) with a small number of parameters. Since the model is large, and the target dataset is smaller, a low learning rate will improve the performance resulting in no overfitting. Fine-tuning works well when the target datasets happen to be significantly non-identical from the base dataset in output labels. Thus, different convolutional layers can therefore be frozen in the pretrained CNN model to enhance performance on the target task based on the data distribution across the source and target domains. Therefore, the primary objective of using TL in classification problems is to deal with smaller target datasets, which is often a matter of concern in real-life scenarios. Figure 10.5 gives an overall view of the concept.

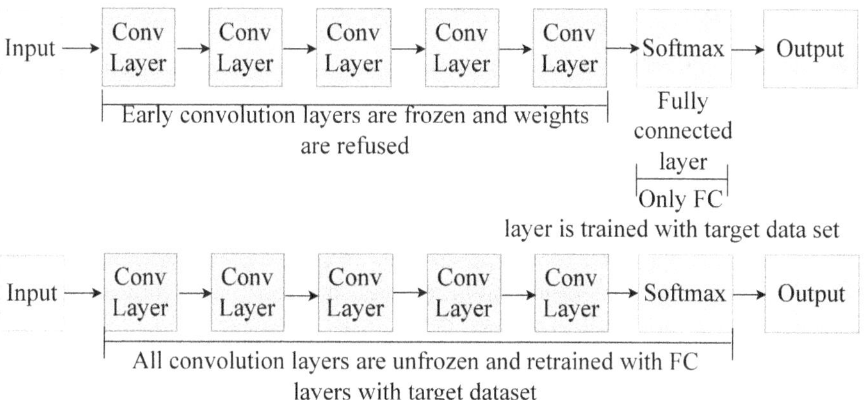

FIGURE 10.4 Feature extraction versus fine-tuning.

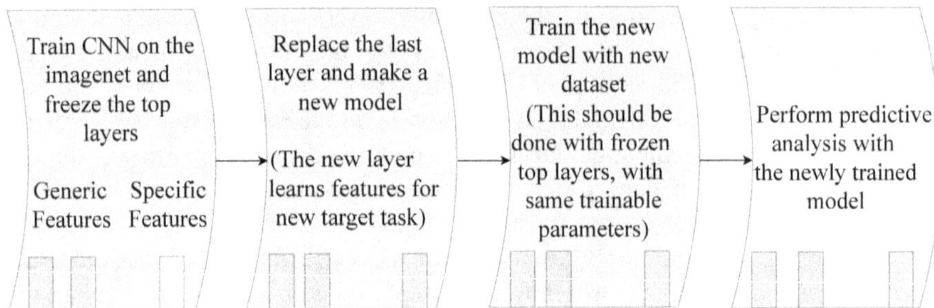

FIGURE 10.5 Steps of transfer learning with pretrained models.

10.3.7 Application of Transfer Learning in Healthcare Domain

Several literary works reveal the extensive application of TL in the healthcare domain. Ravishankar et al. [36] demonstrated the effectiveness of TL applied on CNNs to solve the problem of automatic localization of the kidneys in ultrasound images and have concluded that TL applied on CNN outperforms the state-of-the-art model to achieve a 20% higher performance in general. Samala et al. [37] investigated the training of a deep CNN and proposed a multitask TL to classify malignant and benign masses on mammograms by learning from nonmedical images to medical diagnostic tasks through supervised training and simultaneously learning multiple auxiliary tasks. TL can also be applied to extract CNN-based features with the help of B-mode liver images to perform fatty liver disease classification and determine the level of steatosis in patients [38]. In real-world healthcare applications, the majority of data is imbalanced, which deviates from the classifiers and causes them to generalize patterns observed preferably in the majority class, substantially disregarding the minority class. Data dependence is another issue in classification, especially in deep learning models that require huge amounts of data for improved performance metrics, which are often difficult to collect in healthcare due to the complexity of the ailment, rarity of the disease, heterogeneity of medical data sources, and the cost of accumulation and annotation. With TL, it is possible to mitigate insufficient training data and handle class-imbalanced dataset problems in a given target domain with pretrained models [39]. Farhadi et al. proposed an efficient TL model with structured data using publicly available breast cancer datasets to construct a pretrained model and use the TL concept to predict top-grade malignant tumors in patients [39].

Alghamdi et al. [40] proposed a pretrained deep CNN model for early detection of cardiac attacks, where VGGNET is used for object recognition in order to achieve maximum accuracy as well as a feature extractor by the selection of essential convolutional layers to obtain a clearer representation of ECG data, along with improving the CNN model using augmentation of data. TL may be used to discriminate two classes of skin injuries, which was difficult to accomplish due to a lack of sufficient data through machine learning. Abubakar et al. [41] used three state-of-the-art pretrained CNN models with two approaches commonly applied to TL. In the first, dense and classification layers were replaced with freshly appended layers that were trained using images from the leftover convolutional layers. Support vector machine (SVM), rather than introducing new layers, was employed for classification. TL is effective in the detection of lung carcinoma in patients, using CT images, with three pertained models – VGG19, VGG16, and Xception – with data augmentation and localization for improved performance metrics. Hashmi et al. [42] proposed automatic diagnosis of diseases such as pneumonia with the help of x-ray images of the chest using TL and partial data augmentation techniques were used to increase and hence balance the training dataset along with fine-tuning of the pretrained CNN models to obtain satisfactory performance metrics. TL also solves the problem of overfitting, which is evident in medical images due to insufficient availability of training data.

Pretrained models like InceptionResNetV2 may be used to detect tuberculosis from chest x-ray images, with the help of image preprocessing, augmentation of data, and deep learning classification techniques. Khamparia et al. [43] proposed a modified VGG model implemented on 3D and 2D images of mammograms for early detection of breast cancer, which outperformed the performance metrics of conventional CNNs in the same context and can also help reduce the occurrence of false negatives and false positives in predictions. As stated earlier, it is a cumbersome process to accumulate sufficient training data for certain ailments due to personalized content and cost of collection, such as glucose monitoring in diabetic patients. De Bois et al. [44] proposed a multisource, adversarial, novel TL model that is pretrained on a huge, diverse dataset of diabetic patients.

Srinivas et al. [45] adopted the TL approach to perform brain tumor detection along with data augmentation, preprocessing, and hypothesized hyperparameter integral tuning and observed that out of three pretrained models, namely, Inception-v3, ResNet-50, and VGG-16, the latter renders satisfactory accuracy measures. Alharbi et al. [46] employed image segmentation of pneumonia from x-ray images using BoxENet architecture by incorporating TL from a fusion of SqueezeNet and ImgNet, which is claimed to have outperformed state-of-the-art models of binary as well as multiclass classification. TL is effective in the detection of lung carcinoma in patients, as proposed in [47], using CT images, with three pertained models such as VGG19, VGG16, and Xception, with data augmentation and localization for improved performance metrics.

Ahmad et al. [48] considered a patch selection approach for the classification of breast cancer, from a limited number of histopathological images, adopting a TL approach. Initially, the patches, taken from whole slide images, are put into the CNN model for extraction of significant and primitive features, which gives feature vectors that help to select discriminative patches using a clustered approach. They are once more trained using the Efficient Net architecture, which was previously trained using the ImageNet dataset, and then used to train the SVM classifier for image classification. An interesting work is from Samee et al. [49], who proposed a hybrid technique based on logistic regression and principal component analysis (LR-PCA) for the classification of breast lesions, which is based on CNN architecture, for high-level feature extraction using TL. Using contrast-limited adaptive histogram equalization and pixel-by-pixel intensity correction, pseudo-colored images were created alongside the original grayscale photos in order to enhance the training data. This helps in the extraction of deep features with the help of the TL models VGG, AlexNet, and GoogleNet. The LR-PCA model then selects the most significant components to handle the problem of multicollinearity where the dimensionality is reduced with PCA to generate a low dimensional feature space while retaining the variance of the input data.

Kumar et al. [50] proposed ensemble models for faster diagnosis of COVID-19 using radiographic images, and implemented TL using state-of-the-art pretrained models such as GoogleNet, EfficientNet, and XceptionNet. Altun et al. [51] aimed to detect monkeypox through skin lesions using custom CNNs, supported by hyperparameter optimization and TL pretrained models including VGG19, MobileNetV3-s, and ResNET50. Meena et al. [52] focused on adopting a TL approach to detect the presence of brain tumor in patients and classify it into four categories. Information loss is restricted using a feature fusion method, that allows the integration of course features with fine-grained features for better predictive analysis.

10.4 IMPLEMENTATION OF TRANSFER LEARNING WITH THE APPLICATION OF PRETRAINED MODELS UPON HEALTHCARE DATASETS

The implementation of TL requires well-trained models [53], on large-scale datasets, which can be used to build an intermediate model, which will be further trained on a target dataset. The following section presents a brief implementation of the concept using two well-known pretrained models, i.e., VGG16 and NASNetLarge, extensively used in TL; and two datasets, i.e., Skin Cancer: Malignant vs. Benign and Brain MRI Images for Brain Tumor Detection, which are also discussed in further detail.

10.4.1 Pretrained Model 1: VGG16

VGG16 is the most widely used pretrained model, among several of its contemporaries such as VGG11, VGG13, and VGG19 [55]. This popular CNN-based model [54] was proposed by Karen Simonyan and Andrew Zisserman of the Visual Geometry Group (VGG) Lab of Oxford University in 2014 at the ImageNet Large Scale Visual Recognition Challenge. One of the primary reasons to prefer VGG16 as a pretrained model for experimentation is due to its efficiency in working with moderate-sized datasets as well as its capability to get trained faster in comparison to its contemporaries.

VGG16, as the name suggests, is a 16-layer deep neural network, trained on the ImageNet dataset, that can classify 1000 images with 1000 categories, with a test accuracy of 92.7%. The architecture of VGG16 consists of 13 convolutional layers, 5 max pooling layers, and 3 fully connected layers with very small (3 × 3) convolutional filters for the extraction of features, as shown in Figure 10.6. However, out of these 21 layers, only 16 layers have learnable parameters effectively used to implement the model.

The architecture of VGG16 includes the following components:

Input – The input image size is kept constant at 224 × 224.

Convolutional layers – As mentioned, there are 13 convolutional layers, with a 3 × 3 filter, with a 1 × 1 convolution filter for linear transformation of the input.

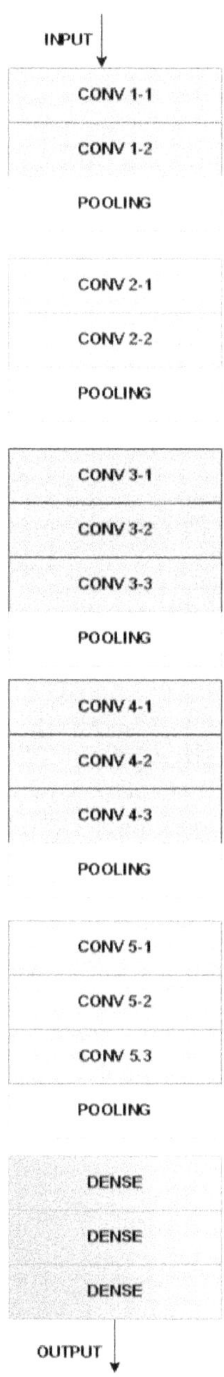

FIGURE 10.6 Basic architecture of VGG16.

ReLU activation – ReLU is a linear function, to render a matching output for positive inputs and a zero output for negative inputs. VGG16 sets a convolution stride of 1 pixel for preserving the spatial resolution once the convolution operation is performed on the input image, which reflects the number of pixels the filter should move/stride to cover the entire image space.

Pooling layers – Convolutional layers are followed by pooling layers whose function is to reduce the dimensionality as well as the number of parameters of the feature map generated in each convolutional layer in the previous steps. Due to pooling, the number of available filters grows from 64 to 512 at the final layers.

Fully connected layers – In the end, VGG16 has three fully connected layers out of which the first two have 4096 channels each and the last one has 1000 channels, each pertaining to one output class.

10.4.2 Pretrained Model 2: NASNetLarge

Another approach to implementing TL is using NASNetLarge [55], a convolutional neural network trained on the ImageNet dataset [32]. NASNetLarge was introduced by Google. It is an effective and efficient CNN framework for a given image dataset that operates on reinforcement learning strategies. It comprises 1000 output classes, which makes it capable of representing the rich features of a variety of images. The default input size of images is 331 × 331 for NASNetLarge, and it is composed of the conv2D layers, BatchNormalization layers, AveragePooling2D layers, and fully connected layers just like a conventional CNN architecture. However, the basic architecture of NASNetLarge is based on cells or blocks, which are predefined by the reinforcement learning search methods, to find the optimal parameters such as filter size, number of strides, number of layers, and the output channel within the given search space. There are two types of cells used in NASNetLarge: normal cells, which are convolutional cells, returning feature maps within the same input dimensions, and reduction cells returning feature maps with a twofold reduction in width and height. The accuracy of the model with the ImageNet dataset was 82.5% with accuracy as the performance metrics. Figure 10.7 shows the architecture of NASNetLarge in detail.

10.4.3 Datasets for Experimentation

The experiments for TL are conducted following the pretrained models mentioned in previous sections using the state-of-the-art datasets as described next.

10.4.3.1 Dataset 1: Skin Cancer: Malignant vs. Benign

The dataset Skin Cancer: Malignant vs. Benign, taken from Kaggle [56], is one of the topmost resources for datasets and code. Having a total of 3297 images, the dataset is divided into train (2637 images) and test (660 images). The latter contains 360 images that are benign and 300 images that fall under the category of malignant. The size of each image is 224 × 224 with high quality. The rights of this dataset

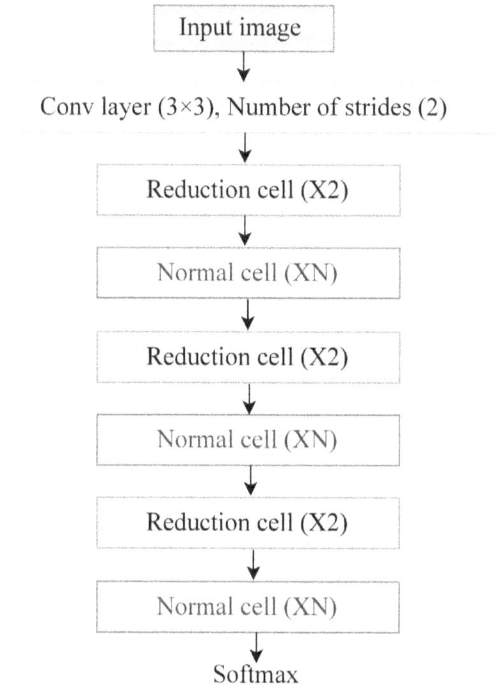

FIGURE 10.7 Basic architecture of NASNetLarge.

TABLE 10.3
Skin Cancer Dataset Description

Parameter	Default Value
Dataset name	Skin Cancer Malignant vs. Benign
Disease to be predicted	Skin cancer
Source	Kaggle2
Total number of images	3297
Images for training	2637
Images for testing	660
Size of each image	224 × 224

are confined to ISIC-Archive. A brief elucidation of the dataset is demonstrated in Table 10.3, and Figure 10.8 depicts a pictorial overview of the dataset.

10.4.3.2 Dataset 2: Brain MRI Images for Brain Tumor Detection

The dataset Brain MRI Images for Brain Tumor Detection, taken from Kaggle [57] as well, has 253 MRI images of brain tumors. Out of these, 98 images are from healthy patients without any ailment, and the remaining 155 are from patients suffering from

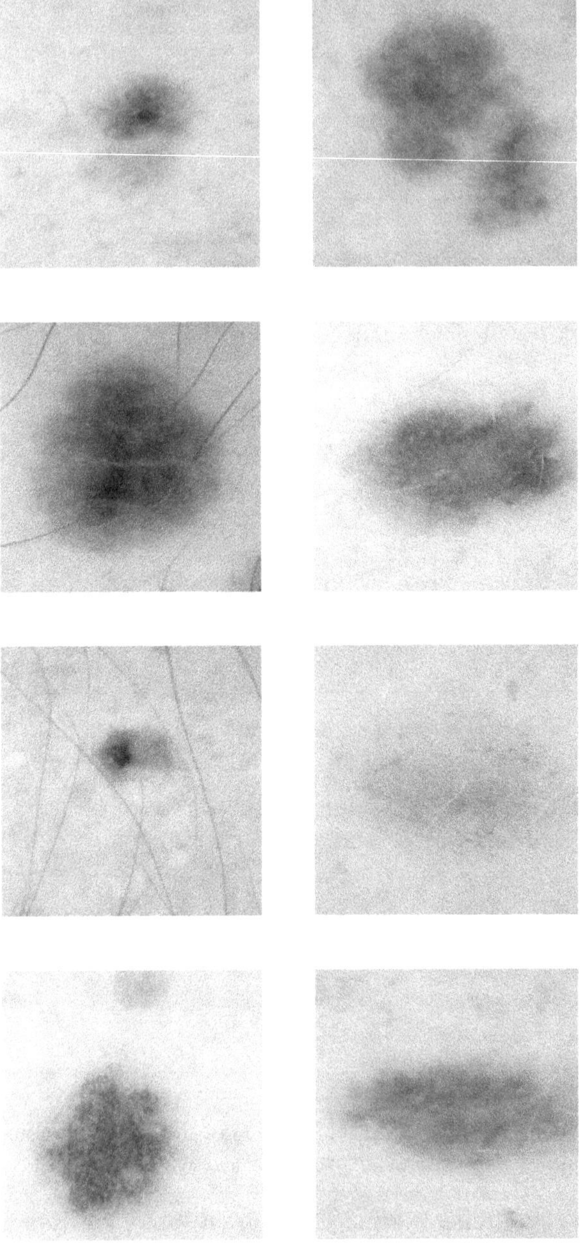

FIGURE 10.8 Images from skin cancer dataset.

TABLE 10.4
Brain Tumor Dataset Description

Parameter	Default Value
Dataset Name	Brain MRI Images for Brain Tumor Detection
Disease to be predicted	Brain tumor
Source	Kaggle3
Total number of images	253
Images for training	226
Images for testing	27
Size of each image	224 × 224

a brain tumor. Out of this, for experimentation purposes, 27 images were taken for testing, whereas the rest were used for training and validation. A brief elucidation of the dataset is illustrated in Table 10.4, and Figure 10.9 depicts a pictorial overview of the dataset.

10.4.4 Experiments and Results on VGGNET16

For experimentation, Python was chosen as the language for coding, and the ML toolkit scikit-learn was used, along with Google Colab as the integrated development environment (IDE). The experiments are conducted in two phases: First, one pretrained model (VGG16) is deployed on two different datasets of diseases (skin cancer and brain tumor) and the respective performance metrics are compared. In the second phase, two different pretrained models (VGG16 and NASNetLarge) are deployed on one dataset (brain tumor) for a similar comparison of accuracies between the two. The second phase enables us to detect the best-performing pretrained model on such small training data, which is the primary purpose of implementing TL over conventional CNN models.

In phase I, for the skin cancer dataset, VGG16 is loaded from the Keras library, and the weights of the trainable parameters of all convolutional layers are frozen, which will be transferred to the next stage (flatten layer) without any retraining. The output layer of the original VGG16 is replaced with a customized dense layer with two neurons, as there are only two outputs to be specified for the binary classification of malignant and benign cancer in this problem. It is observed that out of the total 21,137,729 parameters of VGG16, only 64,23,041 parameters will be trained during TL, whereas the rest of the 14,714,688 parameters will remain frozen and hence untrained in the next stage. The accuracy and loss of the training and validation data obtained upon application of TL are shown in Figure 10.10.

VGG16 is also deployed for the classification of brain tumors where a similar approach is adopted for loading the pretrained model and freezing the weights of the convolutional layers. Here, out of 20,049,473 parameters, only 25,089 will be trainable in the next stage and the remaining 20,024,384 parameters will not be

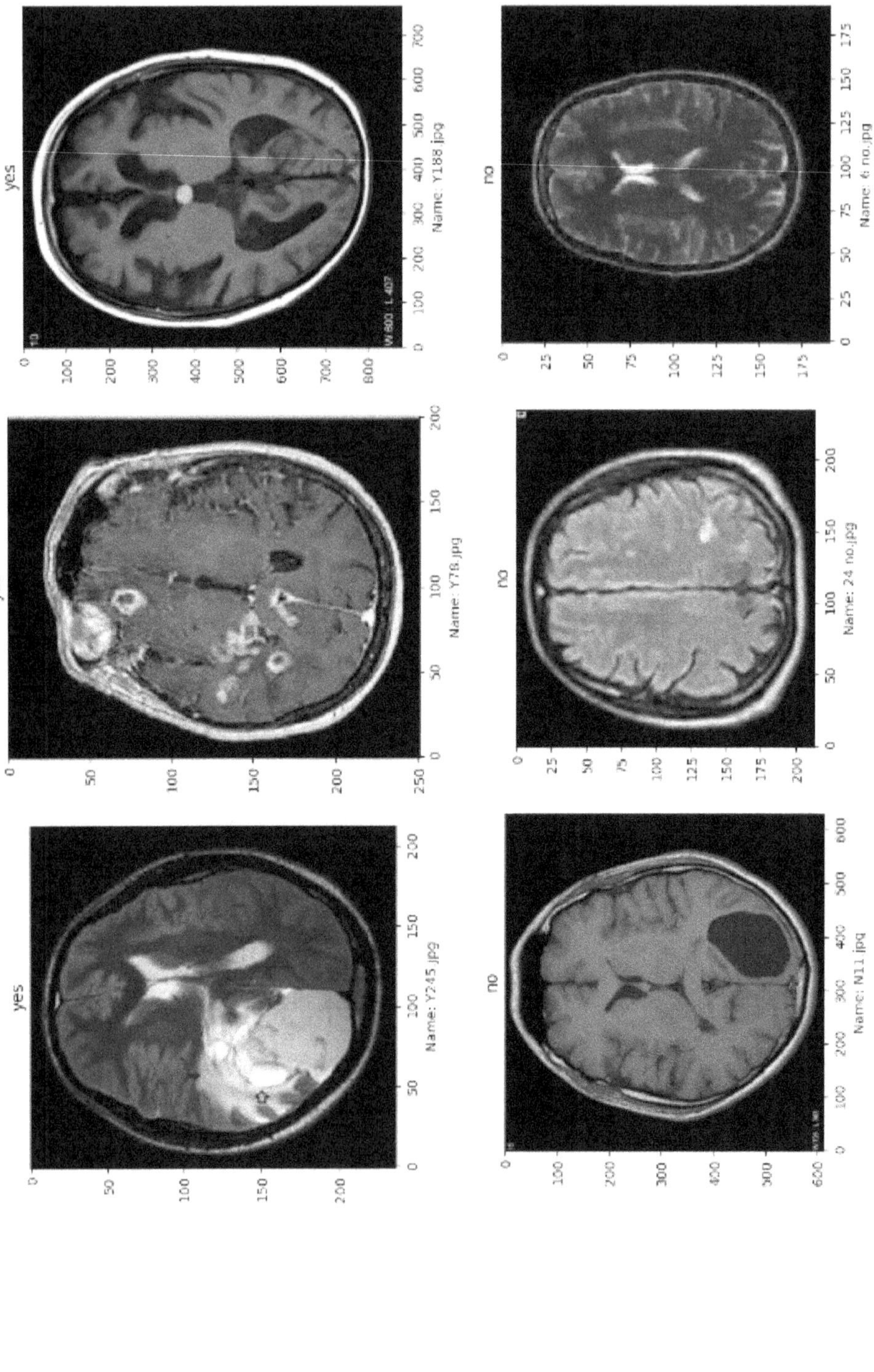

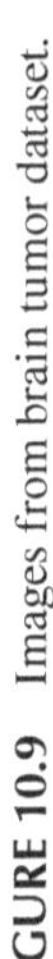

FIGURE 10.9 Images from brain tumor dataset.

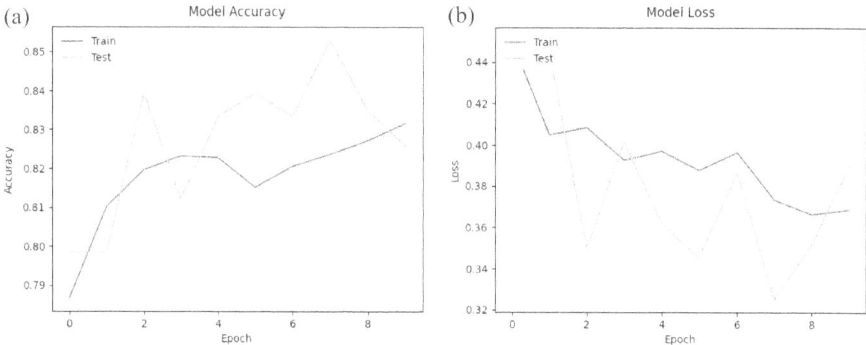

FIGURE 10.10 Model accuracy and loss of VGG16 on skin cancer dataset for transfer learning.

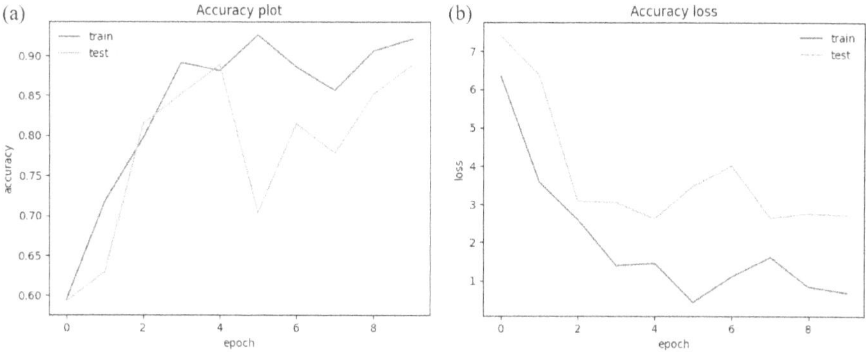

FIGURE 10.11 Model accuracy and loss of VGG16 on brain tumor dataset for transfer learning.

trained during TL. The training accuracy and loss of the final model are shown in Figure 10.11. The accuracy obtained by the brain tumor dataset on VGG16 is 87.5%.

10.4.4.1 Performance Metrics of VGGNET16 on Skin Cancer and Brain Tumor Datasets

In machine learning, there are several performance metrics used to assess the effectiveness and efficiency of classifiers. These include commonly used measures like accuracy, recall, precision, and F-score (F-measure), which researchers often utilize to perform predictive analysis. Out of these, accuracy is the most widely used performance metric that is performed on training, validation, and testing datasets. In our case, the testing accuracies of the VGGNET model on the skin cancer and brain tumor datasets are found to be 82.57% and 87.50%, respectively. However, for a proper understanding of the errors (type I and type II), the results obtained are organized in a confusion matrix (CM), represented as $Cm \times m$ for classification problems with m classes. Figure 10.12 gives a pictorial overview of the confusion matrix in

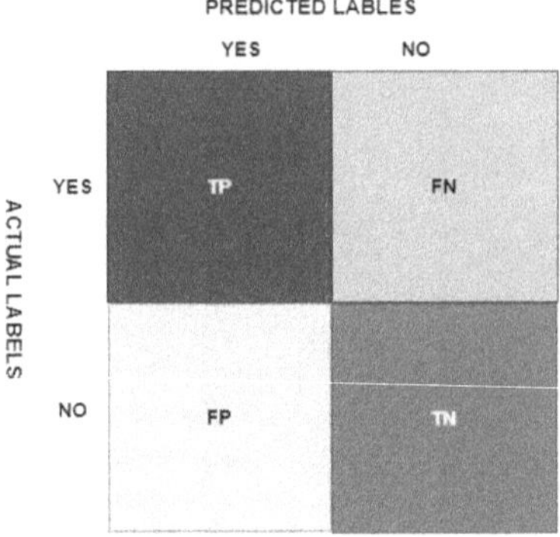

FIGURE 10.12 Basic structure of a confusion matrix.

general. As per standard notions, every element *CMi j* is denoted as the number of instances of class *i*, classified as class *j*. The confusion matrix is designed to have the following values:

- True positives (TP) – The total number of positive instances that are also classified as positive.
- True negatives (TN) – The total number of negative instances that are also classified as negative.
- False positives (FP) – The total number of negative instances that are classified as positive.
- False negatives (FN) – The total number of positive instances that are classified as negatives.

The CM of the VGGNET16 model on the skin cancer and brain tumor datasets is shown in Figure 10.13. Observation reveals that the total number of correctly

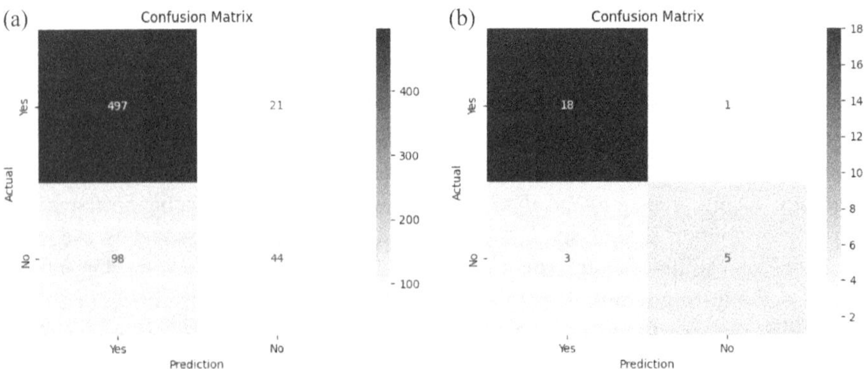

FIGURE 10.13 Confusion matrix of VGG16 on skin cancer and brain tumor datasets.

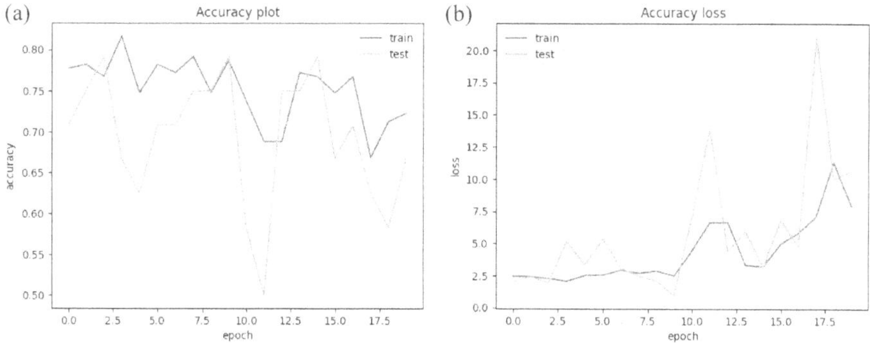

FIGURE 10.14 Model accuracy and loss of NASNetLarge on brain tumor dataset for transfer learning.

identified samples classified by the model is 541 out of 660 in the case of skin cancer, whereas the total number of correctly classified samples of brain tumor stands at 23 out of 27 test data.

10.4.4.2 Performance Analysis on NASNetLarge

In phase II, both VGG16 and NASNetLarge are deployed on one dataset (brain tumor) and TL is conducted likewise. The weights of the convolutional layers of NASNetLarge, obtained upon training with ImageNet, are frozen during training in TL, as done in VGG16. Both models as discussed are deployed on one dataset (brain tumor). Observations reveal that out of 85,404,691 parameters, only 487,873 are trainable for the next stage and the other 84,916,818 parameters remain nontrainable to implement TL with NASNetLarge. Figure 10.14 shows the training accuracy and loss of the NASNetLarge model with the brain tumor dataset. The testing accuracy was found to be 81.48%.

The CM of the NASNetLarge model on the brain tumor dataset is shown in Figure 10.15. Here, the total corrected number of samples is found to be 22 of 27 of the test dataset and the total number of incorrect samples is found to be 5 of 27.

Based on the aforementioned experiments on two state-of-the-art TL models (VGGNET and NASNetLarge), Figure 10.16 shows the comparison of accuracies of both pretrained models (VGG16 and NASNetLarge) on one single dataset (brain tumor). It is observed that the performance of VGGNET16 is comparatively better than NASNetLarge, with an accuracy of 87.50%, which demonstrates the desideratum of TL in deep neural networks. One possible reason for this can be the large size of NASNetLarge, which takes substantial time to be implemented on other datasets. Thus, it can be concluded that the concept of TL can be utilized in the future for better predictive performances on a variety of machine learning as well as deep learning architectures. All the performance metrics (accuracy, precision, recall, and F1-score) for both models (VGGNET16 and NASNetLarge) with both datasets (skin cancer and brain tumor) have been summarized in Table 10.5.

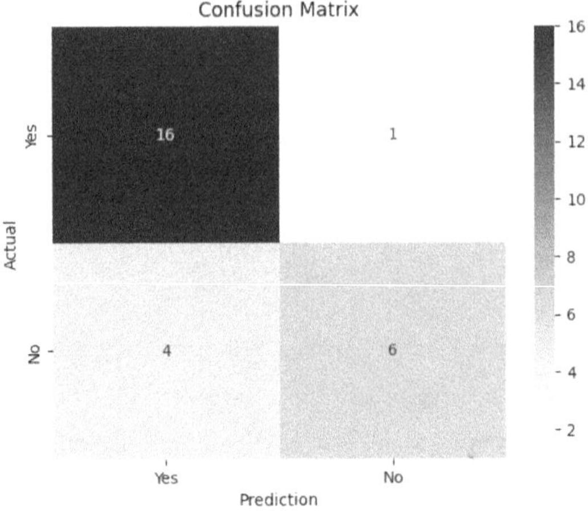

FIGURE 10.15 Confusion matrix of NASNetLarge on brain tumor dataset.

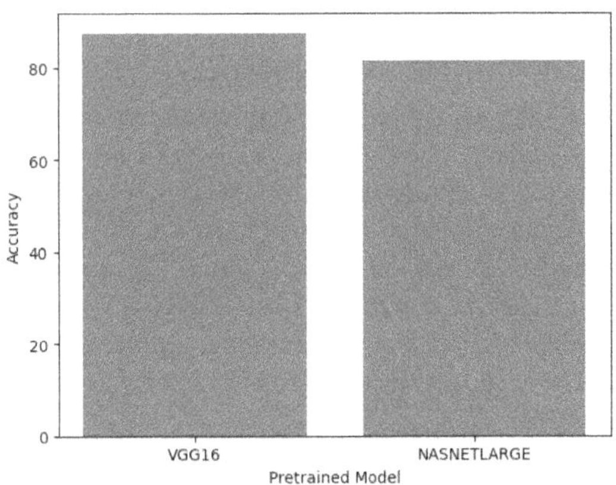

FIGURE 10.16 Comparison of accuracies of VGGNET16 and NASNetLarge on brain tumor dataset.

10.5 CONCLUSION

This chapter furnishes an extensive and elaborate analysis of the impact of TL with an overview of IoT-based healthcare applications. At the onset, a brief overview of the applications in HIoT is given and the contribution of several ML and DL techniques in this domain is surveyed to provide the preliminaries. Next, the concept of TL is presented with basic definitions, and a comparative analysis is made as well with the traditional DL models for better discernment. Since TL is based on deep neural networks trained on large-scale training datasets, a pretrained model is used here that is further reused to train the model partially with a relatively smaller

TABLE 10.5
Summary of Comparative Analysis of Both Datasets with Different Metrics

Performance Metric	Concept	Formula	Skin Cancer VGGNET	Brain Tumor VGGNET	Brain Tumor NASNetLarge
Accuracy	Calculated as the ratio of the total number of correctly predicted instances subject to all given instances	$\frac{TP+TN}{TP+TN+FP+FN}$	82.57	87.50	81.48
Precision (P)	Calculated as the ratio of positive instances classified correctly to the total number of instances classified as positive	$\frac{TP}{TP+FP}$	95.94	94.73	94.11
Recall (R)	Calculated as the ratio of the total number of positive instances correctly classified as positive to the total number of positive data points	$\frac{TP}{TP+FN}$	83.52	85.71	80.00
F-score	Calculated as the harmonic mean of precision and recall	$\frac{2(P*R)}{P+R}$	89.30	90.00	86.48

dataset to solve a new task. Hence, in this chapter, the notion of the pretrained model and CNN is illustrated along with the details of how to incorporate this in order to conduct TL. In addition, potential applications of TL in the healthcare domain are summarized, which renders a cut-above perception of the problem domain as well as the state-of-the-art solutions that can draw further research interest in this domain. Finally, we provide a glimpse of the implementation of TL using the existing pre-trained models, which can provide researchers with the visualization of relevant results to consider as the benchmark for the next level of research.

REFERENCES

1. Bharadwaj, H.K., Agarwal, A., Chamola, V., Lakkaniga, N.R., Hassija, V., Guizani, M., Sikdar, B.: A review on the role of machine learning in enabling IoT based healthcare applications. *IEEE Access* **9**, 38859–38890 (2021).
2. Sharma, S., Dudeja, R.K., Aujla, G.S., Bali, R.S., Kumar, N.: Detras: Deep learning-based healthcare framework for IoT-based assistance of Alzheimer patients. *Neural Computing and Applications*, 1–13 **32**(17) (2020).
3. Naresh, V.S., Pericherla, S.S., Murty, P.S.R., Reddi, S.: Internet of things in healthcare: Architecture, applications, challenges, and solutions. *Computer Systems Science and Engineering* **35**(6) (2020).
4. Pradhan, B., Bhattacharyya, S., Pal, K.: IoT-based applications in healthcare devices. *Journal of Healthcare Engineering*, 1–18 **2021** (2021). 6632599.
5. Chen, M., Hao, Y., Hwang, K., Wang, L., Wang, L.: Disease prediction by machine learning over big data from healthcare communities. *IEEE Access* **5**, 8869–8879 (2017).
6. Ginantra, N., Indradewi, I., Hartono, E.: Machine learning approach for acute respiratory infections (ISPA) prediction: Case study Indonesia. *Journal of Physics: Conference Series* **1469**(1), 012044 (2020).
7. Hadi, M.S., Lawey, A.Q., El-Gorashi, T.E., Elmirghani, J.M.: Patient-centric HetNets powered by machine learning and big data analytics for 6G networks. *IEEE Access* **8**, 85639–85655 (2020).
8. Liu, X., Faes, L., Kale, A.U., Wagner, S.K., Fu, D.J., Bruynseels, A., Mahendiran, T., Moraes, G., Shamdas, M., Kern, C., et al.: A comparison of deep learning performance against health-care professionals in detecting diseases from medical imaging: A systematic review and meta-analysis. *The Lancet Digital Health* **1**(6), e271–e297 (2019).
9. Rahman, M.A., Hossain, M.S., Alrajeh, N.A., Guizani, N.: B5G and explainable deep learning assisted healthcare vertical at the edge: Covid-19 perspective. *IEEE Network* **34**(4), 98–105 (2020).
10. Esteva, A., Robicquet, A., Ramsundar, B., Kuleshov, V., DePristo, M., Chou, K., Cui, C., Corrado, G., Thrun, S., Dean, J.: A guide to deep learning in healthcare. *Nature Medicine* **25**(1), 24–29 (2019).
11. Sarraf, S., Tofighi, G.: Classification of Alzheimer's disease using fMRI data and deep learning convolutional neural networks. arXiv preprint arXiv:1603.08631 (2016).
12. Mohsen, H., El-Dahshan, E.S.A., El-Horbaty, E.S.M., Salem, A.B.M.: Classification using deep learning neural networks for brain tumors. *Future Computing and Informatics Journal* **3**(1), 68–71 (2018).
13. Stephen, O., Sain, M., Maduh, U.J., Jeong, D.U., et al.: An efficient deep learning approach to pneumonia classification in healthcare. *Journal of Healthcare Engineering* **2019** (2019). 4180949.

14. Kourou, K., Exarchos, T.P., Exarchos, K.P., Karamouzis, M.V., Fotiadis, D.I.: Machine learning applications in cancer prognosis and prediction. *Computational and Structural Biotechnology Journal* **13**, 8–17 (2015).
15. Ker, J., Wang, L., Rao, J., Lim, T.: Deep learning applications in medical image analysis. *IEEE Access* **6**, 9375–9389 (2017).
16. Saha, A., Rajak, S., Saha, J., Chowdhury, C.: A survey of machine learning and meta-heuristics approaches for sensor-based human activity recognition systems. *Journal of Ambient Intelligence and Humanized Computing*, 1–28 (2022).
17. Pan, S.J., Yang, Q.: A survey on transfer learning. *IEEE Transactions on Knowledge and Data Engineering* **22**(10), 1345–1359 (2010).
18. Agarwal, N., Sondhi, A., Chopra, K., Singh, G.: Transfer learning: Survey and classification. In: *Smart Innovations in Communication and Computational Sciences. Proceedings of ICSICCS 2020*, pp. 145–155 (2021).
19. Weiss, K., Khoshgoftaar, T.M., Wang, D.: A survey of transfer learning. *Journal of Big Data* **3**(1), 1–40 (2016).
20. Zhuang, F., Qi, Z., Duan, K., Xi, D., Zhu, Y., Zhu, H., Xiong, H., He, Q.: A comprehensive survey on transfer learning. *Proceedings of the IEEE* **109**(1), 43–76 (2020).
21. Tan, C., Sun, F., Kong, T., Zhang, W., Yang, C., Liu, C.: A survey on deep transfer learning. In: *Artificial Neural Networks and Machine Learning–ICANN: 27th International Conference on Artificial Neural Networks*, Rhodes, Greece, October 4–7, 2018, Proceedings, Part III 27, pp. 270–279. Springer (2018).
22. Nanni, L., Interlenghi, M., Brahnam, S., Salvatore, C., Papa, S., Nemni, R., Castiglioni, I., Initiative, A.D.N.: Comparison of transfer learning and conventional machine learning applied to structural brain MRI for the early diagnosis and prognosis of Alzheimer's disease. *Frontiers in Neurology* **11**, 576194 (2020).
23. Albawi, S., Mohammed, T.A., Al-Zawi, S.: Understanding of a convolutional neural network. In: *2017 International Conference on Engineering and Technology (ICET)*, pp. 1–6. IEEE (2017).
24. Kukreja, H., Bharath, N., Siddesh, C., Kuldeep, S.: An introduction to artificial neural network. *International Journal of Advance Research and Innovative Ideas in Education* **1**, 27–30 (2016).
25. Ganji, K., Parimi, S.: Ann model for users' perception on IoT based smart healthcare monitoring devices and its impact with the effect of covid 19. *Journal of Science and Technology Policy Management* **13**(1), 6–21 (2022).
26. Li, Z., Liu, F., Yang, W., Peng, S., Zhou, J.: A survey of convolutional neural networks: analysis, applications, and prospects. *IEEE transactions on neural networks and learning systems* (Jun 10 2021), https://doi.org/10.48550/arXiv.2004.02806.
27. Haq, A.u., Li, J.P., Kumar, R., Ali, Z., Khan, I., Uddin, M.I., Agbley, B.L.Y.: MCNN: A multi-level CNN model for the classification of brain tumors in IoT-healthcare system. *Journal of Ambient Intelligence and Humanized Computing* **14**(5), 1–12 (2022).
28. Soni, M., Khan, I.R., Babu, K.S., Nasrullah, S., Madduri, A., Rahin, S.A.: Light weighted healthcare CNN model to detect prostate cancer on multiparametric MRI. *Computational Intelligence and Neuroscience* **2022**, 11 (2022).
29. Gouda, W., Sama, N.U., Al-Waakid, G., Humayun, M., Jhanjhi, N.Z.: Detection of skin cancer based on skin lesion images using deep learning. In: *Healthcare* **10**(7), 1183 (2022).
30. Guo, T., Dong, J., Li, H., Gao, Y.: Simple convolutional neural network on image classification. In: *2017 IEEE 2nd International Conference on Big Data Analysis (ICBDA)*, pp. 721–724. IEEE (2017).

31. Sahinbas, K., Catak, F.O.: Transfer learning-based convolutional neural network for Covid-19 detection with x-ray images. In: *Data Science for COVID-19*, pp. 451–466. Elsevier (2021).
32. Deng, J., Dong, W., Socher, R., Li, L.J., Li, K., Fei-Fei, L.: ImageNet: A large-scale hierarchical image database. In: (2009 IEEE conference on computer vision and pattern recognition, pp. 248–255. IEEE (2009).
33. Huh, M., Agrawal, P., Efros, A.A.: What makes ImageNet good for transfer learning? arXiv preprint arXiv:1608.08614 (2016).
34. Ribani, R., Marengoni, M.: A survey of transfer learning for convolutional neural networks. In: *2019 32nd SIBGRAPI Conference on Graphics, Patterns and Images Tutorials (SIBGRAPI-T)*, pp. 47–57. IEEE (2019).
35. Yosinski, J., Clune, J., Bengio, Y., Lipson, H.: How transferable are features in deep neural networks? *Advances in Neural Information Processing Systems* **27** (2014).
36. Ravishankar, H., Sudhakar, P., Venkataramani, R., Thiruvenkadam, S., Annangi, P., Babu, N., Vaidya, V.: Understanding the mechanisms of deep transfer learning for medical images. In: *Deep Learning and Data Labeling for Medical Applications: First International Workshop, LABELS 2016, and Second International Workshop, DLMIA 2016*, Held in Conjunction with MICCAI 2016, Athens, Greece, October 21, 2016, Proceedings 1, pp. 188–196. Springer (2016).
37. Samala, R.K., Chan, H.P., Hadjiiski, L.M., Helvie, M.A., Cha, K.H., Richter, C.D.: Multi-task transfer learning deep convolutional neural network: Application to computer-aided diagnosis of breast cancer on mammograms. *Physics in Medicine and Biology* **62**(23), 8894 (2017).
38. Byra, M., Styczynski, G., Szmigielski, C., Kalinowski, P., Michałowski, L., Paluszkiewicz, R., Ziarkiewicz-Wróblewska, B., Zieniewicz, K., Sobieraj, P., Nowicki, A.: Transfer learning with deep convolutional neural network for liver steatosis assessment in ultrasound images. *International Journal of Computer Assisted Radiology and Surgery* **13**(12), 1895–1903 (2018).
39. Farhadi, A., Chen, D., McCoy, R., Scott, C., Miller, J.A., Vachon, C.M., Ngufor, C.: Breast cancer classification using deep transfer learning on structured healthcare data. In: *2019 IEEE International Conference on Data Science and Advanced Analytics (DSAA)*, pp. 277–286. IEEE (2019).
40. Alghamdi, A., Hammad, M., Ugail, H., Abdel-Raheem, A., Muhammad, K., Khalifa, H.S., Abd El-Latif, A.A.: Detection of myocardial infarction based on novel deep transfer learning methods for urban healthcare in smart cities. *Multimedia Tools and Applications* **2022**, 1–22 (2020). 2950699.
41. Abubakar, A., Ajuji, M., Usman Yahya, I.: Comparison of deep transfer learning techniques in human skin burns discrimination. *Applied System Innovation* **3**(2), 20 (2020).
42. Hashmi, M.F., Katiyar, S., Keskar, A.G., Bokde, N.D., Geem, Z.W.: Efficient pneumonia detection in chest Xray images using deep transfer learning. *Diagnostics* **10**(6), 417 (2020).
43. Khamparia, A., Bharati, S., Podder, P., Gupta, D., Khanna, A., Phung, T.K., Thanh, D.N.: Diagnosis of breast cancer based on modern mammography using hybrid transfer learning. *Multidimensional Systems and Signal Processing* **32**(2), 747–765 (2021).
44. De Bois, M., El Yacoubi, M.A., Ammi, M.: Adversarial multi-source transfer learning in healthcare: Application to glucose prediction for diabetic people. *Computer Methods and Programs in Biomedicine* **199**, 105874 (2021).
45. Srinivas, C., NP, K.S., Zakariah, M., Alothaibi, Y.A., Shaukat, K., Partibane, B., Awal, H.: Deep transfer learning approaches in performance analysis of brain tumor classification using MRI images. *Journal of Healthcare Engineering* **2022** (2022). 3264367.

46. Alharbi, A.H., Hosni Mahmoud, H.A.: Pneumonia transfer learning deep learning model from segmented x-rays. *Healthcare* **10**(6), 987 (2022).
47. Humayun, M., Sujatha, R., Almuayqil, S.N., Jhanjhi, N.: A transfer learning approach with a convolutional neural network for the classification of lung carcinoma. *Healthcare* **10**(6), 1058 (2022).
48. Ahmad, N., Asghar, S., Gillani, S.A.: Transfer learning-assisted multi-resolution breast cancer histopathological images classification. *The Visual Computer* **38**(8), 2751–2770 (2022).
49. Samee, N.A., Alhussan, A.A., Ghoneim, V.F., Atteia, G., Alkanhel, R., Al-Antari, M.A., Kadah, Y.M.: A hybrid deep transfer learning of CNN-based LR-PCA for breast lesion diagnosis via medical breast mammograms. *Sensors* **22**(13), 4938 (2022).
50. Kumar, N., Gupta, M., Gupta, D., Tiwari, S.: Novel deep transfer learning model for Covid-19 patient detection using x-ray chest images. *Journal of Ambient Intelligence and Humanized Computing* **14**(1), 469–478 (2023).
51. Altun, M., Gürüler, H., Özkaraca, O., Khan, F., Khan, J., Lee, Y.: Monkeypox detection using CNN with transfer learning. *Sensors* **23**(4), 1783 (2023).
52. Meena, S.D., Bulusu, S.V., Siddharth, V.S., Reddy, S.P., Sheela, J.: Brain tumor classification using transfer learning. In Edited By Tawseef Ayoub Shaikh, Saqib Hakak, Tabasum Rasool, Mohammed Wasid: *Machine Learning and Artificial Intelligence in Healthcare Systems*, pp. 191–209. CRC Press (2023).
53. Basit, A.: Comparison implementation of different pre-trained Keras model for transfer learning. https://medium.com/@AB Niazi/comparison-implementation-of-different-pre- trained-keras-model-for-transfer-learning-ea513d88d3ee (2022).
54. Simonyan, K., Zisserman, A.: Very deep convolutional networks for large-scale image recognition. arXiv preprint arXiv:1409.1556 (2014).
55. https://keras.io/api/applications/.
56. https://www.kaggle.com/datasets/fanconic/skin-cancer-malignant-vs-benign.
57. https://www.kaggle.com/datasets/navoneel/brain-mri-images-for-brain-tumor -detection.

11 Conclusions

Prasenjit Dey

The implications of the Internet of Medical Things (IoMT) and machine learning (ML) in healthcare are substantial, offering an array of potential benefits. Internet of Things (IoT)-enabled wearable devices and sensors furnish a continuous stream of real-time data on patients' vital signs and health metrics. ML algorithms adeptly analyze this treasure trove of information, enabling early anomaly detection and proactive interventions. Consequently, this leads to enhanced patient outcomes and diminished hospital admissions. Moreover, ML-powered diagnostic tools have showcased remarkable accuracy in medical image recognition, augmenting the capabilities of radiologists in disease detection, such as cancer, and the identification of irregularities in medical images. This not only expedites the diagnostic process but also mitigates the scope for human error. Furthermore, ML algorithms scrutinize patient data to formulate personalized treatment plans rooted in an individual's unique genetic, physiological, and lifestyle attributes. This targeted approach amplifies the efficacy of therapies while minimizing potential adverse effects. Predictive analytics, driven by ML, can foresee disease outbreaks, anticipate patient readmissions, and gauge resource requirements. This invaluable foresight empowers healthcare institutions to allocate resources judiciously, strategize for surges in demand, and implement preemptive measures.

Nonetheless, amid these promises lie substantial challenges. Data privacy and security issues loom large, necessitating stringent measures to protect sensitive patient data. Robust data management practices and encryption protocols are paramount in this regard. Additionally, questions surrounding transparency in artificial intelligence (AI) decision-making, algorithmic bias, and accountability must be addressed comprehensively to cultivate trust among both patients and healthcare professionals. Equally pressing is the imperative of ensuring equitable access to IoMT and ML-enabled healthcare solutions, as disparities in technology access could potentially exacerbate existing healthcare inequalities, mandating targeted interventions. Healthcare regulatory bodies must adapt swiftly to the rapid pace of technological advancements, offering clear guidelines for the development and deployment of IoMT and ML within the healthcare sector to ensure patient safety and efficacy.

In conclusion, the full realization of the benefits that IoMT and ML can bring to healthcare hinges on robust collaboration among healthcare professionals, researchers, policymakers, and technologists. The ongoing pursuit of ethical, secure, and equitable integration of these technologies holds the promise of a brighter and healthier future for individuals and societies alike, where healthcare is not just an industry but a dynamic force for positive change and improved well-being.

 DOI: 10.1201/9781003391456-11

While IoT offers tremendous opportunities, it also presents challenges, including security, privacy, scalability, interoperability, and ethical and legal issues. The interconnected nature of IoT devices raises concerns about data security and privacy, making robust cybersecurity measures essential. Similarly, as the number of IoT devices continues to grow exponentially, ensuring scalability and managing vast amounts of data becomes a significant challenge. Devices and systems from different manufacturers must seamlessly communicate and interoperate to unlock the full potential of IoT. IoT data usage, consent, and ownership raise ethical and legal questions that require careful consideration.

In conclusion, the text provides a comprehensive overview of the integration of modern technologies, specifically ML and IoT, in the context of healthcare systems. The overarching goal is to enhance the quality and efficiency of healthcare delivery by harnessing the immense volume of data generated daily in the healthcare sector. The authors emphasize the potential of ML algorithms to analyze healthcare data for optimal prediction and recommendation systems. They highlight the significance of IoT in collecting data from various sensory input devices, which can be further processed through big data architectures to facilitate intelligent decision-making. The combination of ML and IoT, often referred to as the Internet of Medical Things, opens new possibilities for real-time patient monitoring, medical recordkeeping, and disease prediction. However, the text acknowledges the challenges posed by noisy and diverse medical datasets and the need for robust ML algorithms to address them. It underscores the importance of exploring state-of-the-art ML techniques to optimize critical decision-making processes in healthcare.

The chapters provide specific examples of how ML and IoT can be applied to address critical healthcare challenges. Chapter 2 showcases predictive analytics in preventing eating disorders, while Chapter 3 focuses on early-stage breast cancer prediction. Chapter 4 demonstrates the effectiveness of ML and AI in Parkinson's disease diagnosis and care, and Chapter 5 highlights the use of AI in diabetic retinopathy detection. Chapter 6 addresses the transparency issues in medical image retrieval and presents an innovative approach to improving CNN models. Chapter 7 introduces an automated disease detection system for paddy leaf diseases, contributing to agriculture in Asia.

Chapter 8 emphasizes the role of IoT in patient care, administrative efficiency, and patient satisfaction, demonstrating the tangible benefits of IoT in healthcare settings. Chapter 9 presents a practical solution for addressing cost and complexity issues in IoT systems, emphasizing the importance of open-source technologies for intelligent healthcare monitoring. Finally, Chapter 10 highlights Transfer Learning's (TL) key role in addressing data challenges in healthcare. TL transfers knowledge from related domains, improving performance and reducing reliance on specific data. It proves superior to traditional methods, offering potential for optimizing healthcare systems, particularly with IoT-generated medical data.

In summary, this book underscores the immense potential of combining ML and IoT in healthcare to revolutionize patient care, disease diagnosis, and administrative processes. It showcases various applications and research directions, highlighting the ongoing evolution of these technologies and their role in shaping the future of healthcare systems. The convergence of ML and IoT offers promising opportunities to improve healthcare outcomes, and this book contributes valuable insights into this rapidly evolving field.

Index

ABC–LSVM, 15
ABC–QSVM, 15
Accuracy, 27, 38, 41–43, 45–47, 50–52, 97, 99, 102–105, 114, 118–120, 122, 123
ACDC database, 9
Activation function, 5
AdaBoost, 59, 60, 71
Adaptively weighted balance (AWB) loss, 9
Adaptive neuro-fuzzy inference system (ANFIS), 60, 61
AI, *see* Artificial intelligence
AI-assisted surgical procedure, 2
Alexnet, 100, 108, 113, 201
AMIGOS datasets, 14
Anomaly identification, 2
Anorexia nervosa, 19
Arduino IDE, 177
Artificial bee colony algorithm (ABC), 14, 15
Artificial intelligence (AI), 96, 148, 149, 153, 160–163
Artificial neural network (ANN), 64, 65, 67, 68
Automated, 32

Backpropagation algorithm, 6
Batch
 normalization, 128, 136
 size, 103, 106, 114, 118
Bayesian belief network (BBN) classifier, 14
Benign, 202, 204
Bimodal Images, 135
Binge, 19
Biological Information, 48, 49, 52
Biosensors, 2
BITE dataset, 9
Blood oxygen saturation (SpO_2), 166, 174
Bluetooth, 173
BME680, 175
BMI, 23
Brain
 image clustering, 7
 tissue segmentation, 9
 tumor, 205, 207, 209
 tumor classification (MRI) dataset, 117, 119–122
 tumor segmentation, 9
Brainsense headband, 14
Building block, 171
Bulimia nervosa, 19

C4.5, 5
CAD system, 86
Canvas matching method, 9
Capsule Network, 14
Cardiac magnetic resonance (CMR) images, 9
CART algorithm, 5
CBIR Framework, 97, 98, 111, 118, 121–123
Centralized cloud servers, 13
Classification, 3, 39, 40, 42, 44–48, 52, 57–59, 61, 62, 64, 65, 67–69, 71–73, 77, 79, 97, 99, 101, 105, 109, 110, 113, 116–118, 120–124
Classifier, 44, 47–52
Clinical data processing, 6
Cloud-based web service, 13
Cloud computing, 12, 14
Clustering, 7
CNN, *see* Convolutional neural network
CoAP, *see* Constrained Application Protocol
Compliance, 153, 161
Confusion Matrix, 118, 209, 210
Constrained Application Protocol (CoAP), 13
Content-based image retrieval (CBIR), 96–99, 107–109, 111, 116, 118, 121–124
Contrast limited adaptive histogram equalization (CLAHE), 111, 113
Contrast limited adaptive histogram equalization, 111, 113
Controller Application Communication (CAC) framework, 12
Convergence, 7
Convolution, 102, 105, 128
Convolutional neural network (CNNs), 9, 57, 63, 69, 72, 74, 75, 79, 97, 136, 191, 196
Covid-19 radiography database, 98, 117, 119–122
Cross-entropy, 113
Cross-entropy loss, 6, 140
Crossover, 107, 115
Crossover rate, 118
Cross-validation, 117
CT scan, 2

Data, 20
Dataset, 3, 48, 49, 51, 52
Data stream mining, 13
DBD, 87, 91
DE, *see* Differential evolution
Decision support system, 20

Decision tree (DT), 3, 5
Deep belief networks (DBN), 60, 61
Deep brain stimulation (DBS), 55, 62, 63, 69, 70
Deep learning (DL), 21, 55–57, 59, 64, 66, 67, 69–72, 79, 80, 98, 107, 108
Deep neural network (DNN), 9, 56, 57, 59, 61, 63, 66, 69, 70, 99, 108, 109, 128
DenseNet, 106, 109, 113, 119–121, 201
Devices, 147, 148, 150–152, 157, 162, 163
Diabetic retinopathy, 10, 85
Diagnosis, 20
Differential evolution, 97, 107, 109–111, 113–116, 122
Digital, 147, 149, 151
Dimensionality reduction, 7
Disease
  diagnosis, 7
  progression, 6
Distributed system, 13
DREAMER datasets, 14
Dropout, 128
DS18B20, 174

Eating disorder, 21
Eating Disorder Examination Questionnaire (EDE-Q), 22
EHRs, *see* Electronic health records
Electronic health records (EHRs), 1, 11
Email notification, 188
Embedding framework-based transformer model, 9
Embedding pre-sampling module, 9
Ensemble methods, 5
Epoch, 114, 118, 138
ESP32 Do it Kit vl, 172, 173
Estimators, 32
Euclidean distance, 4, 17, 118, 122
Evaluation, 107, 113, 119–121
Experimental set up, 183
Extensible Messaging and Presence Protocol (XMPP), 12

Fl Score, 27, 97, 118, 119, 121, 140
False-negative, 90
False-positive, 90
Feature, 44–52, 98–102
Feature extraction, 57, 65, 66, 76, 78
Feature selection, 5, 56, 59, 65, 68
Feature space, 4
Feedback loops, 6
Feed forward neural network, 6
Fitness evaluation, 113
Fitness function, 113, 116
F-measure, 90
Fog computing, 13, 14
Forecasting, 3
Foster corner detection theory, 9
Foster corner identification principle, 9
Fully connected deep neural network (FCDNNs), 143

Gated Recurrent Units (GRUs), 6
Gaussian blur, 111, 112
Gaussian mixture model (GMMs), 7, 86
General Data Protection Regulation (GDPR), 148, 156
Generation, 107, 113, 116, 118
Generative model, 9
Genetics, 19
Genomic data, 7
Genomics, 1
Glaucoma, 87
Global score, 23
Glucose sensor, 2
GMMs, *see* Gaussian Mixture Model
GoogleNet, 201, 202
GPIO, 172, 173
Gradient-boosted trees, 3
Gradient boosting, 5
Grafana, 181
Grafana Dashboard, 187
GRUs, *see* Gated Recurrent Units

Health, 19
Healthcare, 4.0, 96, 107, 108
  industry, 147, 148, 152, 154, 158, 160, 161
  Internet of Things (HIoT), 190
  providers, 148, 155, 160, 161
  systems, 148, 155, 163
Hierarchical clustering, 7
Histogram equalization, 9
Histogram of oriented gradients (HOG), 75, 127
HOG, *see* Histogram of oriented gradients
Hospitals, 147, 151, 160, 161
HR, 174
Hyper parameters 4, 109
Hyperplane, 3

ID3, 5
Image
  augmentation, 130
  dataset, 97, 108, 110, 111, 114, 117, 118, 122
  descriptor, 109, 110
  histogram, 134
  transformation technique, 130
ImageNet, 197, 198
Imbalanced dataset, 5
InceptionResNetV2, 103, 104, 109, 118–121, 201
Inception-v3, 102, 103, 113, 201

Indian diabetic retinopathy image dataset (IDRiD), 87, 91
Indicator functions, 90
Individual, 99, 113, 114
InfluxDB, 180
Integrate, 147, 154
Intensity inhomogeneity field, 9
Internet of Medical Things (IoMT), 2, 14, 96
Internet of Things (IoT), 1, 96, 97, 166–168
Interpretable Bayesian framework, 9
IoMT, *see* Internet of Medical Things

J48 decision tree, 14

Kaggle, 204
Kaplan–Meier and Cox PH regression, 14
Keras, 198, 207
Kernel function, 4
k-fold cross-validation, 90
K-means clustering, 7, 127
K-nearest neighbor (KNN), 4, 60, 62, 64, 67, 70, 76, 127
Kohonen maps, 8

LeakyReLU, 128
Learning rate, 108, 109, 116, 118
Linear regression, 3
Logistic regression, 3
Logistic regression and principal component analysis (LR-PCA), 201
Long short-term memory (LSTM), 6, 57, 63, 69, 72, 74, 79
LoRa, 188
LoRaWAN network, 15
Loss, 114
Loss function, 6
LSTM, *see* Long short-term memory

Machine learning, (ML), 1, 3, 20, 44–49, 52, 55, 56, 60–66, 70, 71, 75–79, 96
Macular degeneration, 87
Magnetic resonance imaging (MRI), 2, 55, 59, 62, 65, 66, 69, 70, 73
Malignant, 202, 204
MAX30102, 174
Max pooling, 128
Mean squared error loss, 6
Medical imaging, 1
Message Queuing Telemetry Transport (MQTT), 177–179
Messidor, 2, 87, 91
mHealth, 12
Microelectromechanical system (MEMS), 175
ML, *see* Machine learning
ML-fueled drug discovery, 2
MobileNet, 103–105, 113
MobileNetV3-s 202
Morphological operation, 111, 112
MQ-135, 175
MQTT architecture, 179
MQTT client, 171, 179
MQTT protocol, 177
MRI medical image segmentation, 9
MsVRL, *see* Multiscale visual representation self-supervised learning
Multilayer perceptron (MLP), 5
Multiscale visual representation self-supervised learning (MsVRL), 9
Mutant vector, 114, 115
Mutation, 97, 107, 114, 115

NASNetLarge, 211
Near-field communication (NFC), 13
Network, 147, 149–151, 153–155, 157, 159, 160, 162
Neural networks (NNs), 56, 59, 63, 68–70, 73, 74
Neurological disorders, 9
NFC, *see* Near-field communication
NNs, *see* Neural Networks
NodeMCU, 171, 182
Node-RED, 179, 180
Node-RED dashboard, 186
Node-RED flow, 184, 185
Nonlinear mapping, 5

ODLS, *see* One dimensional deep low-rank and sparse network
One dimensional deep low-rank and sparse network (ODLS), 9
Opioid use disorder (OUD), 10
Optimization, 113, 114, 123
Optimized neural network, 97
Original population vectors, 115, 116
Otsu thresholding, 134
OUD, *see* Opioid use disorder
Outliers, 4
Overfitting, 5, 137

Parkinson's disease (PD), 55–80
Parkinson's Progression Markers Initiative (PPMI), 57, 63
Particle swarm optimization (PSO), 59, 60
Patients, 147, 149–151, 153, 154, 157, 159, 160, 162, 163
Performance evaluation, 119–121
PM2.5, 188
PM10, 188
PoE, 172
Pooling, 191, 196
Population, 97, 107, 113, 115, 116, 118

PPM, 186, 187
Precision, 27, 91, 97, 107, 118–120, 141
Predator–prey algorithm, 9
Prediction, 20, 38–40, 42–44, 47–52
Predictive modeling, 6
Preferred Reporting Items for Systematic Reviews and Meta-Analysis (PRISMA), 10
Preprocessing, 110, 128
Pre-trained model, 197, 198, 202–204
Principal component analysis (PCA), 7, 59, 60, 67, 78, 79
Privacy, 148, 156
Proliferative diabetic retinopathy, 87
Providers, 148, 155, 160, 161, 163
Pruning, 5
Purging, 19

Quality of service (QoS), 178
Query image, 110, 111, 116, 122

Radio frequency identification (RFID), 14
Random forest (RF), 3
Raspberry Pi 4, 170, 172
Raspberry Pi IoT server, 171, 185
Real-time monitoring, 6
Recall, 27, 97, 118–120, 142
Recurrent neural networks (RNN), 6, 11, 57, 63
Regression, 3
Reinforced learning, 3
Relay module, 173
ReLU activation, 128
ReLU activation function, 6, 90, 100, 101, 103, 105, 106
Remote patient monitoring, 2, 7
Research, 148, 151–154, 156, 159, 162, 163
ResNet, 50, 102–104, 113, 201, 202
Restriction, 28
RF, *see* Random forest
RFID, *see* Radio frequency identification
RFMiD, 87, 91
Risks, 162, 163
ROC curve, 90

San Francisco COVID 19 dataset, 14
Scaling factor, 115
Sector, 147, 151, 152, 160, 161, 163
Seeded region growing, 9
Segmentation in medical imaging, 7
Selection, 107, 113, 116
Self-organizing maps (SOMs), 8
Sensitivity, 90
Sensor, 1
SHS, *see* Smart healthcare sensors
Sigmoid function, 5
Similarity score, 116–118, 122
Skin cancer, 204, 205
Skin lesion classification, 9
Smart healthcare sensors (SHS), 14
Smart phones, 148, 152, 153, 163
Smart watches, 2
SoC, 160
Softmax, *see* Softmax function
Softmax function, 90, 128
SOM grid, 8
Sparse auto-encoder, *see* Sparse auto-encoder classifier
Sparse auto-encoder classifier, 9
Sparse categorical cross entropy, 113
Sparse reconstruction model, 9
Spatial distance, 112
SqueezeNet, 103, 113
Statistical survival model, 14
Structuring element, 112
Supervised learning, 3
Supervisory control and data acquisition (SCADA), 167, 168
Support vector machine (SVM), 3, 11, 14, 59, 62, 65, 67, 68, 70, 76, 127

Tanh function, 5
t-distributed stochastic neighbor embedding (t-SNE), 7
Technology, 147, 149–154 157, 159, 160, 162, 163
Telemedicine, 12
Temporal network analysis (TNA), 14
Testing, 27
Test set, 117
Time-series data analysis, 6
Time-series forecasting, 3
TNA, *see* Temporal network analysis
TPR, *see* True positive rate
Training, 27, 98, 99, 103, 111, 116, 117
Training data, 3
Training set, 117
Transfer learning (TL), 15, 98, 193–214
Trial vector, 115, 116
True positive rate (TPR), 90
t-SNE, *see* t-distributed stochastic neighbor embedding

UCI Machine Learning Repository, 128
U-Net, 9
Unified Parkinson's Disease Rating Scale (UPDRS), 55, 60, 61, 70, 77, 79
Unsupervised learning, 7
UPDRS, *see* Unified Parkinson's Disease Rating Scale

Validation
  accuracy, 114, 119

loss, 113, 119
set, 114, 117
Vanishing gradients, 6
VGG19, 101, 109, 113, 118–120
VGG16-Net, 86, 207, 209
VGGNET16, *see* VGG16-Net
VGG network, 86
Volatile organic compounds (VOCs), 175

Wi-Fi, 173
Wi-Fi dongle, 176
Wireless sensor networks (WSNs), 14
Wiring diagram, 183, 184
WSNs, *see* Wireless sensor networks

XGBoost, 14, 20, 127
XMPP, *see* Extensible Messaging and Presence Protocol

Yen's thresholding, 130

ZigBee, 15

For Product Safety Concerns and Information please contact our EU
representative GPSR@taylorandfrancis.com
Taylor & Francis Verlag GmbH, Kaufingerstraße 24, 80331 München, Germany

www.ingramcontent.com/pod-product-compliance
Lightning Source LLC
LaVergne TN
LVHW010556110826
845149LV00003B/676

* 9 7 8 1 0 3 2 4 8 9 2 8 5 *